Paediatric & Adolescent Gynaecology

Paediatric & Adolescent Gynaecology

Edited by A S GARDEN MB ChB FRCOG ──────────────
Senior Lecturer in Obstetrics and Gynaecology and Lecturer in Child Health,
The University of Liverpool, Liverpool, United Kingdom

A member of the Hodder Headline Group
LONDON • SYDNEY • AUCKLAND
Co-published in the USA by
Oxford University Press, Inc., New York

First published in Great Britain in 1998 by
Arnold, a member of the Hodder Headline Group,
338 Euston Road, London NW1 3BH

http://www.arnoldpublishers.com

© 1998 Arnold

Co-published in the United States of America by
Oxford University Press, Inc.,
198 Madison Avenue, New York, NY10016
Oxford is a registered trademark of Oxford University Press

Whilst the advice and information in this book is believed to be true and
accurate at the date of going to press, neither the author[s] nor the publisher
can accept any legal responsibility or liability for any errors or omissions
that may be made. In particular (but without limiting the generality of the
preceding disclaimer) every effort has been made to check drug dosages;
however it is still possible that errors have been missed. Furthermore,
dosage schedules are constantly being revised and new side effects
recognised. For these reasons the reader is strongly urged to consult the
drug companies' printed instructions before administering any of the drugs
recommended in this book.

British Library Cataloguing in Publication Data
A catalogue record for this book is available from the British Library

Library of Congress Cataloging-in-Publication Data
A catalog record for this book is available from the Library of Congress

ISBN 0 340 60764 5

Publisher: Georgina Bentliff
Project Editor: Catherine Barnes
Production Editor: Julie Delf
Production Controller: Sarah Kett
Cover Design: Andy McColm

Composition in 10/12 Times and Optima by Phoenix Photosetting, Chatham, Kent
Printed and bound in Great Britain by St Edmundsbury Press, Bury St Edmunds, Suffolk and
Bookcraft Ltd, Bath

Contents

List of Contributors

Marion Cheesbrough BMedSci BM BS MRCPsych
Consultant Child and Adolescent Psychiatrist, Alder Hey Children's Hospital, Liverpool, United Kingdom

M Alison Clarke BA DASS CQSW
Counsellor and Co-ordinator, Arbour–PSS, Liverpool, United Kingdom

Sandra D'Silva MA CQSW
Staff Development and Training Officer, Liverpool Social Services Directorate, Liverpool, United Kingdom

Marion Ferguson RGN, SCM, Family Planning Cert., School Nursing Cert., Formerly Nurse Manager, Community Child Health, Royal Liverpool Children's Hospital, Liverpool, United Kingdom

Alan Fryer BSc MD FRCP
Consultant Clinical Geneticist at the Royal Liverpool University Hospital, Royal Liverpool Children's Hospital and Liverpool Women's Hospital, and Honorary Lecturer in Medicine and Child Health, University of Liverpool, Liverpool, United Kingdom

Anne S Garden MB ChB FRCOG
Senior Lecturer in Obstetrics and Gynaecology and Lecturer in Child Health, University of Liverpool, Liverpool, and Honorary Consultant Obstetrician and Gynaecologist, Liverpool Women's Hospital Trust, United Kingdom

Shirley Y Godiwalla MB MS MD
Herbert Johnston Research Fellow, Royal Liverpool Children's Hospital, Liverpool, United Kingdom

Jennifer Hopwood MB ChB D(Obst)RCOG DipVen MFFP
Colposcopy Co-ordinator, Liverpool Women's Hospital and Wirral Hospital, Liverpool, United Kingdom

Meera Kishen MBBS DGO MD MFFP DipVen
Consultant in Family Planning and Reproductive Healthcare, 'Abacus' Centre for Contraception, North Mersey Community (NHS) Trust, Liverpool, United Kingdom

David A Lloyd MChir FRCS
Professor of Paediatric Surgery, University of Liverpool, and Honorary Consultant Paediatric Surgeon, Alder Hey Children's Hospital, Liverpool, United Kingdom

Paul D Losty MD FRCSI FRCS(Paed)
Senior Lecturer in Paediatric Surgery, University of Liverpool, and Honorary

Consultant Paediatric Surgeon, Alder Hey Children's Hospital, Liverpool, United Kingdom

Annette Lyons TCert BEd(Hons) DipEd MEd
Advisor for Health Education, Education Directorate, Liverpool, United Kingdom

Elizabeth M Molyneux MBBS FRCP(UK) FFAEM DCH DobsRCOG
Associate Professor, College of Medicine, University of Malawi, Malawi, Central Africa

Julia S Nelki MA(Oxon) MBChB DRCOG MRCPsych MSc Family Therapy
Consultant Child and Adolescent Psychiatrist, Alder Hey Children's Hospital, Liverpool, United Kingdom

David Pilling MB ChB DCH DMRD FRCR FRCPCH
Consultant Paediatric Radiologist, Royal Liverpool Children's Hospital and Liverpool Women's Hospital, Liverpool, United Kingdom

Anthony M K Rickwood MA BM BCh FRCS
Consultant Paediatric Urologist, Royal Liverpool Children's Hospital, Liverpool, United Kingdom

W Joan Robson FRCS FFAEM
Consultant in Paediatric and Emergency Medicine, Alder Hey Children's Hospital, Liverpool, United Kingdom

Colin Smith
Senior Lecturer in Child Health, University of Liverpool, and Honorary Consultant Paediatrician, Alder Hey Children's Hospital, Liverpool, United Kingdom

Francis Stewart
Child Psychiatrist, Wolverhampton, United Kingdom

Adrian Sutton BSc MBBS FRCPsych
Child Psychiatrist, The Winnicott Centre, Manchester, United Kingdom

Sam Warner BA MClinPsychol
Clinical Psychologist, Specialist in Child Sexual Abuse, Department of Psychology and Speech Pathology, Manchester Metropolitan University, and Honorary Lecturer, Department of Clinical Psychology, Liverpool University and Honorary Researcher, Department of Research, Ashworth Special Hospital, Liverpool, United Kingdom

Olwen E Willams MBChB FRCP(UK) DipVen(Liverpool) DFFP
Consultant Genito-Urinary Physician, Wrexham Maelor NHS Trust, Wrexham, United Kingdom

Preface and Acknowledgements

When I tell professional colleagues that I have a special interest in Paediatric Gynaecology, their response is usually something to the effect that I can't have many patients requiring my services. A glance at how the Paediatric and Adolescent Gynaecology clinic at the Royal Liverpool Children's Hospital, Alder Hey, has grown over the years will show that is far from the case.

The truth is that Paediatric Gynaecology is poorly understood. Gynaecologists usually do not remember that children are not just small adults – they have different anatomy, physiology and different attitudes and emotions compared to adults. Paediatricians, on the other hand, may forget that sexuality is part of their patients' nature and may feel inadequate to deal with this.

I believe we have the best solution to this dilemma at Alder Hey with gynaecology and paediatric colleagues working together to provide a service for those girls who require it. This book is a tangible product of that co-operation.

When I first became interested in paediatric gynaecology, I approached a colleague who provided such a service elsewhere in the country for some advice. The response I received was that she was self-taught and suggested I went and did the same. I hope that this book will help others begin to do just that.

ACKNOWLEDGEMENTS

Thanks are due, not just to the recognised contributors to this book whose names appear with their chapters, but also to all those colleagues at the Royal Liverpool Children's Hospital, Alder Hey Hospital and at the Liverpool Women's Hospital, for advice, criticism and helpful comments. My thanks also to all those from whom I have begged and cajoled clinical pictures to illustrate the book and who have lent them to me with such good grace. My particular thanks to Mr Paul Nickson, Department of Obstetrics and Gynaecology at the University of Liverpool, for all his help in preparing the photographs for publication.

PART I

GROWTH AND DEVELOPMENT

CHAPTER 1

Gynaecological development

ANNE S GARDEN

This Chapter is intended to provide an overview of the physiological, hormonal and anatomical changes which occur as a girl grows and develops first *in utero*, then in the neonatal, childhood and adolescent years, against which the practice of paediatric and adolescent gynaecology can be practised and understood. It is not intended to be a full review of the subject and readers who wish to learn more of the subject are referred to a more specialised text.

FETAL GROWTH AND DEVELOPMENT (see also p. 50)

The chromosomal sex of a fetus is determined at conception with the fertilisation of the ovum by either an X- or Y-bearing spermatozoon. The gonad first appears around the fourth week of fetal life as a thickening of the coelomic epithelium in the genital ridges on either side of the dorsal mesentery. At this stage it is undifferentiated and consists of a cortex and medulla. At about 6–7 weeks gestation, in the presence of the Y chromosome, the undifferentiated gonad develops into a testis with primitive seminiferous tubules and germ cells. The Sertoli cells of the testis secrete Mullerian Inhibiting Factor (MIF) which inhibits the development of the Mullerian ducts while the Leydig cells, in response to placental human chorionic gonadotrophin (HCG), produce testosterone. In the absence of the Y chromosome and slightly later in development than the testis (Mittwoch *et al.*, 1993), the gonad develops into an ovary. The germ cells migrate from the endoderm of the yolk sac to the cortex of the gonad while the medulla degenerates so that by twelve weeks it consists mainly of connective tissue. (For a fuller description of sex determination, see Chapter 12).

Within the ovary, the germ cells undergo both mitotic and meiotic division initially forming oogonia then oocytes which, at around twenty weeks gestation, are enveloped in granulosa cells to become primordial follicles. They remain in this stage of 'suspended animation' until ovulation which may be over 40 years later! The maximum number of germ cells in the ovary, approximately seven million, are present at around the sixth month of intrauterine life. Thereafter, the numbers drop rapidly with only two million being present by the time of birth and 300 000 at puberty (Baker, 1963).

In the absence of MIF, the Mullerian ducts form the internal female genitalia by fusing in the midline along the lower two thirds to form the uterus, cervix and upper two thirds of the vagina. The unfused portion develops into the fallopian tubes. This process is not dependent on the presence of oestrogen nor is it inhibited by the presence of androgens. Failure of fusion of the Mullerian duct leads to a duplication of the internal female genitalia (Fig. 1.1), which in its most extreme form will present as complete duplication of the vagina, cervix and uterus (Fig. 1.2), each hemi-uterus having one fallopian tube, to the least extreme form which is merely the presence of a septum in the uterine cavity.

The development of the external genitalia, however, is hormone dependent. The external genitalia derive from the genital tubercle, the urethral folds and the labio-scrotal swelling. The presence of androgens cause development into external male genitalia. In the absence of androgens, the genital tubercle develops into the clitoris at about 8 weeks gestation, the labio-scrotal swellings into the labia majora and the urethral folds the labia minora. The lower third of the vagina develops from an upward growth of the urogenital sinus which fuses with the portion developed from the Mullerian duct. This is complete by about 18 weeks gestation.

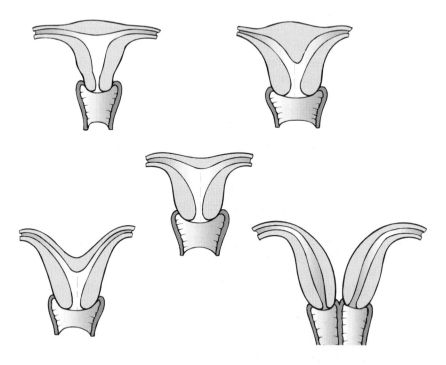

Fig. 1.1   Diagram showing the varying degrees of duplication of the female internal genitalia which may occur due to failure of fusion of the Mullerian duct.

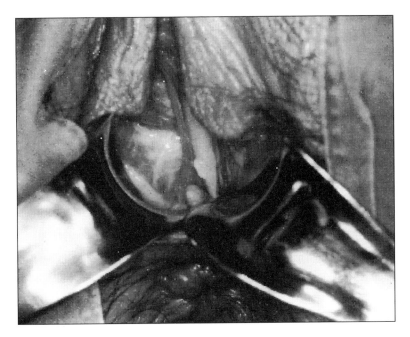

Fig. 1.2 Speculum examination of an adolescent with complete vaginal septum and double cervix. She also had a complete duplication of the uterus.

THE NEONATAL PERIOD

At birth, the appearance of a girl's genitalia is dependent on the circulating maternal hormones. Under the influence of these maternal hormones, particularly oestrogen, the neonate will have enlarged and rounded, often oedematous, labia (Fig. 1.3), a thickened and very prominent hymen and a white, creamy vaginal discharge similar to that normally seen in women during their reproductive years. More rarely, in approximately 10% of girls, there will be withdrawal bleeding similar to a light period and which may last a few days.

Neonatal breasts, of both boys and girls, are also influenced by maternal hormones and at birth show enlargement of the breast tissue and not infrequently, secretion of fluid – colostrum and milk – referred to in some parts as 'witches' milk'.

The responses of the breast and external genitalia to circulating maternal hormones are not so marked in premature girls. Partly because of this, and also because of lack of fat within the labia majora, the clitoris in these girls appears greatly enlarged and may cause concern to parents or clinical staff if they are not aware of the normality of this finding.

The vagina in the immediate neonatal period is lined with a thick layer of squamous epithelium containing many glycogen cells – as is found in the adult woman.

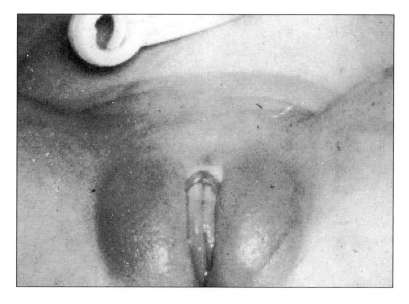

Fig. 1.3   Appearance of the genitalia at birth showing enlarged, rounded, oedematous labia majora and minora.

The uterus is disproportionately large, being approximately the size seen in a 5-year-old girl. The ovaries are also enlarged and may contain follicular cysts.

These changes start receding immediately following birth after withdrawal of the maternal oestrogen. The changes usually have regressed by 1 month of age although they may last up to 2 months.

Hormonal examination, if it were performed in the immediate neonatal period, would show high levels of oestrogen and low levels of the pituitary hormones follicle stimulating hormone (FSH) and luteinizing hormone (LH). As the levels of maternal oestrogen fall, there is an increase in the levels of FSH and LH similar to that which occurs in the post-menopausal period.

GROWTH AND DEVELOPMENT IN CHILDHOOD

Following regression of the effects of maternal hormones, the girl goes into a period in childhood when there is little or no hormonal stimulation and therefore no specific development of the genitalia. The growth of the genitalia is simply in proportion to the general growth of the girl's body.

The labia majora are flattened and the labia minora are thin and attenuated (Fig. 1.4). In the immediate post-neonatal period, the hymen may appear particularly prominent as the effects of the maternal oestrogen on the hymen takes longer to regress and the hymen can appear enlarged for up to two years after birth.

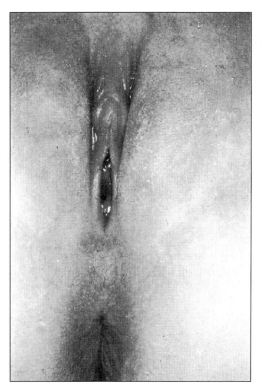

Fig. 1.4   Appearance of the labia of a girl aged seven showing the flattened labia majora, thin attenuated labia minora with the hymenal orifice easily visible without retracting the labia.

The vaginal epithelium becomes thin and loses the glycogen containing cells. The pH of the vagina becomes alkaline and this combination of factors predisposes to recurrent bacterial infections of the vaginal introitus (see p. 107). The uterine size decreases following withdrawal of oestrogen and remains fairly static in size until around the age of 8 when it begins to grow in relation to the girl's growth. The ovaries likewise decrease in size following withdrawal of oestrogen and remain static in size until around the age of 5 years when they begin to grow corresponding to the girl's size. Small follicular cysts may be seen throughout childhood on ultrasound, particularly in early childhood when there are high levels of circulating FSH and LH.

This elevation of FSH and LH mentioned in the section concerned with neonatal development continues to occur over the first 2–3 months of post-natal life and only begins to fall at around 3 years of age. At this time, there is a resetting of what is often referred to as the 'gonadostat' – the mechanism by which the levels of sex steroids is controlled – and the levels of FSH and LH slowly fall. This 'resetting of the gonadostat' represents a maturation of the central mechanism which controls release of gonadotrophin releasing hormone (GnRH) and is thought to be due to a GnRH pulse generator controlled by the higher centres.

GROWTH AND DEVELOPMENT AT PUBERTY

Puberty is the time at which, under the influence of the sex hormones, a child becomes an adult physically, sexually and psychologically. The onset of puberty varies from 8–14 years with an average age in the United Kingdom of around 11 years. The physical events which occur normally do so in an ordered sequence of a spurt in growth, early development of secondary sexual characteristics, the onset of menstruation and finally completion of the development of secondary sexual characteristics and the growth spurt. Tanner and co-workers, who performed the classic studies in puberty in the late 1960s and 1970s estimated that 20% of the normal pubertal growth spurt is completed before the first appearance of breast budding or pubic hair development (Marshall and Tanner, 1969; Tanner *et al.*, 1976) (Fig. 1.5). These changes occur under the influence of the ovarian sex steroids controlled by the pituitary gonadotrophins which themselves are controlled by GnRH from the hypothalamus.

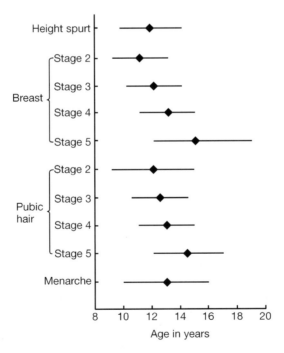

Fig. 1.5   Diagram of the sequence of events at puberty (redrawn with permission from Marshall and Tanner, 1969).

While the exact mechanisms by which the hypothalamic–pituitary–ovarian axis is 'switched on' and the various feedback mechanisms developed are not known, the changes in levels of gonadotrophins, adrenal and ovarian hormones have been well studied. Pulsatile secretion of GnRH from the hypothalamus causes release of the gonadotrophins, FSH and LH, from the anterior pituitary. FSH and LH stimulate release of oestrogens from the ovary. The hypothalamic release of GnRH is controlled, as in the adult, by poorly understood mechanisms in the cortex of the brain but which include nutrition, general health, stress, environmental and hereditary factors.

Hormonal Control of Puberty

The first hormonal sign of the onset of puberty occurs around the age of 6–9 years and is an increase in the pulsatile release of GnRH during sleep. This results in an increase in release of FSH and LH from the anterior pituitary gland.

As the girl becomes older, the increase in pulsatile release of GnRH during sleep increases with concomitant increased pulsatile release of FSH and LH. The latter causes the release of the oestrogen precursor, androstenedione, from the theca lutein cells of the ovary. Androstenedione is converted to produce oestradiol by aromatases released under the influence of FSH. FSH as its name suggests also increases follicle growth. Increased levels of oestrogens produce the changes in the internal and external genitalia and the breast associated with puberty.

The final hormonal event in puberty is the development of the positive feedback mechanism. Prior to this time, the hypothalamic–pituitary–ovarian axis had been under the control of a negative feedback mechanism by which release of small amounts of oestrogen from the ovary had an inhibitory effect on the release of GnRH, FSH and LH. At puberty, however, a positive feedback mechanism develops by which release of small amounts of oestrogen stimulates the release of FSH and LH. Rapidly rising levels of oestrogen trigger a steep rise in LH and FSH levels which in turn trigger ovulation.

Adrenarche

The first physical sign of puberty is the development of the breast bud followed by growth of sexual hair, initially in the pubic area and, approximately 1 year later, in the axilla. Stimulation of this hair growth is not by oestrogens but by the adrenal androgens from the zona reticularis – particularly dehydroepiandrosterone (DHA), dehydroepiandrosterone sulphate (DHAS) and androstenedione – under the control of adrenocorticotrophic hormone (ACTH). The release of adrenal androgens, with subsequent hair growth, is known as andrenarche and occurs from around the age of 8 and is complete by the age of about 15 years. The control of this process is unknown.

The first sign of pubic hair growth can be seen as a sparse growth of straight hair along the edge of the labia majora. As the girl develops, this hair becomes coarser and more curly and appears on the pubic area. Thereafter, the hair spreads initially across the mons pubis and then onto the medial aspects of the thighs. The development and stages of pubic hair growth were described by

Marshall and Tanner in their study of pubertal development in 192 schoolgirls (Marshall and Tanner, 1969) (Fig. 1.6).

As pubic and axillary hair development is controlled by adrenal androgens, those girls with absent or non-functioning ovaries will have a normal adrenarche. Girls with complete androgen insensitivity (see p. 142) have poor pubic and axillary hair growth. Girls with constitutional delay in puberty will have a delayed adrenarche as well as a delay in the oestrogen-driven aspects of pubertal development.

The Effects of Oestrogen on Pubertal Development

PUBIC HAIR

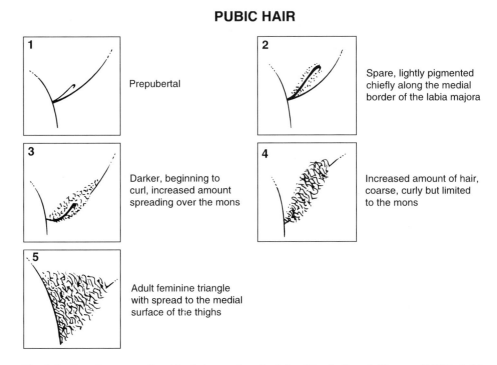

1   Prepubertal

2   Spare, lightly pigmented chiefly along the medial border of the labia majora

3   Darker, beginning to curl, increased amount spreading over the mons

4   Increased amount of hair, coarse, curly but limited to the mons

5   Adult feminine triangle with spread to the medial surface of the thighs

Fig. 1.6 Development of pubic hair as described by Marshall and Tanner (1969) (with permission).

Breast development

The first sign of oestrogenisation is the development of the breast bud seen as an elevation of the breast tissue from the chest wall, with elevation of the nipple and enlargement of the areola. This is usually first seen in girls at around the age of 10–11 years and is referred to as thelarche. Breast development is caused by proliferation of the ductal and alveolar system with specific deposition of fat within the ductal system, both of which occur under the stimulation of oestrogen. Thereafter, over a period of around four years, the breast grows by enlargement of the breast, areola and nipple. Early in development, the contours between the constituent parts are smooth, but later in development, there is elevation of the areola and nipple from the breast tissue. In the final stages, the nipple alone is elevated above the surrounding breast and areolar tissue. The stages of breast development were initially described in the classic work of Marshall and Tanner (1969) (Fig. 1.7). Breast development is complete in most girls by the age of 18, although further development of the alveolar lobules of the breast will occur during her first pregnancy.

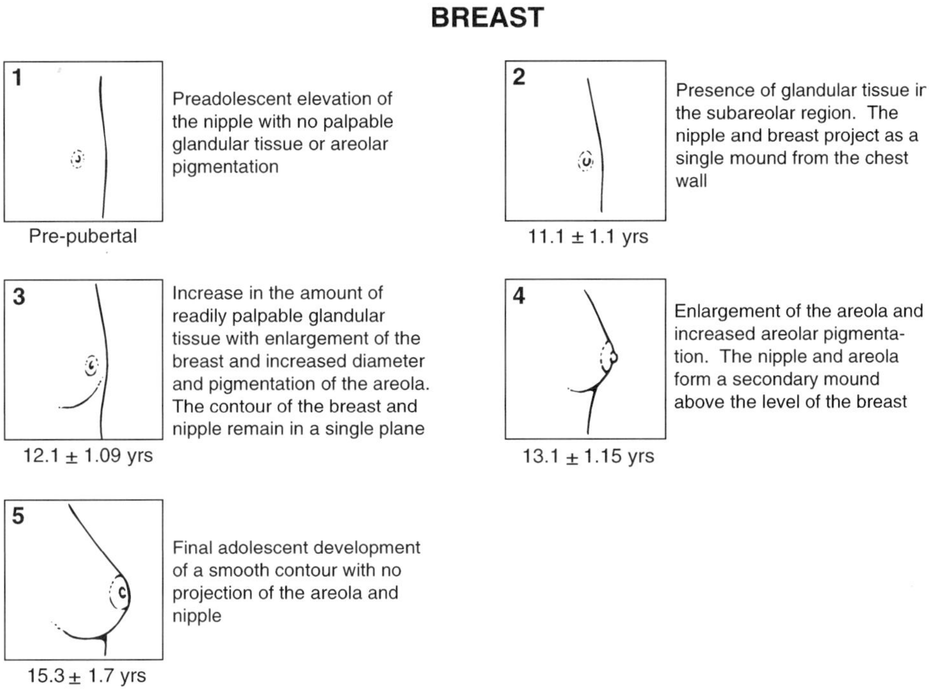

BREAST

1
Preadolescent elevation of the nipple with no palpable glandular tissue or areolar pigmentation

Pre-pubertal

2
Presence of glandular tissue ir the subareolar region. The nipple and breast project as a single mound from the chest wall

11.1 ± 1.1 yrs

3
Increase in the amount of readily palpable glandular tissue with enlargement of the breast and increased diameter and pigmentation of the areola. The contour of the breast and nipple remain in a single plane

12.1 ± 1.09 yrs

4
Enlargement of the areola and increased areolar pigmentation. The nipple and areola form a secondary mound above the level of the breast

13.1 ± 1.15 yrs

5
Final adolescent development of a smooth contour with no projection of the areola and nipple

15.3 ± 1.7 yrs

Fig. 1.7 Development of the breasts as described by Marshall and Tanner (1969) (with permission).

It is not unusual for initial breast development to be asymmetric with one breast developing before the other, or with one breast developing larger than the other. In most girls, the difference in size is negligible by the end of puberty, although in a minority of girls, corrective surgery may be required.

Absence of breast development by the age of 14 is abnormal and should be investigated. Breast development before the age of eight should be considered as precocious puberty and investigated accordingly. Interestingly, girls with precocious breast development may not have increased levels of oestrogen as measured by a standard assay.

It is suggested that testosterone has a specific inhibitory effect on breast development although the mechanism for this is not understood. This absence of an inhibitory effect has been postulated as the reason for good breast development in girls with androgen insensitivity despite the low levels of circulating oestrogen.

Development of the external genitalia

While growth of the hair on the external genitalia is dependent on the adrenal androgens, the development of the external genitalia themselves is oestrogen-dependent. Under the influence of oestrogens, the labia majora and labia minora increase in size and thicken. It is not well documented at what stage in pubertal development this occurs, but it is complete before the onset of menstruation.

While there is rarely any significant difference in size between the labia majora, wide variation in the size of the labia minora is common, both in terms of an individual girl having labia minora of differing sizes (Fig. 1.8) and a variation in size of labia minora within the population. Unfortunately, girls at this stage of their development are very sensitive about this part of their anatomy and

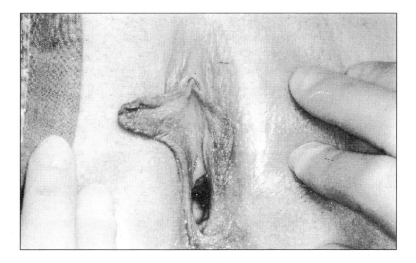

Fig. 1.8   Wide variation in size of the labia minora in an adolescent girl for whom it was causing extreme distress and who presented with a request for surgery.

often present with a request for reduction in the size of one or both labia minora. (Interestingly, I have never been asked to augment the size of labia). Every effort should be made to convince adolescent girls that variation in size is normal but such advice is rarely heeded. If surgery is performed, it is essential that this is delayed until growth of the labia is complete.

Along with growth of the labia is the development of the hymen. Under oestrogenic stimulus, the hymen thickens and the hymenal orifice enlarges to the adult size of 10 mm. The glands on the vestibule – Skene's glands around the urethra and Bartholin's glands in the inner aspect of the posterior third of the labia – begin to produce secretions.

The clitoris undergoes general enlargement at this time. It is thought that androgens also contribute to the development of the clitoris, but the extent to which this occurs is not known.

Vaginal development

Under the influence of oestrogen, the vagina lengthens, develops a thicker epithelial lining and begins to secrete mucus. The vagina begins to develop at around the same time as the breast and the final adult length of the vagina of about 10 cm is reached around the time the adolescent girl reaches her final height.

In the pre-pubertal girl, the vaginal epithelium is red and shiny in appearance whereas in the post-pubertal girl it is much thicker and pink in colour with the formation of folds or rugae. This change is due to thickening of the vaginal epithelium with cornification of the superficial layers caused by oestrogen. Vaginal smears with subsequent cytological examination to visualise these changes used to be performed to assess oestrogenisation prior to the widespread use of serum hormone estimation.

Along with the anatomical and histological changes, which occur in the vagina under oestrogen stimulation, is a change in function. The vaginal epithelium begins to secrete mucus and the pH of the vagina is reduced. Both of these mechanisms increase the resistance of the vagina to infection. The secretion of mucus causes the adolescent girl to develop a white vaginal discharge which is physiological but which may cause her some consternation if she does not know that this is likely to occur.

Uterine development

Uterine growth starts with the production of oestrogen. The first change is an increase in the length of the uterus so that the pre-pubertal ratio of uterus : cervix of 1 : 2 is reversed to 2 : 1. Thereafter, there is a thickening of both the myometrium, due to both myometrial hyperplasia and hypertrophy, and the cervix. These changes begin to occur around the age of nine and are complete at around the same time that breast development is complete. Changes in uterine size can be detected using ultrasound.

Prior to oestrogen stimulation, the endometrium of the uterus is a single layer of cuboidal cells. Under the influence of oestrogen the endometrium becomes columnar and multilayered. The thickness of the endometrium depends on the level and duration of oestrogen stimulation.

The columnar cells in the ectocervix begin to secrete mucus which add to the vaginal discharge experienced by adolescent and adult women.

Menstruation

The final obvious sign of puberty and the one which is particularly regarded as a rite of passage is the onset of menstruation or menarche which occurs in adolescents in the United Kingdom at around the age of 12.8 years and when a girl has attained Tanner stage 4–5 of breast development.

It has already been mentioned that the endometrium grows under the influence of oestrogen. During the follicular part of the cycle, or in early puberty, oestrogen only is being produced by the ovary. This causes proliferation of the endometrium. With rising or continuing oestrogen stimulus the endometrium thickens until it attains a thickness which is too great for its blood supply causing it to be shed in menstruation. This is likely to be the pattern for anything up to the first two years following menarche and explains why for many girls their periods in the early years are likely to be irregular (Apter, 1978). Depending on the levels of oestrogen or the length of stimulation before the endometrium is shed, these initial periods may also be extremely heavy.

With the maturation of the hypothalamic–pituitary–ovarian axis and the development of the positive feedback mechanism, ovulation occurs. Following ovulation, the follicle from which the ova is released becomes the corpus luteum and begins to secrete progesterone. During this second or luteal phase of the cycle, the proliferative endometrium undergoes secretory changes and becomes much more stable. The fall in progesterone levels which occurs when the corpus luteum involutes, however, causes the endometrium to shed. The onset of regular ovulation, therefore, brings about regular menstruation as well as being the final step in puberty – the achievement of fertility.

In summary, therefore, an knowledge of the anatomical and endocrine changes which occur as a girl grows from a baby to adolescence is extremely helpful in understanding some of the gynaecological disorders which she may present with.

REFERENCES

Apter VR, 1978: Hormonal patterns of adolescent cycles. *Journal of Clinical Endocrinology and Metabolism* **47**, 944–954.
Baker TG, 1963: A quantitative and cytological study of germ cells in human ovaries. *Proceedings of the Royal Society of London (Biological Sciences)* **158**, 417–433.
Marshall WA, Tanner JM, 1969: Variations in the pattern of pubertal changes in girls. *Archives of Disease in Childhood* **44**, 291–303.
Mittwoch U, Burgess AMC, Baker PJ, 1993: Male development in a sea of oestrogen. *Lancet* **2**, 123–124.
Tanner JM, Whitehouse RH, Hughes PCR, Carter BS, 1976: Relative importance of growth hormone and sex steroids for the growth at puberty of trunk length, limb length and muscle width in growth hormone-deficient children. *Journal of Pediatrics* **89**, 1000–1008.

CHAPTER 2

Psychosexual development

JULIA NELKI AND FRANCIS STEWART ———————————

Before Anneli is aware of her own sexual identity she knows which areas of life
are masculine. She's 20 months old and can say 'man talk', 'man drive car', 'man
motorbike', 'man kissie', 'woman nothing on', 'woman cleaning'

There's a good girl
Grabucker, 1988

INTRODUCTION

How does a girl get a sense of being female and what does being female mean?
Is it something we innately know or something we learn and copy from those
around us? Or is it a combination of the two?

Psychosexual development is a complex area that can be broken down into
component parts to incorporate gender identity, by which is meant a person's
concept of themselves as female or male; sex-typed behaviours which are those
behaviours that appear to differentiate the sexes and sexual activities, interests
and orientation which refer to sexual relationships, fantasies and feelings (Rutter,
1980). It is achieved through the complex interplay of anatomical, physiological,
developmental and psychological factors in the context of family, society and
culture and is central to one's identity. From very early on, one thinks of oneself
and of others as female or male. It is very hard to think of oneself simply as a
person. Psychosexual development is a lifelong process with no definite end
point. It is an aspect of development and a part of one's life. From a notion of
femaleness or maleness, the origins of which are uncertain, the infant gradually
develops a more complex understanding of what it means to be a woman or a
man. The interplay between biological factors such as anatomical, physiological
and hormonal influences and environmental ones that include parental projections, sex-role projections, cultural expectations and personal experiences is
complex but adds up over the years to help us define our sense of ourselves in
relation to our gender. Although the anatomical distinctions between women and
men are usually clear-cut, the psychological ones are less so. Jung (1961)
described 'biological bisexuality' by which he meant that we all have feminine
and masculine traits within us. Socialisation pressures and genetic sex differences lead to a trend for the more feminine traits to be developed in women and
masculine ones in men. The 'other' is, however, according to Jung, always

present and part of each of us. Whatever the origins, the characteristics and traits associated with being female or male tend to be reflected in the roles assigned to them, with women often put in a subordinate position and excluded from major decision-making positions as if this was a 'given'. The evidence does not support such a rigid view.

The following pages look at the different influences at different ages and give an idea of the complexity of the process; the difficulty of disentangling different components and the increasing body of knowledge supporting flexibility of roles for women and men acknowledging the particular importance of social factors.

BEFORE BIRTH

There is some evidence that later sexual behaviour and gender identity, not only physical changes, are, to some extent, determined by hormone activity while the fetus is developing (Rutter, 1980). The development of the brain is altered by the presence or absence of the male sex hormones in the fetus and there may be some gender differentiation even at this stage. Prenatal hormones that are out of keeping with chromosomal sex affect sex-typed behaviours though not gender identity (Yalom *et al.*, 1973). In girls with congenital adrenal hyperplasia (CAH) where there is excessive androgen production *in utero* or in pregnancies when synthetic progestogen has been given to prevent miscarriage, there is increased 'tomboyish' behaviour in girls and marked differences in types of play in relation to controls but gender identity is unaffected (Money and Ehrhardt, 1972). A comparison between sisters and controls showed that those with CAH had more homosexual and bisexual fantasies and less sexual relationships than their sisters but all had a strong sense of being female (Dittmann *et al.*, 1992). It may be that hormones affect the developing brain in ways that facilitate the learning of opposite gender behaviours but many other factors are obviously involved and male/female behaviors are not polarised and totally separate. Stoller (1976) suggests that core gender identity, a precursor of gender identity, starts in the fetus, with the help of sex hormones, anatomy and physiology. Social and psychological factors have an influence, even at this early age, as the prospective parents begin a relationship with their baby, together with their hopes, fears, expectations and assumptions about femaleness and maleness. A relationship with a fantasy baby exists that has to be modified when the baby is born. There is some evidence that a mother's hopes and fantasies influence initial responses to infants (Kestenberg, 1976) and that once parents know the sex, whether before or after the birth, they react in different ways depending on the sex of the child (Tyson and Tyson, 1990). Their own experiences as a baby are usually triggered as parenthood approaches and, depending on their nature and how these experiences have been resolved, integrated and understood, parents will respond differently to a girl or boy.

PRESCHOOL: 0–5 YEARS

The appearance of the external genitalia at birth are usually the main determinant of sexual assignment. Naming the sex at birth is often a powerful moment for the parents. Core gender identity incorporates knowing what gender one is and understanding that gender is stable over time and cannot change. It is influenced by the relationship a child has with its mother and 'the mother's acceptance and acknowledgement of the baby's sex at birth' (Welldon, 1988). It will also depend on other relationships, particularly that with the baby's father, siblings and extended family or those closely involved in the child's upbringing. Although anatomical features are important, the assigned gender and parental rearing are of greater importance in the development of core gender identity which is normally established by the age of 3 years (Rutter, 1980). If a firm core gender identity has been established, it is difficult to make changes after the age of 3 years. Hormones given post-natally can affect the later sex drive of the child (Money and Ehrhardt, 1972) but do not ordinarily make a difference to the acquisition of gender identity unless there are major physical changes and an already weak gender identity. When physical appearances are ambiguous, the core gender identity is often less certain and there are many accounts of successful changes in sexual identity after this time.

Gender identity as a broader concept can be taken to be a psychological configuration that includes personal identity and biological sex (Tyson and Tyson, 1990). It will include masculine and feminine components from all the influences on a child as she or he develops together with body image, a basic concept of a person's relationship to her/his self.

Sex-typed behaviours are the differences in behaviours, play and actions between the sexes. 'Masculine' activities are described as those being more rough and tumble, outdoor and mechanical in contrast to those described as 'feminine' which are considered as being more artistic, creative and indoor. Behavioural differences between girls and boys are noted from early on and their origins are the centre of many debates.

The biological view (Diamond, 1965) holds that genetic and hormonal influences determine sex differences and that the environment has little effect. Prenatal hormones do influence both gonad formation *in utero* and later sexual behaviour (Money and Ehrhardt, 1972) but there is plenty of evidence for other influences as well. The shift towards 'boyish' behaviour is not found in all girls exposed to pre-natal androgens and certainly 'boyish' and 'girlish' behaviours are seen in all children. It is also possible that hormonal influences are not the only variables in these children and that parental attitude may differ with the androgenised children from the others.

Cognitive-developmental approaches (Kohlberg, 1966) state that children move through different stages of development which represent increasingly detailed ways of thinking and understanding their environment. Gender is used from very early on, initially based on physical attributes, to understand the self, others, attitudes and behaviours. The construction of stereotypes leads to sex-typed behaviours. Values and behaviours develop out of a need to behave in ways which are consistent with a child's concept of herself as female or himself as male. After these values are acquired, the desire to be masculine or feminine leads to identification with male or female role modes. Knowledge of gender stereotypes is thought to precede sex differences in behaviour. An example of this would be:

- Observation related to gender – 'she has long hair and is a girl'
- Inference – 'she has long hair because she is a girl'
- Stereotype – 'she has long hair, doesn't play with trains, is soft etc because she is a girl'
- Sex-typed behaviours – 'girls have long hair, are soft etc.'
- Gender identity – 'I must have long hair, be soft, not play with trains etc.'

In support of this, Martin and Little (1990) looked at the relationship between gender understanding, sex-typed preferences and gender-stereotypes in 3–5-year-olds over time and found that once children recognised their own gender, they would begin to behave in sex-typed ways and choose gender-specific toys and activities. Gender consistency understanding did not have to be established for this to happen but they concluded that a basic idea of gender begins early and precedes sex-typed behaviours.

In contrast, social learning theories (Mussen and Eisenberg-Berg, 1977) propose that identification and imitation lead to a sense of being female or male. No particular knowledge about gender is required and sex-typed preferences are thought to be determined by the responses they elicit. Cognitions are not thought to play a major role in sex-typing. Children will copy others if they associate themselves with them, are capable of copying them and if there are sufficient available incentives.

Early on, family models are the most important. Later, peer group, media pressures and cultural expectations have more influence. While there is evidence to support the importance of modelling in psychosexual development, and this would provide an explanation for societal variation, it is not on its own sufficient. Children often have opposite sex role models and their behaviours do not mirror very closely that of adults. Nevertheless, social learning is very important as illustrated by Maccoby (Maccoby, 1993) who showed that sex-typed behaviours are socially determined and minimal when children are observed individually. By looking at the play of pairs of previously unacquainted 3-year-olds, she found that children played much more when playing with same sex children than with the opposite sex and that sex differences in behaviour were only apparent when playing with opposite sex partners. Girls became much more passive when playing with boys and boys became much more dominant and unresponsive to their female partners than their male ones. Children preferred same sex playmates from preschool times and this became much more marked by the age of 6.

Gender schema theory is a cognitive theory that allows for the influence of social factors (Serbin *et al.*, 1993). It states that infants develop gender schemas, by which is meant networks of characteristics associated with females or males.

They begin as naive concepts that gradually become more complex as the understanding of what constitutes femaleness or maleness deepens. Environmental factors are thought to influence the content of the schemas and therefore individual differences, taking into account particular experiences, are possible. Children do preferentially remember information consistent with gender role which supports this theory and children's knowledge of sex-typing as regards toys, behaviours and even occupations is evident even at primary school (Serbin *et al.*, 1993). Serbin *et al.* (1993) found that the level of cognitive maturity determined children's knowledge of sex-typed stereotypes but that the influence at home was also important. Sex-typed preferences for activities, occupations and peers related to attitudes at home. Cognitive factors were also important in that children who believed gender stereotypes to be flexible were less sex-typed in their choices. The review by Serbin *et al.* (1993) of the studies of gender stereotyping found that, throughout middle childhood, children use gender stereotypes to make inferences about others but become less rigid as they get older. Although sex differences in activities and interests develop early, flexibility in terms of gender stereotyping develops more slowly. It is a function of cognitive maturity but is also influenced greatly by paternal education and presence in the home, maternal occupation and parental modelling (Serbin *et al.*, 1993). Resistance to categorising was a normal feature of development too, as if to counter the strong wish to categorise at an earlier age.

There are many psychoanalytic views which focus on the unconscious and what the child brings from its internal world to its relationships with others. Infantile sexuality was described first by Freud (1905) in his 'libido theory' which states that the infant relates to others only for the relief of biological needs. The child is presumed to pass through a series of psychosexual stages – oral, anal and phallic – which will determine later sexuality and personality depending on how these stages are managed. Freud's phallocentric view focused on the central importance of the discovery of genital difference in the phallic stage at around 4, and that the awareness of the presence or absence of the penis was the determining factor in differentiating the psychosexual development of girls and boys (Freud, 1926, 1931). This view has been challenged by many and the idea of 'primary femininity' proposed by Stoller is supported by many analysts (Sayers, 1991). The mother–daughter relationship is a complex one, and the developing girl struggles with both identifying with her mother and needing to separate and find her own identity. The father can have an important influence on a girl's growing sense of femininity, particularly around the age of 2, when separation is a major task. A girl often forms a new and intimate relationship with her father at this time (Samuels, 1985; Tyson and Tyson, 1990).

It is to be expected that development may proceed differently in boys who can visualise and feel their genitals and see that it is like their daddies', though smaller, from girls who can feel their vagina but only imagine their womb and later developing breasts like their mummies. Both can only imagine the later function their bodies can have and it is only in middle childhood that children recognise that their gender is fixed and will not change. Boys can form discrete concrete mental representations of their genitals. Girls cannot. Symbolisation may play a greater part in development for a girl than a boy (Bernstein, 1990) though what the implications of this might be is not known.

Patterson (1992) notes that psychoanalytic and social learning theories emphasise the importance of children having both heterosexual female and male parents. Cognitive developmental theories do not and are, therefore, supported by studies showing that being brought up in a homosexual or transsexual household has no particular influence on psychosexual development (Green, 1978; Golombok *et al.*, 1983; Javaid, 1993).

Sexual activity is noted in the first year in both sexes in terms of interest in their genitals. About 36% of 1-year-olds are reported to show genital play (Newson and Newson, 1963) and this increases over the years.

From an early age, children are interested in sex and where babies come from. Their questions and understanding are in line with their cognitive development and they will tend to have a concrete understanding in this period, imagining that babies are made by eating certain foods, or come out from the anus, or by being cut out of the tummy. Most 5-year-olds do not understand how a baby is born even if they have seen pictures.

MIDDLE CHILDHOOD: 5–11 YEARS

This is a time of transition to the outside world where there are enormous changes in social relationships, intellectual and other skills, physical development and the development of a social conscience. This period is crucial for forming the basis of relationships with the same and opposite sex and with persons in positions of authority and for the development of a sense of self in relation to others. Freud (1926) described this as the latency period believing it to be a time when psychosexual interest declined and oedipal concerns faded. It is, however, a time of great sexual interest and exploration with a strong need for identification.

Sex-typed behaviours are more marked during this time with a lot of interest in peer group relationships and the learning of social roles and rules. Although children know what sex they are before this stage and that their sex will not change, they are less clear about other children and apparently it is only by about 7 years that they reliably use genital cues and only by 11 that they are fully aware that the genital difference is the prime difference (Rutter, 1980).

A few children experience pubertal changes through this time and it can be a hard time for those that have, particularly for girls. For boys, it is often harder to be a slow developer and smaller than your peers though for girls the reverse is true. Competitive peer relationships, social interactions and the learning of sex-typed stereotypes can mean that stereotyping is more marked during this time with exaggerated feminine behaviour by some girls and 'tomboyish' behaviour in others depending on their identifications and preoccupations at the time.

ADOLESCENCE: 12–18 YEARS

Adolescence is the transitional period from childhood to adult autonomy and psychosexual development with the acquisition of secondary sexual characteristics and adult reproductive capacities is a crucial element of this stage. The physical changes of puberty have been dealt with on p. 8 and cannot be considered in isolation from the psychosocial perspective. Biological factors are seen by some as the guiding force behind young people's alterations in behaviour, moods, thinking and relationships although others place greater emphasis on family, society and cultural influences. S. Freud's (1924) views of an upsurge of instinctual drive energies at puberty which have to be channelled away from parents on to peers and coping mechanisms depending on early experiences of drive satisfaction were further expounded by A. Freud (1969). She described the attempts of the adolescent to manage anxiety-provoking increases in sexual feelings by denial or sublimation into creativity, asceticism or intellectual pursuits. Swings from consideration for others to self-centredness, from hope to despair, from love to aggression and from dependence to independence, she considered to be part of the young person's coping process. Adolescence marks a second step towards individuation, the first having happened around the second year, when the child begins its fight for autonomy (Blos, 1962). The adolescent further develops her/his sense of identity by rebelling against emotional ties to parents, with the acknowledgement that sexual and emotional needs should also be met outside the family. Loneliness, isolation and confusion can result as well as the stress of new sexual feelings.

Erikson (1959) proposed a series of life span stages, each characterised by a major conflict which has to be resolved for satisfactory progress towards maturity. He described the main task of adolescence as the formation of identity: a coherent sense of self, based on commitment to present and future roles, ideology and values regarding future relationships. The parental role in this is to loosen ties held on the young person.

The psychological effects of the physical changes are thought to come about by the interplay between direct hormonal effects and the perception of the meanings attributed to these changes by family, peers and society. Eccles *et al.* (1988) found oestrogen levels to be related to positive mood in adolescent girls but there is other evidence that alterations in hormone levels are associated with depression and decreased impulse control (Brooks-Gunn and Warren, 1985). Early onset of puberty appears to have an effect on well-being and adjustment with an increased risk of poor body image (Blyth *et al.*, 1985; Duncan *et al.*, 1985), poor educational progress and behavioural problems in school (Hyjer Dyk, 1993). These physically mature girls attract opposite sex interest and have to cope with the stresses of puberty while being emotionally less mature than later developers. There is, however, apparently no long-term effect (Peskin, 1967). Generally, responses to menarche are found to be related to preparedness which, in turn, is associated with attitudes in the family, with peers and in educational settings. 20% of girls interviewed within 2–3 months of menarche rated the experience positively and 20% negatively. McGrory (1990) found no difference in the self-esteem of pre- and post-menarcheal girls.

Many adolescent girls are dissatisfied with their body appearance (Lerner *et al.*, 1976) particularly weight. Schonfeld (1969) reported 70% of girls wanted to be thinner with the most popular girls most concerned about their weight. He described family factors as important, such as when family members make a fuss about changes in appearance and place a high value on beauty; or when parents project their own anxieties about sexuality onto their children. Anorexia nervosa can sometimes develop and is characterised by 'the relentless pursuit of thinness' (Bruch, 1978), amenorrhoea and a distorted body image (Boocock and Trethewie, 1981). Cultural and media images linking beauty and desirability to thinness contribute to the strong association in the minds of young girls between self-esteem and body size. Other authors relate anorexia to an unconscious flight from sexual maturity with a return to a child-like body and the cessation of menstruation when weight decreases below a certain level (Kessler, 1966). Family influences are described by Minuchin *et al.* (1978) who views anorexia as a way of coping with over-controlling and disunited parents. Where a family exerts heavy demands for conformity and achievement, control over food intake and weight can be a means of re-establishing some feeling of control of self and others. Clearly, sexuality within the cultural and family contexts has an important place in the development of this life-threatening condition.

The characteristics attributed to gender identity develop further in adolescence with an increase in the acquisition of ideas of attractiveness of the self and the opposite sex, and with values and attitudes to sexuality. Gender role relates largely to cultural values which incorporates behaviour attributed as feminine by society. Its acquisition is a vital part of the adolescent task of identity formation and achieving autonomy. The development of the cognitive ability to evaluate, in the mind, the consequences of one's own actions and those of others is held to be a prerequisite for the integration of value systems (Colby and Kohlberg, 1987).

Marcia (1966) elaborates this theory by relating the examination of attitudes in personal, social and sexual domains to identity formation. There are many models, values and attitudes available to young girls from family, peers, school, the media, culture and religion. Peer influences are generally found to be more significant than those of the family (Thornton and Camburn, 1987), and the rejection of parental values may be a necessary step towards identity formation.

Although choice of sex object plays an important part in adolescence, it is unlikely to be consolidated until early adulthood. Orientation includes sexual interest, fantasies and behaviour. Uncertainty and confusion about orientation occurs frequently in adolescence. Family upbringing is not thought to exert an influence on orientation whereas there is some evidence that there may be a familial tendency (Bailey and Bell, 1993). Peters and Cantrell (1991) found no correlation between early sexual traumas or negative heterosexual experiences and homosexuality though this is a controversial area. Certainly, sexual abuse, particularly incest, has major effects on the self and social functioning (Cole and Putnam, 1992). Adjustment to a lesbian identity can be stressful and lengthy, particularly because of stigma and a lack of information. Many girls go through a period of anxiety about their sexual identity for which support and exploration of their feelings can be helpful.

Adolescent girls report less masturbatory experiences than boys. It may be that sex drive is displaced onto close friendships and crushes, or that gender role expectations play a part in this lower sex interest (Dusek, 1991). Circulating hormones have an unclear role in female sexual interest and arousal but social factors seem to be of greater significance (Udry *et al.*, 1986).

The average age of first sexual intercourse for girls is 17 with a steady progression over 2 years from first dating through kissing and petting to sexual intercourse. Most girls report planning their first intercourse to satisfy curiosity and deepen the relationship with a partner whom they are likely to have known for some time. Social pressure exerts a strong influence (Davis and Harris, 1982). Early maturity, homelessness and lack of family support or closeness are all associated with early sexual activity. This may occur through attempts to achieve independence, to enhance low self-esteem and to meet non-sexual needs for closeness.

The change in age of first sexual intercourse over the past decades and in different cultures reflects the influence of cultural factors such as the increasing acceptance of female sexuality, the assertion of women's rights and needs, the acceptance of pre-marital and extra-marital sexual activity and the availability of contraception.

Adolescence can be a turbulent time which, if negotiated successfully, results in a young woman developing a sense of her own identity and moving towards emotionally mature, sexually intimate relationships with the capacity for long-term relationships and motherhood.

Healthy psychosexual development is the likely result of a combination of constitutional and environmental factors. An interactional model is probably the most useful with different factors assuming more or less importance depending on age. A girl's sense of identity, a sense of herself as female results from the interplay between physical appearance, hormonal influences, parental attitudes and expectations, cultural and social settings, and personal experiences and relationships.

No theory alone would be able to account for the whole process of psychosexual development. Studies that show interactions, such as the link between cognitive factors and influences in the home (Serbin *et al.*, 1993) or where behaviour is markedly different depending on the gender of the person one is with (Maccoby, 1993), are exciting but at an early stage. Women and men have traditionally been assigned to particular roles and behaviours and Chodorow (1974) believes female subordination to be universal. Schlegel (1977) in her cross-cultural studies differentiated between sexually stratified societies where, by custom or law, women cannot have positions of power, from sexually inegalitarian ones where it is possible but difficult. She also found cultures where women have higher status than men primarily because they are responsible for childcare. However, no roles other than childbearing, and to some extent early childrearing, are invariant and flexibility is possible.

SUMMARY

A girl develops her identity and sense of herself as female through a combination of her physical appearance, hormonal influences, parental attitudes, cultural expectations and her own particular experiences. The cultural and social setting, as well as parental expectations, will determine opportunities and roles for women and what value is attributed to particular behaviours and achievements. Biological differences between the sexes are likely to account for some of the sex-typing though it is clear from the wide variation across cultures that many aspects are acquired rather than biologically determined. Cognitive, psycho-analytic and social theories ascribe prime importance to different features – stage of cognitive capacity, intrapsychic development or the impact of the environment. Biological and cognitive development follow similar lines for all children allowing stability and consistency across the population and through generations while psychoanalytic, gender schema and social learning ideas contribute to our understanding of how individual differences are established.

Differences between the sexes are obvious, necessary and to be welcomed though rigidity of roles and systems that attribute lower value and status to certain areas, such as childcare, than to others, such as work outside the home, can lead to competition, resentment and low self-esteem rather than creativity and a working together for the mutual benefit of children and society.

REFERENCES

Bailey JM, Bell AP, 1993: Familiality of female and male homosexuality. *Behavior Genetics* **23**(4), 313–322.

Bernstein D, 1990: Female genital anxieties, conflicts and typical mastery modes. *International Journal of Psycho-analysis* **71**, 151–165.

Blos P, 1962: Introduction: Puberty and adolescence. In *On adolescence: A psychoanalytic interpretation*. New York: Free Press, 1–15.

Blyth DA, Simmons RG, Zakin D, 1985: Satisfaction with body image for early adolescent females: a developmental perspective. *Journal of Youth and Adolescence* **14**, 207–226.

Boocock RM, Trethewie KJ, 1981: Body image and weight relationship in teenage girls. *Proceedings of the Nutrition Society of Austrialia* **6**, 166–167.

Brooks-Gunn J, Warren MP, 1985: Measuring physical status and timing in early adolescence: a developmental perspective. *Journal of Youth and Adolescence* **14**, 163–189.

Bruch H, 1978: *The golden cage*. London: Open Books, ix.

Chodorow N, 1974: Family structure and feminine personality. In Rosaldo MZ, Lamphere L, (eds), *Women, culture and society*. Stanford University Press, 43–66.

Colby A, Kohlberg L, 1987: *The measurement of moral judgment. Theoretical foundations and research validation*. New York: Cambridge University Press, **1**, 1–60.

Cole P, Putnam F, 1992: Effect of incest on self and social functioning: a developmental psychopathology perspective. *Journal of Consulting and Clinical Psychology* **60.2**, 174–184.

Davis SM, Harris MB, 1982: Sexual knowledge, sexual interest and sources of information of rural and urban adolescents from three cultures. *Adolescence* **17**, 471–492.

Diamond M, 1965: A critical evaluation of the ontogeny of human sexual behaviour. *Quarterly Review of Biology* **40**, 147–175.

Dittmann RW, Kappes ME, Kappes MH, 1992: Sexual behaviour in adolescent females with congenital adrenal hyperplasia. *Psychoneuroendocrinology*, **17**(2–3), 153–170.

Duncan P, Ritter P, Dornbusch S, Gross R, Carlsmith J, 1985: The effects of pubertal timing on body image, school behaviour and deviance. *Journal of Youth and Adolescence* **14**, 227–236.

Dusek JB, 1991: *Adolescent development and behaviour.* New York: Prentice-Hall, 252–292.

Eccles JS, Miller CL, Tucker ML, *et al.* 1988: Hormones and effect at early age adolescence. In Brooks-Gunn J, (chair), *Hormona; contributions to adolescent behaviour.* A Symposium conducted at the second biennial meeting of the society for Research on adolescence. Alexandria, V.A.

Erikson E, 1959: Identity and the life cycle. *Psychological Issues* **1**, 1–71.

Freud A, 1969: Adolescence as a developmental disturbance. In Caplan G, Lebovici S, (eds), *Adolescence: psychosocial perspectives.* New York: Basic Books, 5–10.

Freud S, 1905: *Three essays on the theory of sexuality.* SE7, London: Hogarth, 1953, 130–134.

Freud S, 1924: *The dissolution of the Oedipus complex,* SE19, London: Hogarth, 1961, 173–182.

Freud S, 1926: *The question of lay analysis.* SE20, London: Hogarth, 1959, 183–250.

Freud S, 1931: *Female sexuality.* SE21 London: Hogarth, 1961, 225–243.

Golombok S, Spencer A, Rutter M, 1983: Children in lesbian and single-parent households: psychosexual and psychiatric appraisal. *Journal of Child Psychology and Psychiatry* **24**, 551–572.

Grabrucker M, 1988: *There's a good girl.* Women's Press, 29.

Green R, 1978: Sexual identity of 37 children raised by homosexual or transexual parents. *American Journal of Psychiatry* **135**, 692–697.

Hyjer Dyk P, 1993: Anatomy, physiology and gender issues in adolescence. In Gullotta T, Adams G, Montemayor R, (eds), *Adolescent sexuality.* London: Sage, 35–56.

Javaid GA, 1993: The children of homosexual and heterosexual single mothers. *Child Psychiatry and Human Development* **23**, 235–248.

Jung C, 1989: *Memories, Dreams & Reflections.* Fontana, 210–212.

Kessler J, 1966: *Psychopathology of childhood.* Englewood Cliffs, New Jersey: Prentice-Hall, 108–110.

Kestenberg JS, 1976: Regression and reintegration in pregnancy. *Journal of the American Psychoanalytic Association* **16**, 213–250.

Kohlberg, 1966: Cognitive stages and preschool education. *Human Development* **9**, 5–17.

Lerner RM, Orlos JB, Knapp JR, 1976: Physical attractiveness, physical effectiveness and self concept in late adolescence. *Adolescence* **11**, 313–326.

Maccoby EE, 1993: Gender and relationships. *American Psychologist* April, 513–520.

Marcia J, 1966: Development and validation of ego identity status. *Journal of Personality and Social Psychology* **3**, 551–558.

Martin CL, Little J, 1990: The relation of gender understanding to children's sex-typed preferences and gender stereotypes. *Child Development* **61**, 1427–1439.

McGrory A, 1990: Menarche: Responses of early adolescent females. *Adolescence* **25**(98), 265–270.

Minuchin P, Rossman B, Baker L, 1978: The anorectic family. *Psychosomatic families: Anorexia nervosa in context.* Cambridge, MA: Harvard University Press, 51–73.

Money J, Ehrhardt AA, 1972: *Man and woman, boy and girl.* Johns Hopkins University Press, 1–24, 95–114.

Mussen PH, Eisenberg-Berg, 1977: Culture and prosocial behaviour. In *Roots of caring, sharing and helping.* San Francisco: Freeman, 47–63.

Newson J, Newson E, 1963: *Four years old in an urban community.* London: Penguin, 375–383.

Patterson C, 1992: Children of lesbian and gay parents. *Review of Child Development* **63**, 1025–1042.

Peskin H, 1967: Pubertal onset and ego functioning. *Journal of Abnormal Psychology* **72**, 1–15.

Peters DK, Cantrell PJ, 1991: Factors distinguishing samples of lesbian and heterosexual women. *Journal of Homosexuality* **21**, 1–15.

Rutter M, 1980: Psychosexual development. In Rutter M, (ed.), *Scientific foundations: developmental psychiatry.* Heinemann, 322–338.

Samuels A, 1985: *The father. Contemporary Jungian perspectives.* Free Association Books, 1–45.

Sayers J, 1991: *Mothering psychoanalysis.* Penguin, 92–99.

Schlegel A, 1977: *Sexual stratification. A cross-cultural view.* Columbia University Press, 1–37.

Schonfeld WA, 1969: The body and the body image in adolescents. In Caplan G, Lebovici S, (eds), *Adolescence: psychosocial perspectives.* New York: Basic Books, 27–53.

Serbin LA, Powlishta KK, Gullap J, 1993: The development of sex typing in middle childhood. *Monographs of the Society for Research in Child Development* **58**(2), 1–99.

Stoller RJ, 1976: Primary femininity. *Journal of the American Psychoanalytic Association* **24**, (suppl), 59–78.

Thornton A, Camburn D, 1987: The influence of the family on premarital sexual attitudes and behaviour. *Demography* **24**, 323–340.

Tyson P, Tyson R, 1990: Psychoanalytic theories of development. In *Gender.* Yale University Press, 249–294.

Udry JR, Talbert LM, Morris NM, 1986: Biosocial foundations for adolescent female sexuality. *Demography* **23**(2), 217–230.

Welldon E, 1988: *Mother, Madonna, Whore.* Free Association Books, 45.

Yalom I, Green R, Fisk N, 1973: Prenatal exposure to female hormones. *Archives of General Psychiatry* **28**, 554–561.

CHAPTER 3

Anatomical development assessed by ultrasound

DAVID PILLING

INTRODUCTION

The rapid development of ultrasound in the 1980s enabled the uterus and ovaries of children to be studied non-invasively for the first time. Much of this work has been correlated with the postmortem anatomical work available, particularly the work of Krantz and Atkinson (1967).

ULTRASOUND EXAMINATION

The best ultrasound examinations are undertaken using high frequency transducers and real time equipment. In the neonate and infant 7.5 megahertz (mHz) is appropriate with 5 mHz being used in the older children and adolescents. The pelvic organs can only be satisfactorily imaged if the urinary bladder is full. In the neonate and infant, this is obviously a matter of chance but in a well hydrated patient and with some patience, a satisfactory examination can be obtained. In older children a full bladder, but not an overdistended one, enables the uterus to be demonstrated in all patients and the ovaries in the majority of patients.

MEASUREMENT

Measurement of ovarian and uterine size is most accurately undertaken using calculated volumes. This makes the assumption that each of these organs is an ellipsoid with a volume calculation made using three linear diameter measurements, the volume being calculated from the formula length $\times$ width $\times$ height $\times$ 0.5. In some studies only, linear measurements have been available (Willi, 1992) and while this may be acceptable for the length of the uterine body, this cannot be accurate enough for the assessment of the ovaries.

UTERINE APPEARANCE IN THE NEONATAL PERIOD

The uterus in the neonate has a prominent endometrium (Fig. 3.1) and in its long axis measures 3.5 to 5 cm with a mean volume of 3.0 ml (Haber and Mayer, 1994). Over the first 3 months of life, the endometrial prominence resolves and the shape of the uterus converts to the infantile type, with a mean volume of 1.0 ml. The uterine shape in the neonatal period is more adult like with thick myometrium and endometrium, the body being larger than the cervix, the so-

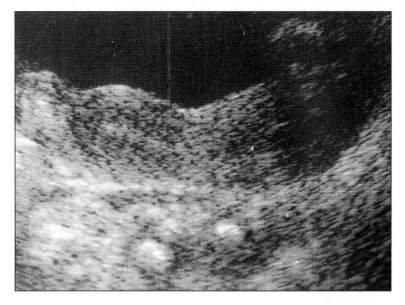

Fig. 3.1   Neonatal uterus showing 'pear shape' and prominent endometrium.

called 'pear shape'. When the hormonal stimulus has resolved, the uterus reverts to the infantile type with reduction in the myometrium of the body and relative prominence of the cervix. This has been described as the 'tear drop' shape but in reality is usually more cylindrical (Fig. 3.2). The uterine volume and appearances remain virtually unchanged up to the age of about 8 years when the uterine volume starts to increase with physical growth and further rapid increase occurs at around the time of puberty, due to the hormonal stimulus of the uterus. At this stage, the uterine shape changes from the rather cylindrical appearance of the infantile uterus to the more 'pear shape' appearance characteristic of the adult. The endometrium also takes on a slightly thickened appearance in response to hormonal stimulus. By the age of 16 years, the uterine volume has risen to a mean of 20 ml.

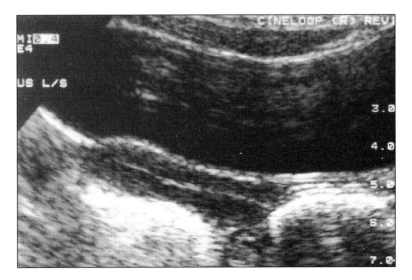

Fig. 3.2 Normal uterus in an 8-year-old girl. Note the thin endometrium and relative prominence of the cervix.

OVARIAN APPEARANCE

The ovaries can be difficult to image due to their variable position (Figs 3.3 and 3.4). The internal iliac vessels are a good marker as the ovary is normally just medial to the vessels although this is not invariable. The appearances of the ovary are static during the early years of life. The mean ovarian volume is about 0.7 ml from birth to 7 years of age (Bridges *et al.,* 1993). Some authors have suggested that there is an increase in size with age, the volume rising to 2.0 ml at 12 years. Others have suggested that ovarian volumes increase following hormonal stimulus but about 2 years after the start of increase in uterine volume (Haber and Mayer, 1994). Small cystic elements are frequently seen within the ovaries of children, with larger cysts being commoner in asymptomatic older children (Fig. 3.5). This is thought to be due to low level intermittent gonadatrophin secretion. As well as the overall ovarian volume increasing with hormonal change, the number of follicles increases. This can give the appearance of a 'multicystic' ovary in the adolescent which should not be confused with a pathological ovary. If follicles enlarge, they can produce cysts which are very obvious on ultrasound. Many authorities would suggest that if a 'cyst' is unilocular, echo free and less than 5 cm in diameter it is unlikely to require treatment. Observation will usually confirm resolution with time. Difficulty in excluding such a lesion as a cause of the patient's symptoms leads to difficulty in management.

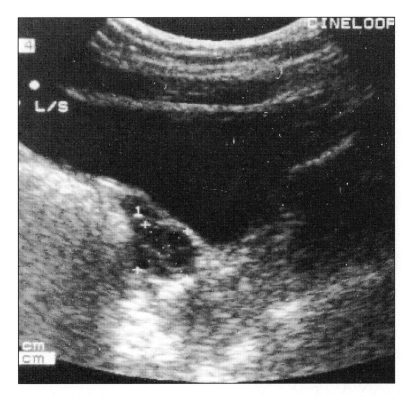

Fig. 3.3 Longitudinal section of normal ovary at 10 years of age. Note mixed echo pattern due to multiple small follicles.

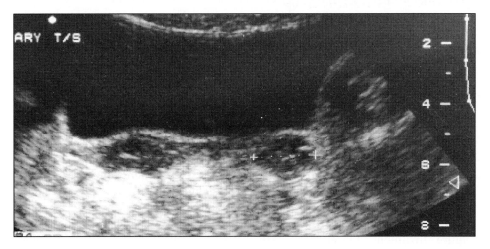

Fig. 3.4 Transverse section of normal ovaries of the same patient. (left marked **) showing similar characteristics.

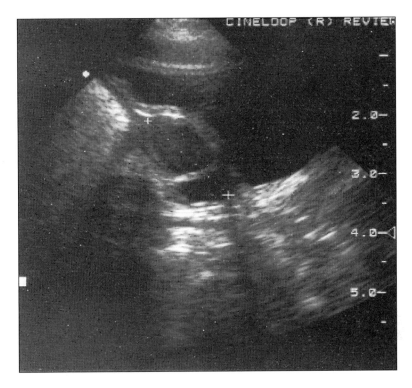

Fig. 3.5 Longitudinal section of ovary in a girl age 14 years. Note two small cysts which were entirely asymptomatic.

OTHER PELVIC ORGANS

The small bowel is frequently identified in the pelvis. If fluid loaded, this is easy to identify with its mixed echo appearance and peristalsis being obvious. Collapsed, empty small bowel has a soft tissue density and is difficult to separate from the other pelvic organs. Large bowel is seen predominantly on the left as a mixed echo structure but with brighter than average soft tissue due to gas and faeces mixed in the bowel. The large bowel frequently obscures the left ovary making it difficult to identify. Free fluid in the Pouch of Douglas is a normal finding if small in amount. This appears as an echo free appearance of irregular shape behind the uterus. The fallopian tubes cannot be identified if normal by trans-abdominal scanning.

SUMMARY

In normal infants, the uterus is quite prominent during the first month of life with a decrease in volume and reduction in endometrial thickness following the withdrawal of maternal hormonal stimulation. Growth of the uterus is very limited up to about the age of 8 years when there is only a slight increase in growth prior to the pubertal growth which is stimulated by increasing hormone levels.

The ovaries, in contrast, remain relatively static in size from birth to about 8 years of age. They then show some increase in size, but this is less spectacular than the uterine changes. Irregularities of ovarian texture are common; particularly around the age of puberty, and these must not be interpreted as pathological findings.

REFERENCES

Bridges NA, Cooke A, Healy MJR *et al.,* 1993: Standards for ovarian volume in childhood and puberty. *Fertility and Sterility* **60**, 456–460.

Haber HP, Mayer EI, 1994: Ultrasound evaluation of uterine and ovarian size from birth to puberty. *Pediatric Radiology* **24**, 11–13.

Krantz KE, Atkinson JP, 1967: Gross anatomy. *Annals of the New York Academy of Sciences* **142**, 551.

Willi UV, 1992: Pediatric gynaecologic problems. In Schulz RD, Willi UV, (eds), *Atlas of pediatric ultrasound*, Thieme 148.

CHAPTER 4

Gynaecological examination in childhood and adolescence

W JOAN ROBSON

INTRODUCTION

Gynaecological examination is part of the assessment of babies, children and adolescents who present in many different ways. They may have definitive gynaecological problems or non-specific symptoms. Some, in all age groups, will be suspected victims or will have disclosed sexual abuse. Others will need a gynaecological examination as part of the investigation of a congenital abnormality or a disease in another system.

These assessments must be done in appropriate surroundings. A quiet, comfortable room with good lighting is essential. Suitable toys, books, magazines and games must be available during the waiting periods before the patients are seen by doctors. However, delays must be minimised to reduce anxiety in the adolescents and to improve co-operation in the younger age groups.

All staff in contact with the family must be good at communicating with babies, children and adolescents. They must introduce themselves by name and explain their roles. Doctors who do the assessments must be experienced in consultations with children, adolescents and their families. They must have knowledge of the changes in the anatomy and physiology of females which occur at different ages. The ability to recognise normal variants is also important. Training in basic general paediatrics and in gynaecological examination is essential for those undertaking this work. Children should be given the option of being examined by a doctor of the same gender if one with appropriate experience and training is available.

Relevant consent must be obtained first. Next a full history is taken. Following this a full general examination and a gynaecological examination are undertaken.

Forensic specimens may be necessary if sexual abuse has occurred recently. Microbiological specimens are taken if viral, bacterial or fungal infections are suspected or threadworms may be present. Blood tests are necessary if chromosome abnormalities, endocrine or metabolic disorders are in the differential diagnosis and pregnancy tests will also be needed sometimes. Radiological investigations are used and examples include plain X-rays to assess bone age, and ultrasound scanning for abdominal masses, including pregnancy.

At the end of the assessment decisions must be made on the diagnosis, immediate management and any follow-up which is necessary. These are communicated to the family.

Clear, legible, contemporaneous medical records must be made including diagrams where appropriate. Photographs may be helpful to enhance the records. This potential advantage must be balanced against the possible embarrassment for the adolescent if photographs of the genitalia are produced in court proceedings.

Letters and reports should be written promptly. Remember that specific consent is needed for some reports.

CONSENT FOR EXAMINATION

Apart from exceptional circumstances a doctor may not undertake examination of any person without consent. A failure to obtain consent may lead to civil action for damages or to criminal proceedings for assault or indecent assault (McClay, 1990; Hendrick, 1993).

Implied consent means that the patient has come voluntarily or has been brought by someone with parental responsibility (Children Act, 1989) to be seen by a doctor. The doctor will then examine as much of the child as is felt necessary. For most paediatric practices, this will involve full examination of the child following a verbal request to do so. When examination involves invasion of the body cavities, or the handling of the external genitalia, express consent should be obtained. This is a formal request to the person to be examined. This may be given orally or in writing. Ideally oral-expressed consent should be witnessed by a third party.

A mentally sound person over the age of 16 can give full consent. Below that age, permission must be sought from a person with parental responsibility. In addition, a young person who is sufficiently mature to be aware of the purposes of the examination should give his or her own permission. If the person being examined is detained in custody under the Police and Criminal Evidence Act of 1984 and is a juvenile, i.e. a person who is, or appears to be, under the age of 17, then consent must be given by an appropriate adult (Clause 5). An appropriate adult may be a parent, guardian, care authority, organisation social worker or a responsible adult who is not a police officer or employed by the police.

Since the Gillick ruling in 1987 young women under the age of 16 years can have consultations for contraceptive advice and for pregnancies without the consent of parents. Doctors working in these clinics should refer to Hendrick (1993) for detailed guidance.

Those suffering from a mental disorder may be able to give satisfactory consent depending on the nature of the disorder. If there is any doubt about the patient's ability to understand the nature of the examination or proposed procedures then consent should be obtained from a relative or other appropriate adult. Please note that a person under the influence of drugs or alcohol cannot be regarded as fit to give informed consent.

An unconscious patient is incapable of giving consent and the doctor must act in the best interests of the patient. Consent may be sought from relatives or guardians when they can be found but this must not delay any treatment of the patient. The same applies if the patient presents with a life-threatening emergency situation.

Consent to examination does not extend to permission to take forensic specimens or to provide reports to third parties. Specific informed consent should be taken for each of these situations. Reports for child protection may be given to social services without consent following a recommendation of the General Medical Council Standards Committee in 1987 (see Working together under the Children Act, 1991) but every possible effort should be made to obtain consent before disclosure of confidential information.

After consent for the medical assessment is obtained, older children and adolescents are asked whom they wish to accompany them for the taking of the history and the examination itself. If a girl chooses to have a trusted adult present, a further opportunity to talk in private to health professionals should be offered at the end of the consultation. The same facility should be available to each parent or relevant care giver.

HISTORY

The initial medical history must cover all aspects of the life and health of the girl. Most of the information will be obtained from parents but the older girl should be encouraged to contribute. Adolescents should be asked to give the history of their present condition and answer the questions in the systemic enquiry themselves. Some may wish to do this in private rather than with a third party present. This should be respected, although at the beginning of the consultation a clear indication must be given that if any abuse is disclosed which needs action then the doctor has a duty to share that information with social services (see Working together under the Children Act, 1991).

History of the Present Condition

Few patients who present with gynaecological problems have life-threatening situations. Therefore a full history can normally be taken before any treatment is needed. Initially, each older girl, or adolescent and a parent, should be asked to give details of the present problems. These should be free recitals without interruptions. Any clarification should be sought after each person has finished talking. The doctor should listen very carefully and record all details as much useful information can be gained by this method of consultation. The relationships between those present can be assessed at this stage and noted. These will be added to the record of the examination.

A systematic enquiry should then made for symptoms which have not been mentioned in the introductory discussion. These should cover the cardiovascular, respiratory, gastrointestinal, urogenital, central nervous and musculo-skeletal systems and any abnormalities of the skin.

Personal History

Information should be obtained on the nursery or school which the girl attends or any childminders who are involved in her care. Older girls and adolescents should be asked about their use of drugs, alcohol and cigarettes, and about any prescribed drugs they may take, particularly those containing hormones. The state of immunisation and any known allergies should be recorded.

For older girls and adolescents, a picture of the use of leisure time should be built up. The girl should be asked about relationships outside the family, both those that are enjoyable and those which cause pressure.

Past History

The life of the girl from conception to the present time is important when assessing gynaecological problems. A full history of the pregnancy, birth, neonatal period and developmental milestones should be taken. Some of the questions on the pubertal stages of development will have come into the systemic enquiry but it is useful to summarise the developmental history at this stage, including the thelarche and the menarche.

Details should also be obtained of all previous illnesses and accidents, and specific enquiries made about any treatment with hormones or other drugs which are likely to affect the urogenital system.

Family History

The relationships within the family should be discussed first. Blood relatives and those coming into the family through marriage or re-marriage of one or both parents should be included. In addition, other members of the household who are not related to the girl should be recorded. This part of the history may be complex and all questions must be asked in a sensitive manner. If those present do not wish to disclose details of relationships, the general practitioner or health visitor should be approached for this information. All details of the family and social history are important in diagnosing congenital abnormalities, possible abuse and diseases which may have a genetic base.

A family tree is helpful. If disorders have occurred in several members of a family then a pattern will be clearer using this method of recording.

The parents should be asked about present or past illness in close family members. These may have a bearing on the medical diagnosis or may have led to psychological disturbance in a girl or adolescent which is contributing to the presenting symptoms.

GENERAL EXAMINATION

When a full history has been obtained, the doctor can do a general examination. This should be from head to toe, examining all systems simultaneously in each area of the body. For the purposes of this Chapter, the examination will be described in sections but in practice, examination is done progressively downwards from head to feet.

Babies can be undressed for the general examination, leaving only a nappy on while older girls should undress one area at a time so that once the examination of that area has been completed, the girl can put her clothes over that area and undress the adjacent one. Girls feel very vulnerable if they are totally exposed, even if they are underneath a blanket or sheet. They feel much more comfortable if they remain partially dressed throughout the examination.

Growth and Development

The head circumference, length and weight of babies, and the height and weight of older girls should always be measured and charted within standard growth charts. If any abnormality of growth is suspected then growth velocities must also be calculated.

A brief developmental assessment of the girl should be made which includes her behaviour and the relationships between the girl and the care givers present.

The absence or presence of secondary sexual characteristics should also be noted. The appearance of the breast bud, is, as a rule, the first sign of puberty in the female, though the appearance of pubic hair may sometimes precede it.

The pubic hair stages are described below (Tanner, 1955):

Stage 1   Pre-adolescent: the vellus over the pubes is not further developed than that over the abdominal wall, i.e. no pubic hair.

Stage 2   Sparse growth of long, slightly pigmented downy hair, straight or only slightly curled, appearing chiefly along the labia.

Stage 3   Considerable darker, coarser and more curled hair. This spreads sparsely over the junction of the pubes.

Stage 4   Hair now resembles the adult in type, but the area covered by it is still considerably smaller than in the adult. No spread to the medial surface of the thighs.

Stage 5   Adult in quantity and type with distribution of the horizontal (or classically *'feminine'*) pattern (Dupertuis *et al.*, 1945). The spread is to the medial surface of thighs but not up to the linea alba or elsewhere above the base of the inverse triangle.

In about 10 per cent of women, the pubic hair spreads further into one of the patterns called sagittal, acuminate or disperse (Dupertuis *et al.*, 1945) but this takes some time to occur after Stage 5 is reached. Often it is not completed till the mid-twenties or later, beyond the more concentrated period of adolescence.

Axillary hair usually first appears some two years after the beginning of pubic hair growth, i.e. when pubic hair is just reaching Stage 4. However, in a few girls axillary hair appears first. Circumanal hair, which arises independently of the spread of pubic hair down the perineum, appears shortly before axillary.

Breast development is also recorded using the Tanner classification (Tanner, 1955) (see also p. 4, Chapter 1).

Stage 1 Pre-adolescent: elevation of nipple (papilla) only.

Stage 2 Breast bud stage: a little development of the breast bud which appears as a small mound beneath an enlarged areola.

Stage 3 Further enlargement and elevation of breast and areola with no separation of their contours.

Stage 4 Nipple and areola enlarge to a greater extent than the rest of the breast tissue forming a secondary mound above the level of the remainder of the breast.

Stage 5 Mature stage: projection of nipple only, due to recession of the areola to the general contour of the breast.

Note that some girls do not go through Stage 4 but go directly from Stage 3 to Stage 5.

The average times at which these stages are reached are indicated in Fig. 4.1. The transition from Stage 2 to Stage 5 takes about four years on average but may be completed as quickly as two years in some children and prolonged up to six years in others.

Physiological breast development in the adolescent may be unequal in the early stages. Breast shrinkage may occur as a result of profound weight loss such as in anorexia nervosa. This can give the overlying skin and nipple a wrinkled appearance.

In some babies born at term, both male and female, there is transient breast enlargement which is a physiological response to passive hormone stimulation which has reached the child across the placenta. This breast enlargement usually lasts a maximum of two weeks then disappears completely.

Skin

The skin must be examined very carefully. Accurate records must be made of any bruises, swellings, lacerations or marks which appear to be teeth marks or

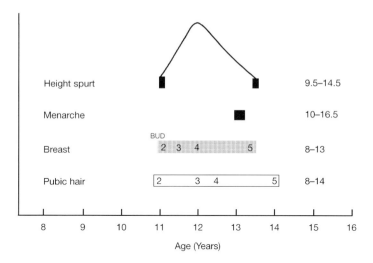

Fig. 4.1 Diagram of sequence of events at adolescence in girls. An average girl is represented. The range of ages within which some of the events may occur is given by the figures placed on the right.

abrasions. If present they must be measured and notes made on their anatomical site. Hair over the lower spine may be a pointer to spina bifida occulta and associated spinal cord dysraphism.

Diseases of the skin such as acne, lichen sclerosis et atrophicus, psoriasis and eczema are important in the differential diagnosis of gynaecological abnormalities. Signs of infection must be sought, particularly of the herpes simplex virus, human papilloma virus and fungal infections.

Systemic Examination

A general examination will reveal signs of anaemia, enlarged lymph glands and other swellings. Evidence of dehydration, weight loss or rapid weight gain should be sought. The thyroid gland should be inspected and palpated before listening for a bruit.

The eyes, ears, nose, mouth and throat should be examined, looking for congenital abnormalities, infection and trauma. Note any hoarseness or abnormal pitch in the voice. The cardiovascular and respiratory systems should also be examined in detail.

The abdomen should be inspected and palpated as this is helpful in examining for lesions in the bladder, uterus and ovaries. In addition pathology in the gastrointestinal tract, liver, kidneys and spleen may be apparent.

The limbs, spine and limb girdles should be inspected carefully for signs of any abnormality followed by a basic neurological assessment of the cranial nerves, motor and sensory systems.

GYNAECOLOGICAL EXAMINATION

A natural progression should occur from the general examination to the examination of the external genitalia, pelvis and anus. For this, girls under 3 years are
more comfortable lying on their mother's lap. Older girls and adolescents can be
examined lying on a couch in the '*frog-legged*' position, i.e. lying supine with
the hips flexed and the soles of the feet touching. Adolescents can be examined
in the 'frog-legged' position or if necessary the lithotomy position. If there is a
problem in visualising the posterior margin of the hymen adequately this may be
more easily examined by the girl being in the prone knee chest position but many
find this very uncomfortable.

Younger girls prefer to be able to see what is going on but older girls like to be
covered during this part of the examination with a sheet over the abdomen and
legs and the examiner looking beneath this. The doctor should be sitting down
and have good lighting to illuminate the genitalia and anus.

External Genitalia

The female external genitalia are commonly referred to as the vulva. They
include the mons pubis, the labia majora and minora, the clitoris and the
vestibule (Fig. 4.2).

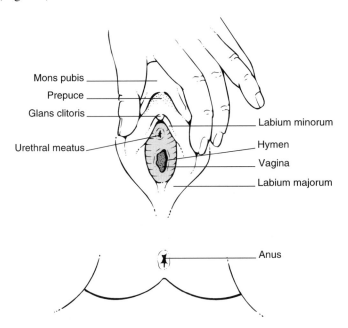

Fig. 4.2 Anatomy of the normal prepubertal girl's external genitalia (from Paradise JE,
Pediatric and adolescent gynecology. In Fleischer G, Ludwig S, (eds), *Textbook of pediatric
emergency medicine*, 2nd edn. Baltimore, MD, Williams & Wilkins, 1988).

The labia majora are two folds of skin covering adipose tissue on each side of the vaginal opening. Anteriorally they fuse to form the mons pubis. Posteriorly they merge with the perineum, which is the area between the vagina and the anal canal. From puberty the outer surfaces of the labia majora are covered with coarse hair. The inner surfaces are smooth but have numerous sebaceous glands.

The labia minora are two small vascular folds of skin containing sebaceous glands which lie within the labia majora. They are devoid of adipose tissue and are not well developed before puberty. Anteriorly, they are divided into two to form the prepuce and frenulum of the clitoris. Posteriorly, they fuse to form a fold of skin called the posterior fourchette.

The clitoris is a small erectile structure. The body of the clitoris is attached to the inferior border of the pubic rami. The cutaneous nerve supply is highly developed and the body of the clitoris contains erectile tissue. Therefore it is a very sensitive organ.

The glans clitoris in pre-menarchal children should not exceed 3 mm in length or 2 mm in width. The clitoral index is the glans length multiplied by the width in mm^2; an index over 6 mm^2 is clitoromegaly. After puberty the clitoris is about 2.5 cm long and 2–4 mm in width (Cowell, 1981).

The vestibule is the area between the labia minora into which open the urethra, the vagina, the para-urethral (Skene's) ducts and the ducts of the greater vestibular (Bartholin's) glands.

Inspection should be done first with the labia in their normal position. The thumbs are placed on the labia majora which move laterally and downwards to expose the hymen and urethra. This must be done with gentleness or tearing of the posterior fourchette can occur. Improvement in assessment of detail may be obtained using an otoscope lens with the speculum removed which gives a $\times 5$ magnification.

The groins, labia majora, labia minora, clitoris, vestibule, urethra, posterior fourchette, hymen and what is visible of the vagina should be inspected and the absence of any structure and variants or abnormalities documented. Labial adhesions should be recorded. If there are rugae or fusion of the labia majora the child may have been exposed to a source of androgen. A particular note should be made of the size of the clitoris – virilisation should be suspected if there is hypertrophy. Skin problems, signs of infection, active bleeding or dried blood and signs of recent or old injuries should be sought.

The groins and labia majora should be palpated. If masses are present these may be gonads, either ovaries in normal females or testes in hermaphrodites.

Vagina and Hymen

The vagina is a fibromuscular tube which extends postero-superiorly from the vestibule to the uterine cervix. The size varies with age (Cowell, 1981). In the newborn it is 4 cm long, increasing to 8 cm in late childhood. At puberty it measures 10–12 cm in length and is more distensible, the mucosa becoming moist and thick.

The hymen is a thin fold mucous membrane across the entrance of the vagina. In normal girls there are usually one or more openings in it. If the membrane is not perforated then at menstruation the blood collects behind forming a haematocolpas. The shape of the hymenal orifice has many normal variants. The common appearances are annular, crescentic (posterior rim), and fimbriated (frilly) (Fig. 4.3). The size of the hymenal opening varies during inspection, even if this is only for a few seconds. The maximal size should be assessed. Some physicians use glass rods to assess the hymenal size but this is not generally recommended as the tissue is dynamic and elastic, rendering measurement in this way unreliable. Glass rods or bulbs (Glaister Keen rods) as shown in Fig. 4.4 are useful in enabling the edge of the hymen to be examined to reveal previously undetected splits in the hymen. They can be used also to confirm that a hymen is imperforate.

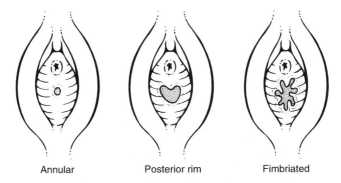

Annular   Posterior rim   Fimbriated

Fig. 4.3   Variations in configuration of the hymen (Report of the Royal College of Physicians, 1991).

The appearance of the hymen changes with age (see Report of the Royal College of Physicians, 1991). At one year of age it is often sleevelike, fleshy and redundant. At around three years of age there may be a longitudinal fold anteriorly with flaps of redundant hymen. With increasing age the hymenal membrane becomes thinner. As puberty approaches the hymen assumes a sleevelike or flowerlike appearance (fimbriated variety). Vaginal septal remnants may remain as a projection or smooth non-scarred bump on the hymen.

In some centres a colposcope is used which has been adapted for examination of the external genitalia and hymen, with an in-built measuring device and camera. However, care should be taken in interpreting the colposcopic findings. The use of the colposcope in childhood sexual abuse examinations is well described by McCann (1990).

Digital examination of the vagina is not indicated in young children. If they require investigation for bleeding or recurrent discharge due to a possible foreign body then examination under general anaesthesia should be done.

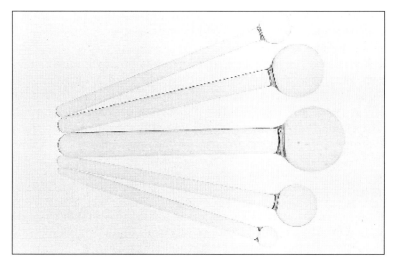

Fig. 4.4   Glaister Keen rods.

Uterus, Cervix, Fallopian Tubes and Ovaries (see also p. 13 and p. 28)

The uterus is a muscular organ which varies with age (Cowell, 1981). At birth it is 4 cm long and has no axial correction. Within 8 weeks there is regression but the neonatal size is regained at the age of five years. The main growth is then in the body of the uterus, the ratio of body to cervix changing from 1 : 1 to 2 : 1. During puberty anteflexion occurs.

The cervix in young children is flush with the vault of the vagina. The knob-like protrusion into the vagina occurs during puberty.

The uterine or fallopian tubes are two oviducts going from the cornu of the uterus along the upper margins of the board ligament. They end in the peritoneal cavity close to the ovaries. The abdominal end of the tube is fimbriated forming a trumpet-shaped lateral portion of the tube.

In childhood the ovaries are small and situated near the pelvic brim. During puberty they descend to the adult pelvic position. At adolescence they are almond-shaped, solid and greyish pink in colour, each measuring 3 cm in length and 1.5 cm in width and they are 1 cm thick. Each ovary is attached to the cornu of the uterus by the ovarian ligament and at the hilum to the broad ligament by the meso-ovarian ligament which contains the vessels and nerves. Laterally, each ovary is attached to the suspensory ligament with folds of peritoneum. Ova are first shed around the time of onset of menstruation and ovulation is usually established within a couple of years. Some of the signs of pathology in the uterus, tubes and ovaries can be revealed in the abdominal examination, for example, tenderness and a mass arising out of the pelvis. Additional information can be gained from a bimanual examination.

In babies and young children gentle pelvic examination can be done with one finger in the rectum and the other hand examining the abdomen. This is useful when a pelvic tumour is suspected.

Post-pubertal girls can have a bimanual examination by insertion of one finger slowly and gently into the vagina with the other hand palpating the abdomen. This should be done after rectal bimanual examination.

Adolescents who are sexually active can have a normal bimanual assessment. A vaginal speculum can be used if inspection of the vaginal wall or the cervix is indicated or high vaginal swabs are needed.

Examination of the Anus

The relationship of the anus to the vagina is recorded during the examination of the genitalia. Discharge of meconium or faeces from the vagina indicates a congenital abnormality or an acquired recto-vaginal fistula.

The anal and perianal areas are inspected in the '*frog-legged*' position in a young girl. For a clear view the older girl and adolescent will need to lie in the left lateral position, curled up with hips and knees flexed and the head resting on a pillow. The buttocks are gently separated using both hands. This will reveal signs of inflammation, injury or venous congestion. Threadworms may be seen crawling around the perianal area. During observation for about thirty seconds, gradual opening of the anus will occur as the external sphincter relaxes. In significant reflex anal dilatation the internal sphincter also relaxes so that the rectal mucosa is visible. This '*reflex*' is present in many conditions so interpretation of the significance of this finding in relation to child abuse must be with caution.

Gentle palpation of and traction on the anal verge allows assessment of tone of the external sphincter and inspection of fissures or sentinel tags where fissures have healed. A digital examination of the anus is not necessary unless it is part of a bimanual examination or there is an allegation of chronic anal abuse.

INVESTIGATION DIAGNOSIS AND MANAGEMENT

The details of these will be covered in relevant Chapters. A few general principles apply. Investigations should be done and the results made available as soon as possible to minimise the anxiety of parents and adolescents. Some system should be in place for sharing of the results of investigations early by letter or through the general practitioner if the follow-up appointment is several weeks or months ahead.

Diagnosis and management should be discussed with the parents and with patients who are old enough to understand, using language which is at an appropriate level for each person. Some adolescents will ask for part, or all, of the information to be kept confidential to them. This confidence should be respected unless child protection issues are present, in which case social services must be involved (see Working together under the Children Act, 1991).

REFERENCES

Cowell CA, 1981: The gynecological examination of infants, children and young adolescents. *Pediatric Clinics of North America* **28**, 247–266.

Dupertuis CW, Atkinson WB, Alftman H, 1945: Sex differences in pubic hair distribution. Human Biology **17**, 137–142.

Hendrick J, 1993: *Child care law for health professionals*. Oxford and New York: Radcliffe Medical Press.

McCann J, 1990: Use of the colposcope in childhood sexual abuse examinations. *Pediatric Clinics of North America* **37**, 863–880.

Mcclay WDS, 1990: *Clinical forensic medicine*. London and New York: Pinter Publishers.

Report of the Royal College of Physicians – Physical Signs of Sexual Abuse in Children. 1991: The Royal College of Physicians of London.

Tanner JM, 1955: *Growth at adolescence*. Oxford: Blackwell Scientific Publications.

Working together under the Children Act, 1991: HMSO, 12.

PART II

GYNAECOLOGY IN CHILDHOOD

CHAPTER 5

Problems identified at birth and in the neonate

ANTHONY MICHAEL KENT RICKWOOD AND SHIRLEY Y GODIWALLA

Gynaecological problems are unusual during the newborn period, accounting for only a small fraction of neonatal surgical practice. A few encompass minor functional complaints but a much larger proportion are made up of congenital anomalies, the greater part of them occurring in association with other major malformations. A minority present with symptoms, some frankly gynaecological but more often from the consequences of hydrometrocolpos, while a majority have either an evident gynaecological abnormality as part of a more major malformation or have some occult condition detected by virtue of a known association with another complex or syndrome. Lastly, an appreciable proportion of congenital gynaecological abnormalities, notably vaginal agenesis, pass unnoticed at birth, and often on to menarche, usually from a combination of rarity, absence of symptoms and lack of immediately obvious physical signs.

Table 5.1 summarises the various conditions recognisable neonatally which have gynaecological associations.

Table 5.1 Gynaecological associations of other congenital anomalies recognisable neonatally

Anomaly	Gynaecological associations			
	Clitoris	Vagina	Uterus	Gonads
Anal imperforation/ cloaca/persistent urogenital sinus	— — —	Duplication Occlusion Hydrocolpos	Duplication (occasional)	—
Vesical exstrophy	Duplication	Duplication (occasional)	Duplication (occasional)	—
Cloacal exstrophy	Duplication Absence	Duplication Absence	Duplication Absence	Absence (unilateral, occasional)
Turner's syndrome	—	—	Hypoplasia	Streak ovaries Absence (unilateral, occasional)

SEXUAL AND GENITAL DEVELOPMENT
(see also p. 3)

Most congenital gynaecological anomalies can be explained from a knowledge of sexual and genital development.

In summary, until 9 weeks' gestation the gonads are indistinguishable and the external genitalia are undetermined although both the Mullerian and Wolffian ducts are formed by this time (Jost, 1972) Gonadal differentiation proceeds according to the sexual karyotype, if XX to a normal ovary, if XO to a streak gonad. Thence, in the absence of Mullerian inhibitory factor (MIF), produced by the testicular Sertoli cells (Grumach and Conte, 1981), the Mullerian ducts develop to form the fallopian tubes, uterus and proximal vagina.

The cloaca arises from the hindgut at 4 weeks' gestation and by the seventh week fuses with the cloacal membrane. The developing urorectal septum separates caudal hindgut from ventral urogenital sinus. Similarly, the cloacal membrane separates to form the dorsal anal and ventral urogenital membranes. The point of entry of the Wolffian ducts into the primitive urogenital sinus divides this structure into a cranially disposed urethrovesical canal and a caudal urogenital sinus proper (Marshall, 1978).

By the sixth week of gestation, the Mullerian ducts have developed from the coelomic epithelium of the urogenital ridges (Felix, 1912) and, extending caudally, pass lateral to the Wolffian ducts then towards each other, fusing as a single midline structure, the uterovaginal canal, which adjoins the urogenital sinus at the Mullerian tubercle. Proximally, the separated Mullerian ducts form the fallopian tubes. This entire process is completed by 10 weeks' gestation.

Subsequently, the uterovaginal canal retracts cranially, and mesoderm between its extremity and the urogenital sinus thickens to form a solid vaginal cord. Meanwhile, during the tenth week of gestation, the sinovaginal bulbs proliferate, producing the vaginal plate, which first infiltrates and next replaces the vaginal cord, then canalises so that the uterovaginal canal communicates with the urogenital sinus. The latter becomes progressively shallower and ultimately the Mullerian tubercle comes to surface level to produce separate urethral and vaginal orifices.

The vulva itself represents remnants of the urogenital sinus and the hymen the junction between the sinus and the canalised vaginal plate. Unfused urethral plates form the labia minora and the genital swellings the labia majora. The urogenital groove remains open to form the vestibule.

VAGINAL OCCLUSIONS AND AGENESIS

General

The various forms of congenital vaginal obstruction may be complete or incomplete and, almost without exception, only the former come to notice neonatally.

Apart from imperforate hymen, which may be noted in its own right, other forms of complete obstruction present neonatally only when complicated by hydro-metrocolpos or when associated with some other more evident malformation (or, sometimes, both together).

Hydrometrocolpos (see also p. 246)

With vaginal occlusions, secretory hydrometrocolpos develops prenatally as the cervical and vaginal glands respond to circulating maternal oestrogens (Hahn-Pederson *et al.*, 1984). The condition occurs in approximately 1 in 16 000 female births (Westerhout *et al.*, 1964) and is easily recognisable on fetal ultrasonography beyond 30 weeks' gestation (Hill and Horsch, 1989). The retained fluid may be clear, milky or mucinous and, on histological examination, contains desquamated epithelial cells and leucocytes.

The distension is largely confined to the vagina with the uterine component modest if present at all. Occasionally the fallopian tubes are involved and very rarely the fluid may leak into the peritoneal cavity to produce a plastic peritonitis (Cetallos and Hicks, 1970). Because the vaginal component is all-important, it follows that the complication will not occur where there is proximal vaginal atresia, with or without atresia distally, and hence that this condition will scarely ever be discovered neonatally unless having a recognised association with some other more obvious anomaly.

As a rule, the vaginal distension causes no more than a lower abdominal mass, arising from the pelvis, but occasionally there is more massive enlargement, even to the extent of causing dystocia or respiratory distress. The vaginal enlargement elongates and angulates the urethra, causing urinary retention, sometimes leading, in turn, to hydroureteronephrosis, a complication recognisable on fetal ultrasonography (Davis *et al.*, 1984). Compression of adjacent structures can also cause intestinal obstruction or venous stasis of the legs.

In the absence of any obvious vaginal obstruction, hydrometrocolpos is distinguishable from most other causes of pelvic mass neonatally by rectal examination, when the tense cystic vaginal mass is palpable anteriorly or, in high lesions, antero-superiorly, and by failure of the mass to resolve following urethral catheterisation. Nowadays the issue is usually determined by ultrasonography (Fig. 5.1), an examination particularly helpful where hydrometrocolpos occurs in the presence of anal imperforation.

Massive hydrometrocolpos, usually associated with high vaginal obstruction, constitutes a neonatal surgical emergency and newborns with respiratory distress due to elevated diaphragms may require endotracheal intubation and ventilation. In the very ill, the situation is retrievable by construction of a temporising cutaneous vaginostomy via a short midline abdominal incision. Urinary drainage must be established via a urethral catheter. Occasionally, and presumably on account of extreme urethral distorsion, a catheter cannot be passed, a situation requiring either placement of a catheter suprapubically or establishment of a temporary cutaneous vesicostomy.

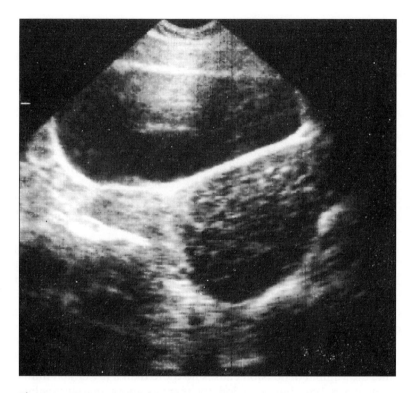

Fig. 5.1 Hydrocolpos. Sagittal ultrasound image of the pelvis showing a full bladder anteriorly and the hydrocolpos posteriorly. The normal uterus is seen superior to the hydrocolpos.

Embryology

The various forms of congenital vaginal occlusion are explicable from the organ's dual origin from the Mullerian system and from the vaginal plate, plus the embryological conjunction of these structures and of the vaginal plate to the urogenital sinus, and finally from the process of canalization of the vaginal plate. Indeed, the possible combinations and permutations of embryological maldevelopment are such that most anomalies can be explained in more than one way and similarly that vaginal occlusion can occur along almost any length and at any level.

Hymenal imperforation, for example, is often considered to be due to failure to establish continuity between vaginal plate and urogenital sinus and higher septa from similar failure between the vaginal plate and the Mullerian system. Some, however, take the view that all transverse septa occur from partial failure of canalisation of the vaginal plate and Antell (1952) maintained that with imperforate 'hymen', the hymen proper is recognisable as a separate structure distal to the obstructing membrane. Again, high vaginal obstruction, with persistent complete urogenital sinus and a high transverse septum, may be explained either by failure of the Mullerian ducts to join the urogenital sinus or by failure of development of the vaginal plate.

Imperforate Hymen

Hymenal imperforation is much the commonest form of congenital vaginal obstruction, occurring in approximately 1 in 2000 female newborns. The condition has no association with other congenital anomalies.

Presentation neonatally may be either with noticeable bulging of the hymenal membrane between the labia (Fig. 5.2) or with a degree of hydrocolpos which is seldom severe.

Treatment is simply by cruciate incision of the membrane, covered peroperatively and for a few days after by antibiotic prophylaxis. Where there is only modest hydrocolpos, the bulge of the membrane can be accentuated for incision by anterior pressure from a finger in the rectum.

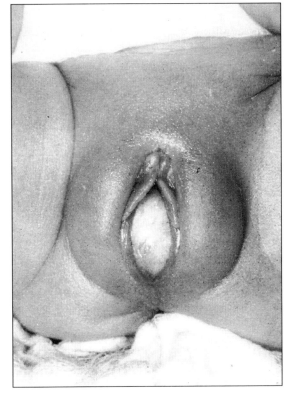

Fig. 5.2 Imperforate hymen in a neonate.

Transverse Vaginal Septum

Transverse septa, of varying thickness, and occasionally multiple, can occur at any level above the hymen, most commonly at the junction of the middle and upper thirds of the vagina. The septa may be complete or incomplete, with the former more common distally. Only completely obstructing septa complicated by hydrometrocolpos present neonatally and require treatment at this time.

The introitus is normal but the uterine cervix is not visible on vaginoscopy. The thickness of the obstructing membrane is determinable by ultrasonography or by computerised axial tomography.

Low, thin membranes can be safely incised transvaginally. Such an approach risks damage to surrounding structures, the urethra particularly, with higher, thicker membranes. In this situation, laparotomy is advisable. With the abdomen open, the anterior wall of the vagina is incised and the fluid within it removed by suction. The septum can then be safely divided under guidance from within.

High Vaginal Obstruction

This anomaly tends more than any other to be complicated by massive hydrometrocolpos and is characterised by a complete urogenital sinus with the urethra entering its apex (Fig. 5.3). The condition may be inherited as an autosomal recessive trait (McKusick *et al.*, 1964; Chitayat *et al.*, 1987). Associated congenital anomalies are common and include polydactyly (Kaufman *et al.*, 1972), heart defects and malformations of the upper urinary tracts (Tran *et al.*, 1987).

The external genitalia appear superficially unremarkable and the anus is sited in its normal position. On separation of the labia there is a single vulval orifice, typical of urogenital sinus, and catheterisation returns urine.

If the general condition of the infant is compromised by massive hydrometrocolpos or by some associated anomaly, usually cardiac, formation of a cutaneous vaginostomy is advisable followed by definitive reconstruction later. Otherwise advantage may be taken of the massive vaginal dilatation to undertake reconstruction neonatally (Ramenofsky and Raffensperger, 1972).

The procedure is performed with the infant in lithotomy position, the bladder catheterised and the abdomen and perineum prepared in a single field. The abdomen is opened via a low midline or transverse incision to expose the distended vagina with the uterus at its apex. The vagina is dissected from the bladder anteriorly so that it can be opened low in the pelvis.

A 'V' skin flap is raised on the perineum, based posteriorly and with its apex immediately behind the urogenital sinus. With downward pressure exerted via the pelvic incision in the vagina, the posterior wall of the vagina is approached through the perineal incision and is mobilised from the rectum posteriorly (Fig. 5.4) until reaching the skin flap without tension. The vagina is opened at this

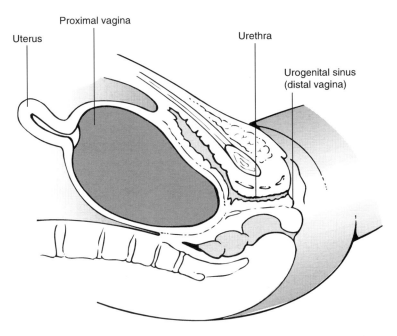

Fig. 5.3 Diagrammatic view of high vaginal obstruction with hydrocolpos.

point and sutured around the perineal flap and to the posterior wall of the urogenital sinus. In some cases where the vagina is more than usually mobile and capacious, it is possible to mobilise its posterior wall to the perineum, without need of a skin flap, where, after incision, it can be sutured immediately posterior to the urogenital sinus. The procedure, which is completed by closure of the pelvic incision in the vagina and the abdominal wall, separates the genital and urinary tracts and leaves the urogenital sinus as the urethra. Postoperatively, periodic dilatation under general anaesthetic is advisable until the distal vaginal anastomosis has stabilised.

Vaginal Agenesis (Mayer–Rokitansky Syndrome)

This anomaly, representing maldevelopment of the Mullerian system caudally, is usually associated with a uterus which is hypoplastic or absent and less often the proximal fallopian tubes are similarly affected. The ovaries are normal. As a rule the vagina is entirely absent, with the orifice represented by a shallow pit between the labia minora, but occasionally the distal third of the organ, of separate embryological origin, is normally formed.

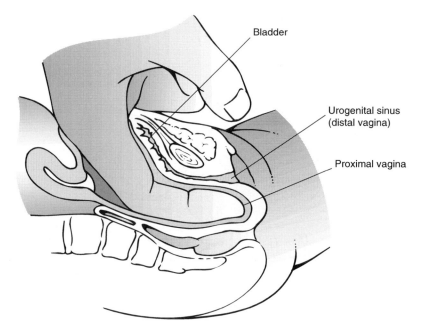

Bladder

Urogenital sinus
(distal vagina)

Proximal vagina

Fig. 5.4   Surgery of high vaginal obstruction. The vagina has been opened anteriorly and
mobilised downwards to the perineum.

Presumably because of the close association of the Mullerian and Wolffian
systems, abnormalities of the upper renal tracts are common and include unilateral renal agenesis, horseshoe kidney and pelviureteric junction obstruction.
These conditions, which are rarely symptomatic neonatally, or necessarily later
either, are nowadays often detected by prenatal ultrasonography and in females
so affected close vulval inspection neonatally is recommended. Full consideration of this anomaly is to be found in Chapter 8.

Vaginal Atresia

Distal vaginal atresia presumptively results from maldevelopment of the vaginal
plate although in practice the atretic segment usually extends more proximally
than this embryological explanation would suggest. Hydrocolpos is rare so that
the anomaly is detected neonatally only if associated with another malformation,
most commonly imperforate anus.

Vaginal Occlusion and Duplication

The various forms of vaginal occlusion can occur in one half of a duplication
anomaly, especially in the cloacal deformity. Treatment depends upon the location and extent of the obstruction and may involve vagino-vaginostomy.

DUPLICATION AND MISCELLANEOUS ANOMALIES OF MULLERIAN DEVELOPMENT

Duplication Anomalies

General

Such anomalies result from some degree of failure of fusion of the paired Mullerian ducts. Some occur in isolation among which a small number are complicated by obstruction unilaterally. These latter tend to present with pain from haematocolpos at menarche rather than with hydrocolpos neonatally, although a few come to light fortuitously at an earlier stage by virtue of an association with renal agenesis ipsilaterally (Tridenti *et al.*, 1988).

Otherwise the various forms of duplication are discovered neonatally only as being part of a more major malformation, cloacal exstrophy (almost universally), vesical exstrophy, cloaca (often), other forms of anal imperforation and persistent urogenital sinus (although rarely when as a feature of an intersexual state). Except when complicated by obstructive hydrocolpos, they require no treatment at this stage although it is usually convenient to deal with them, if necessary, as part of the definitive reconstruction of the primary anomaly.

Classification

Longitudinal vaginal septum occurs from partial fusion failure of the distal Mullerian ducts or from incomplete canalisation of the sinovaginal bulbs (or both) and results in a septum which partly or completely divides the vagina. Partial septa may extend from the cervix downwards or from the hymen upwards and the uterus may also be bicornuate or septate. Complete septation is always associated with duplication of the cervix and uterus. Vaginal duplication arises from complete failure of Mullerian fusion and is found in most cases of cloacal exstrophy. Partial, proximal, duplication is an occasional feature of the cloacal deformity. Complete duplication of the vagina otherwise, each half having its separate mucosa, lamina propria and muscular coat, is an exceptionally rare deformity and in extreme cases there is also complete duplication of the entire genitourinary tract, bladder, urethra, clitoris and vulva.

Uterine duplication anomalies, with or without associated vaginal septation or duplication, comprise uterus didelphys, bicornuate uterus and septate uterus (Buttran and Gibbons, 1979) and result from some degree of fusion failure of the Mullerian ducts more proximally. Unicornuate uterus results from partial unilateral arrest of Mullerian development cranially. The rudimentary horn and its fallopian tube may join the main body of the uterus, or may be quite separate from it, and may or may not contain functional epithelial lining. The ipsilateral upper renal tract is often absent (Beazley, 1974). As well as occurring in association with the anomalies previously listed, these various uterine deformities may result from fetal exposure to thalidomide or to diethylstilboestrol, or may be the result of a familial predisposition (Beninshka, 1973; Gilsany and Cleveland, 1982; Elias *et al.*, 1984).

Miscellaneous Anomalies

Uterine agenesis is an exceptionally rare malformation (Dehner, 1975) and in 75% of cases is associated with vaginal agenesis (Koram *et al.*, 1979). The fallopian tubes and ovaries are almost always present and normal (Koram and Mrouch, 1978).

Uterine hypoplasia is found in association with various forms of gonadal maldevelopment (Grover *et al.*, 1970), Turner's syndrome, pure gonadal dysgenesis, mixed gonadal dysgenesis and true hermaphroditism, and is also a consistent feature of the Mayer–Rokitansky syndrome.

Cervical agenesis and cervical atresia are both exceptionally rare anomalies in isolation and may or may not be associated with a normal uterus (Geary and Weed, 1973). In the former instance, successful pregnancies have followed establishment of uterovaginal continuity (Walker *et al.*, 1988).

UROGENITAL SINUS ANOMALIES

General

Persistent urogenital sinus, in its various forms, can exist as an isolated anomaly, as part of a cloacal deformity or as a feature of some intersexual state. The first two forms are characterised by the presence of a single, unusual, vulval orifice, resembling neither a normal urethral meatus nor a normal vaginal orifice (Fig. 5.5). Despite this clear-cut sign, and presumably on account of their great rarity, isolated urogenital sinus anomalies are apt to pass unnoticed neonatally unless complicated by urinary hydrocolpos.

The urogenital sinus deformity associated with intersexual states differs from others in having no association with anomalies of other systems and, usually, in being compounded by some clitoral enlargement and masculinisation of the urethral plate so that the orifice resembles more or less exactly that of a male hypospadiac, typically perineal but sometimes more distal and very occasionally glanular.

With isolated urogenital sinus the anus is frequently anteriorly ectopic and this anomaly, along with cloaca, occupies a continuum of congenital deformities also including all forms of anal imperforation. As such, there is a consistent pattern of association with congenital anomalies of other systems, notably of the upper urinary tracts, the spinal column, sacral agenesis in particular, the female genital tract and, less often, of the upper gastrointestinal tract or heart. Those of the female genital tract relate principally to defects of Mullerian development, mainly in the form of duplication, less often occlusion, including occlusion unilaterally in a duplicated system.

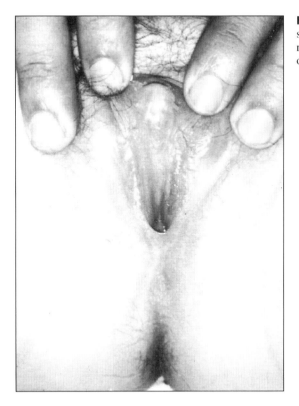

Fig. 5.5 Urogenital sinus. The single vulval aperture resembles neither a normal urethral nor vaginal orifice.

Isolated urogenital sinus and cloaca may be complicated neonatally by hydrocolpos and here the retained fluid is predominantly or entirely urine. Although the resulting vaginal distension rarely approaches the extreme degrees sometimes occurring with vaginal occlusion, it is usually evident in the form of a lower abdominal mass and is often sufficient to cause a degree of urinary retention, occasionally with secondary changes in the upper renal tracts. Untreated, the pooled urine in the vagina may become infected, with resulting septicaemia. Urinary sepsis proper may also ensue if the bladder is obstructed and which can lead, in turn, to permanent renal damage if there is vesicoureteric reflux.

In the absence of some form of complete vaginal obstruction, the cause of the hydrocolpos in these cases is somewhat mysterious since it is only seldom that the urogenital sinus or its orifice is so stenotic as to be evidently obstructive.

Anatomy

The anatomy of these lesions, although often complex, can be considered in five general categories. In the most straightforward varieties, the urethro-vaginal confluence can be low (Fig. 5.6) or high (suprasphincteric (Fig. 5.7)). In both types the urogenital sinus proper is of comparatively small calibre, more

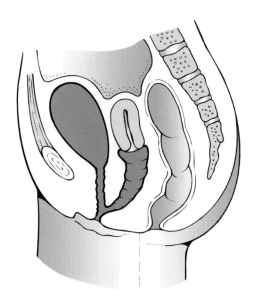

Fig. 5.6 Persistent urogenital sinus with low urethro-vaginal confluence.

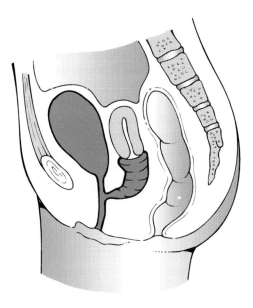

Fig. 5.7 Persistent urogenital sinus with high urethro-vaginal confluence.

resembling a 'urethra' than a 'vagina' and, in the high forms, is always employed as the urethra in reconstruction. In intersexual states, the deformity is almost always modified by clitoral enlargement, with masculinisation of the urethral plate, and, as a general rule, the greater the degree of virilisation, the higher the urethro-vaginal confluence. With isolated urogenital sinus, the anus is frequently anteriorly ectopic and here, as with the cloacal deformity, the labia minora are typically high riding and somewhat hypoplastic.

Urovaginal confluence represents an uncommon variant of isolated persistent urogenital sinus (Fig. 5.8). Here the bladder neck, which is usually totally incompetent, is confluent at a high level with vagina. Uniquely among these deformities, the distal common channel is wide and will form the vagina after reconstruction.

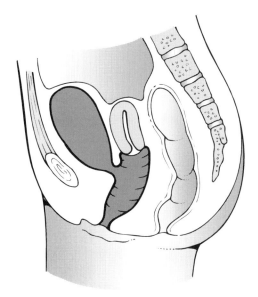

Fig. 5.8 Urovaginal confluence.

In the most complex of urogenital sinus deformities, cloaca, the level of confluence of urethra, vagina and rectum may also be low (Fig. 5.9) or high (Fig. 5.10). In a few instances the level of confluence is asymmetrical, nearly always with low urethral but high rectal confluence. Once again the common channel is of comparatively small calibre and, with high anomalies, will come to form the urethra during reconstruction. As the complexity of urogenital sinus anomalies increases, so also the risk of associated malformations. Congenital anomalies of the urinary tracts were detected in upwards of 50% of patients in one series of cloaca (Rich *et al.*, 1988) and, as a general rule, the higher the level of confluence the greater the chance of sacral agenesis and defects of Mullerian development.

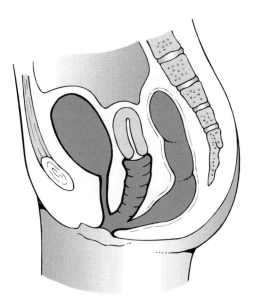

Fig. 5.9 Cloaca with low confluence of urethra, vagina and rectum.

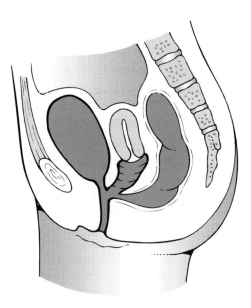

Fig. 5.10 Cloaca with high confluence of urethra, vagina and rectum.

Treatment Neonatally

Treatment of the newborn is necessary only where faecal or urinary drainage is impaired. Those with a cloacal deformity are best managed by a loop sigmoid colostomy, the proximal limb providing faecal drainage, the distal limb serving as an outlet for any urine pooling in the colon inferiorly.

The management of hydrocolpos, with or without bladder retention, can be more problematical. Dilatation of the common tract or a cautious posterior meatotomy is worthwhile only in the occasional case where there appears to be true organic obstruction. In a proportion of patients otherwise, satisfactory drainage can be established by intermittent catheterisation of the common channel four or five times daily. Over a period of a few weeks the vagina shrinks to normal dimensions and, once this has occurred, the system drains adequately without need for further catheterisation. Where this stratagem fails, the problem is usually soluble by creation of a temporising cutaneous vesicostomy, with the stoma apically in the bladder to minimise risk of prolapse. In the occasional case where hydrocolpos still persists, perhaps because of some form of vaginal occlusion, cutaneous vaginostomy is necessary also.

Definitive Treatment

General

Because this is not undertaken neonatally only the general principles are outlined.

As a preliminary, the anatomy of the lesion must be defined, mainly by a combination of endoscopy and radiological contrast studies. Magnetic resonance imaging (MRI) may also be helpful, especially with more complex deformities. The principal concerns are the length and calibre of the common channel and the presence or otherwise of complicating factors, notably duplication anomalies of the genital tract. Both with isolated urogenital sinus anomalies and cloaca, the nature and timing of reconstruction may be materially influenced by two further factors, the state of the upper renal tracts and the presence or otherwise of any spinal anomaly, most commonly sacral agenesis, likely to cause neuropathic bladder and bowel dysfunction. This is probable when two or more sacral segments are absent but interpretation of X-rays in this area can be difficult during infancy and as a clinical rule of thumb any readily palpable defect in the sacrum distally will almost certainly be associated with pelvic neuropathy. It has also become appreciated that occult spinal cord lesions may co-exist with the complex of anal imperforation (Sheldon *et al.*, 1981) and in some centres MRI is routinely undertaken to exclude these as far as possible.

Reconstruction in the presence of neuropathy is nearly always best deferred until bladder dysfunction can be accurately assessed and the child is old enough to co-operate with any necessary treatment, usually intermittent self-catheterisation.

Anomalies of the upper urinary tracts are less often influential but occasionally it is advisable to correct an obstructive uropathy or, less often, vesico-ureteric reflux, prior to reconstruction.

Low urethro-vaginal confluence

This deformity is almost always amenable to reconstruction by posterior skin flap vaginoplasty (Mundy, 1994). In cases of intersex, with clitoral hypertrophy, this procedure can be combined with clitoral reduction and undertaken at just a few months of age.

High urethro-vaginal confluence

Correction of this deformity poses considerably greater difficulties and although early reconstruction, during infancy, is widely advocated in order to minimise emotional disturbance, the reported long-term results are not always impressive and in one series only 21% had a satisfactory vaginal canal when examined at puberty (Bailez *et al.*, 1992). The authors' preference is for reconstruction later in childhood, approaching puberty.

Various procedures have been described, including use of combined anteriorly and posteriorly based perineal skin flaps (Mundy, 1994), or buttock flaps (Donahoe and Powell, 1993), and which may need to be combined with a trans-abdominal dissection to achieve sufficient downward mobilisation of the vagina. Where the vagina is severely deficient, an intestinal segment may be required for distal reconstruction.

Urovaginal confluence

Here the problem is one of urethral rather than vaginal reconstruction. In the occasional case where the bladder neck is competent this can be effected by tubularisation of a strip of anterior vaginal wall; the resulting vaginal defect is covered by a skin flap inlaid from the perineum (Hendren, 1980). Where the bladder neck is incompetent, the initial stage of any reconstruction comprises separation of bladder neck from vagina via an abdominal approach. Various types of neourethral reconstruction are described, Mundy (1994) employing a tubularised anterior bladder flap, based lateral to the bladder neck, and around which is placed an American Medical Systems (AMS) artificial urinary sphincter to ensure continence.

Cloaca

This is approached sagittally (Pena and de Vries, 1982) by a midline incision extending from the sinus orifice anteriorly to the sacrum posteriorly and deepened strictly via the midline of the pelvic muscle complex to expose the posterior aspect of common channel and its confluence with the rectum. First the rectum is severed from the common channel and mobilised from the vagina anteriorly then similarly the vagina from urethra. Both vagina and rectum, and vagina and urethra share common walls for some distance inferiorly and from which only mucosa can be separated before they definitively part company. Separation of vagina from urethra can prove to be especially trying and once this has been achieved it may still be necessary to deal with vaginal septation, duplication or occlusion.

The site of confluence in the common channel is closed and this conduit now forms the urethra anteriorly. At this point, the vagina may be of sufficient length to reach the perineum comfortably. If not, further mobilisation of the viscus transabdominally may achieve a satisfactory outcome. Where the vagina is unusually deficient, distal reconstruction using an intestinal segment, usually ileal, is necessary. The procedure is completed by pulling through the trimmed rectum to its normal site with the pelvic and sphincteric musculature sutured accurately around it.

Miscellaneous Related Anomalies

Urethralisation of the female phallus

Less than 50 examples of this deformity have been recorded worldwide. The most immediately obvious feature is clitoral hypertrophy but with two genitourinary orifices, one terminally on the glans clitoris, the other, typical of urogenital sinus, in the perineum (Fig. 5.11). The anus is anteriorly ectopic and the perineal body and the labia are deficient. The usual anatomy is shown in Fig. 5.12. In a few cases, there has been a cloacal deformity and in one example of these the common urogenital sinus was absent with voiding via an unusually wide phallic urethra (Tam *et al.*, 1990). In all other cases the clitoral urethra was very fine with voiding entirely via the common urogenital sinus. Some cases have been complicated neonatally by hydrocolpos.

Possibly the condition is caused by a combination of incomplete Mullerian descent and failure of differentiation of the pericloacal mesoderm (Howard and Hinman, 1951). The clitoral hypertrophy has been ascribed to the presence of the phallic urethra preventing completion of the normal female chordee (Bellinger and Duckett, 1982).

Correction of the deformity is achieved by combining posterior skin flap vaginoplasty and reduction cliteroplasty. Formal excision of the phallic urethra is unnecessary.

Female hypospadias

This uncommon anomaly, bearing not the least embryological or anatomical correspondence with its male counterpart, is nearly always asymptomatic and only comes to light neonatally, or at any other time, when bladder catheterisation is attempted.

The ectopic urethral orifice enters the vagina anteriorly, within 1 cm of the introitus, and the deformity is distinguishable from urogenital sinus anomalies

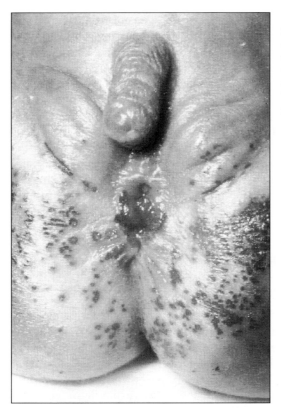

Fig. 5.11 Urethralisation of the female phallus. There is a small urethral orifice upon the glans of the enlarged clitoris. Posteriorly is situated a wide urogenital sinus orifice with the anteriorly ectopic anal orifice immediately behind it. Labia majora and labia minora are both deficient.

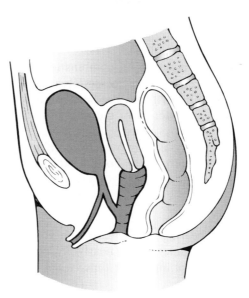

Fig. 5.12 Diagrammatic representation of the anatomy typical of urethralisation of the female phallus.

proper in that the vagina distal to the confluence is normal (Fig. 5.13) and so too its orifice.

Very occasionally there is stenosis of the urethral meatus, causing urinary difficulty, and which usually responds to a single dilatation. Otherwise no treatment is required.

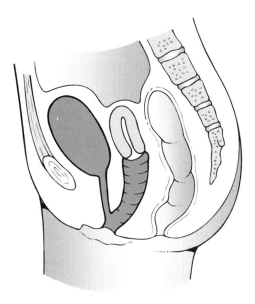

Fig. 5.13 Female hypospadias.

Imperforate anus

As described previously, isolated persistent urogenital sinus and the cloacal deformity come within the general continuum of anal imperforation, and other forms of the anomaly affecting females (perineal fistula, vestibular fistula, low vaginal fistula, anorectal agenesis without fistula) deserve mention here in that they too are apt to be associated with developmental anomalies of the female genital tract, with the chance increasing with the severity of the primary deformity.

In a series of 223 such cases seen in Helsinki, 34 (15%) had associated genital tract anomalies (22 uterine and/or vaginal duplication, six distal vaginal atresia, six utero-vaginal agenesis) (R. Rintala, personal communication).

Bilateral single ectopic ureters

This exceptionally rare anomaly also deserves mention because in a proportion of affected females it is combined with isolated persistent urogenital sinus, nearly always with low urethro-vaginal confluence. The ureters terminate ectopically in the urethral channel. The bladder neck and sphincteric mechanism are wholly incompetent and the bladder itself is hypoplastic. The ureters are dysmorphic and the kidneys are dysplastic, usually with a degree of renal insufficiency from birth.

Reconstruction of the genital deformity is compounded by the need to combine sphincteric reconstruction with augmentation cystoplasty, all against a background of chronic renal failure.

EXSTROPHIC ANOMALIES

General

Although most gynaecological abnormalities associated with this rare complex are evident enough neonatally, they are usually consequential only during adult reproductive life, although it is possible that the quality of early treatment influences the later risk of gynaecological complications (Canning and Gearhart, 1993).

The commonest variant, classical vesical exstrophy, occurs in 1 : 10 000 to 1 : 50 000 live births and in a male to female ratio of 2.7 : 1. The least severe anomaly, epispadias, is approximately one fifth as common, with a male–female ratio of 3.5 : 1 and the most severe, cloacal exstrophy, one twentieth as common with a 1.6 : 1 male–female preponderance (Canning and Gearhart, 1993).

Embryology

The defect fundamental to all exstrophic anomalies is failure of primitive streak mesoderm to invade the allantoic extension of the cloacal (infraumbilical) membrane so that ectoderm and endoderm remain abnormally in contact in the developing lower abdominal wall without intervening mesoderm. In this unstable state, disintegration of the infraumbilical membrane follows and the pelvic viscera are laid open upon the surface of the lower abdomen. The abnormally extensive cloacal membrane acts as a wedge, holding apart the developing lower abdominal wall, and is responsible for the pubic separation characteristic of these anomalies and, cranial to the bladder, for a wide linea alba or even an exomphalos. This effect similarly causes failure of fusion of the paired genital tubercles, or of the Mullerian ducts, leading to partial or complete separation of the clitoris, of the female genital tract or of both.

The form of exstrophic anomaly is determined by the extent of the allantoic expansion of the cloacal membrane and upon the timing of its dehiscence. Classical vesical exstrophy follows breakdown of an extensive membrane, after completion of the urorectal septum, while a less extensive infraumbilical membrane, limited to the pubic area, leads to epispadias without exstrophy. Cloacal exstrophy represents the same basic anomaly but where breakdown of an extensive infraumbilical membrane occurs earlier, before formation of the urorectal septum, so that there is a central bowel field between the separated halves of the exstrophied bladder.

Classical Vesical Exstrophy

The bladder, of variable size, lies completely open upon the lower abdominal wall (Fig. 5.14) and the umbilical vessels emerge from its apex. At either side there is diastasis of the pubic bones, the extent of which tends to increase with the size of the bladder. In females the urethra is short, occasionally almost absent, and is almost always completely epispadiac. The vaginal orifice lies immediately posterior to the urethral plate or, in a few severe cases, may enter the plate inferiorly, and is almost always somewhat stenotic though never to an extent causing hydrocolpos. Finally the anus is anteriorly ectopic and, occasionally, stenotic.

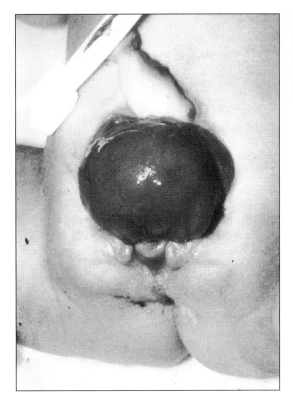

Fig. 5.14 Classical vesical exstrophy in a female neonate. In this instance the exstrophic bladder is large. The umbilical vessels emerge from its superior aspect and inferiorly are seen the separated hemi-clitori. The anus is anteriorly ectopic.

The clitoris is bifid and the labia are separated anteriorly so that the vaginal orifice is more than usually evident. Complete duplication of the female genital tract is rare but partial septation of the vagina and bicornuate uterus are relatively common. The fallopian tubes and ovaries are normal.

In sagittal section (Fig. 5.15), the distance between umbilicus and anus is considerably foreshortened with both urethral and vaginal orifices displaced anterosuperiorly, even to the extent, in a few cases, to occupy the lower abdominal wall

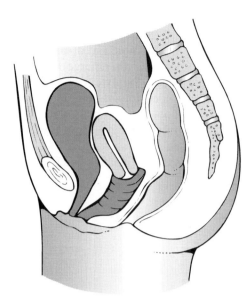

Fig. 5.15 Bladder exstrophy in sagittal section. Urethral, vaginal and rectal orifices are displaced anteriorly and the vagina pursues an almost horizontal course posteriorly with the cervix entering its anterior wall.

rather than the perineum. The vagina itself pursues an almost horizontal course posteriorly with the cervix lying more upon the anterior wall than the vault. Additionally, the internal genitalia and anorectum lack the normal support of the endopelvic fascia and pelvic floor muscles so that both procidentia and rectal proplasus are apt to occur, the former usually during adult life, the latter most commonly during infancy.

Despite the severity of the primary anomaly, neonates with vesical exstrophy are otherwise nearly always healthy and associated abnormalities are rare. In particular the upper urinary tracts are normal. There is very occasional association with congenital cardiac lesions and with myelomeningocele.

Details of reconstruction are beyond the scope of this Chapter but, in summary, primary reconstruction is undertaken neonatally except in the rare case with an unusually small, non-invertible bladder or with some other more major anomaly, usually cardiac. The bladder is circumcised from the surrounding skin and mobilised first from the recti on either side and then extraperitoneally. The urethral plate is similarly defined and mobilised on either side. These manoeuvres enable bladder and urethra to be closed vertically in the midline; at this stage no attempt is made to create a competent sphincteric mechanism. The procedure is combined with pelvic osteotomy which allows the pubic bones to be approximated anteriorly and with them the lower abdominal wall and the two halves of the clitoris.

Further measures, to produce continence, are deferred until the child is older and able to co-operate, usually between 5 and 8 years of age. Where the bladder has useful capacity, 50 ml at a minimum, some surgeons have obtained good results by bladder neck repair alone although it has been more common experience to find this procedure followed either by persistent sphincteric incompetence or by outflow obstruction with overflow incontinence from a distended bladder, sometimes with secondary upper renal tract complications in the form of obstruction or vesicoureteric reflux. Currently, preferred practice is to construct an overcompetent sphincteric mechanism by tubularisation of the trigone, with reimplantation of the ureters at a higher level in the bladder, and to combine this with simultaneous augmentation cystoplasty using a detubularised bowel segment. Voiding is by urethral self-catheterisation or, where this is not accepted, by catheterisation of a continent abdominal stoma, usually constructed from the appendix (Mitrofanoff procedure). Using this approach, complete urinary continence is almost always achieved without recourse to permanent urinary diversion.

As a rule, correction of any stenosis of the vaginal orifice is best deferred until puberty and, because of the risk of procidentia, should be limited to a cautious vertical episiotomy, sutured transversely, the minimum necessary for the purposes of sexual intercourse. Any degree of vaginal septation can be treated, if necessary, at the same time. Once through puberty, the vaginal orifice may be unusually and displeasingly evident by virtue of its anterior ectopia and lack of pubic hair in the midline of the lower abdominal wall. This problem can be disguised, rather than corrected, by excision of the non-hair-bearing area of skin and approximation of hair-bearing flaps in the midline.

Almost all females with repaired exstrophy enjoy normal sexual activity and the great majority appear to have unimpaired fertility (Shapiro *et al.*, 1984). Pregnancy is apt to be complicated by cervical or uterine prolapse (Krisiloff *et al.*, 1978). It has been suggested that risk of this complication can be minimised by Caesarean section and it is also possible that it occurs less frequently where the initial reconstruction incorporated repair of the pelvic ring (Canning and Gearhart 1993; Blakely and Mills, 1981).

Complete procidentia may also occur spontaneously and should be dealt with not by hysterectomy but by a sling procedure anchoring the uterine cervix to the sacrum posteriorly (Woodhouse, 1991) and, usually, by rectopexy to reduce the risk of rectal prolapse or rectocele.

Epispadias

The urethral plate lies open anteriorly and widens proximally to enter a clearly incompetent bladder neck (Fig. 5.16). The clitoris is bifid, rather than duplicated, and at either side there is a minor degree of pubic separation with a wide linea alba above. The vaginal orifice is slightly ectopic anteriorly, but is otherwise normal, while duplication anomalies of the vagina proper or uterus are exceptional.

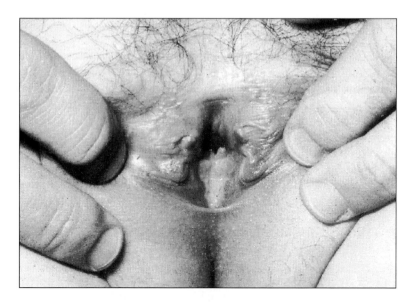

Fig. 5.16   Female epispadias. There are separated hemi-clitori and the open bladder neck is visible at the apex of the urethral strip.

Even though female epispadias is evident enough on inspection, it is sometimes overlooked neonatally, doubtless on account of its extreme rarity.

The lesion is repaired by tubularisation of the urethral plate and it is usually advisable to narrow this proximally. The thin skin lying between the separated mons veneris is excised and fat from the mons may be employed to cover the urethral repair and obliterate space behind the pubic symphysis. The two halves of the mons are closed together in the midline and so too the bifid clitoris.

This repair may itself increase urethral resistance sufficient to secure urinary continence. If not, formal bladder neck repair is necessary and is more likely to be successful than with exstrophy since with, isolated epispadias, bladder capacity and function are nearly always normal.

So far as is known, the gynaecological and obstetric problems occurring in adult females with repaired exstrophy are not encountered in these with pure epispadias.

Cloacal Exstrophy

The anatomy of this most extreme form of exstrophy is illustrated diagrammatically in Fig. 5.17 and a clinical example is shown in Fig. 5.18. In practice many variations occur upon this basic theme (Hurwitz *et al.*, 1987).

From a gynaecological viewpoint, there are usually two widely separated hemi-clitori. Occasionally there is absence of one or both and rarely they exist as

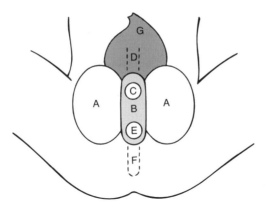

Fig. 5.17 Diagrammatic representation of the typical features of cloacal exstrophy. Between the two bladder plates (A) is situated the central bowel field (B), representing the ileo-caecal area, and which has two orifices, the upper (C) leading from the ileum (D), the lower (E) leading to the blind-ending colon (F). Superiorly there is an exomphalos (G) of variable size.

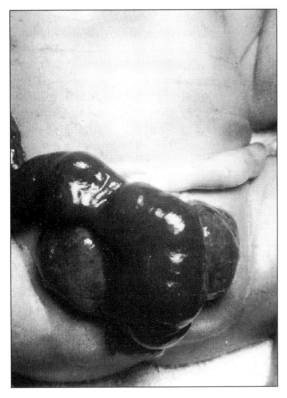

Fig. 5.18 Cloacal exstrophy. Two hemi-bladders are situated at either side and in the midline small bowel prolapses from the central bowel field. Unusually, in this case there is no exomphalos and the umbilical vessels emerge from the superior aspect of the lesion.

a single midline structure. As a rule the ovaries are normal. Abnormalities of Mullerian development are almost always present, with uterine duplication in 95% of cases, vaginal duplication in 65% and vaginal absence in 25% (Hurwitz *et al.*, 1987). Utero-vaginal agenesis, with fusion of fallopian tubes to the distal ureters, has also been described (Hurwitz *et al.*, 1987).

In contrast to other forms of exstrophy, associated anomalies of other systems are common, notably of the gastrointestinal tract (short bowel, malrotation, duplication), upper urinary tracts (renal agenesis, multicystic dysplasia, ureteric obstruction), spinal column (hemi-vertebra, sacral agenesis) and central nervous system (myelomeningocele) (Soper and Kilger, 1964; Mitchell *et al.*, 1990). Cardiovascular and pulmonary anomalies are comparatively rare.

Reconstructive procedures for this anomaly pose considerable practical difficulties and, sometimes, even more intractable ethical dilemmas. Where active treatment is considered advisable, the form this takes is determined by the various features obtaining in any individual case, in particular the length of small bowel proximally, the size of the hemi-bladders and the presence of a neurological defect from myelomeningocele or from sacral agenesis.

In general terms, reconstruction commences neonatally, in one or two stages, beginning with closure of the exomphalos. Depending upon the length of the small bowel, the gastrointestinal malformation is usually dealt with either by detachment and tubularization of the central bowel field, with approximation of the hemi-bladders in the midline, or by detachment of ileum and colon from the central bowel field, restoration of gastrointestinal continuity by the ileo-colonic anastomosis and leaving the bowel field in situ to act, in effect, as an endogenous bladder augmentation. In either case, the colon distally is brought out as a terminal colostomy. Once this part of the repair is complete, anterior reconstruction of the bladder, combined with pelvic osteotomy, follows along the lines described for classical vesical exstrophy, either immediately or at a second stage a month or so later. A pull-through procedure to correct the anal imperforation is worth considering only in the absence of any neurological lesion. Otherwise a permanent terminal colostomy is preferable.

It is usually possible to at least partly correct the gynaecological malformation at the time of bladder and pelvic ring closure. The two halves of the clitoris, if present, can often be sutured together to form a single midline structure. Again, it is often possible to approximate the distal half to one-third of the two vaginas and which are incised medially and sutured together to form a single tube distally in the midline. The resulting orifice is sutured to the surrounding perineal skin immediately behind the reconstructed urethra. An alternative approach, especially where genital tract development is asymmetrical, is to retain the better developed of the two vaginas, discarding the other along with its associated uterus and fallopian tube (Lund and Hendren, 1993). In cases where vaginal development is absent or severely hypoplastic, anatomically satisfactory reconstruction has been achieved using split skin grafts (Braren, 1994). Alternatively, an ileal segment can be employed for this purpose provided that this does not compromise the length of small bowel remaining.

The long-term results of these various gynaecological reconstructions are, as yet, largely unknown. As would be expected, there is no recorded example of successful pregnancy in a female with cloacal exstrophy.

Although males predominate among cases of cloacal exstrophy, it is only seldom that they have more than rudimentary penile development and which typically takes the form of two small epispadiac hemi-phalli arising from each pubic bone. Occasionally there is a single midline structure, with or without epispadias, but still small and, rarer still, there are no recognisable external genitalia.

Apart from the exceptional case with good phallic development, attempts to construct a functioning penis of adequate dimensions have been uniformly unsuccessful and for this reason there has been a strong trend in recent years to undertake gender reassignment and to rear these infants as females. Naturally a decision of this magnitude necessitates careful and sympathetic discussion with the parents, yet should be determined definitively as soon as is possible. At least under English law, the infant's birth and name must not be registered until the decision is made one way or the other.

Where reassignment is decided, the testes, if present, are excised and the two halves of the scrotum are reduced in size, by excision of vertical ellipses of skin, to resemble labia majora. This is undertaken during the first or second stage of neonatal reconstruction. At the same time it is usually possible to mobilise the two haemophalli sufficiently to bring them together in the midline, above the urethral reconstruction, to form a 'clitoris'. Vaginal reconstruction follows later using a bowel segment where practicable or employing conjoined gracilis myocutaneous flaps (Mundy, 1994).

Although this quite recent policy of gender reassignment seems eminently reasonable, desirable even, it remains to be seen whether children so managed will grow up to be adequate females any more than did their predecessors adequate males.

OVARIAN LESIONS

Ovarian Absence

Except where the condition is bilateral, ovarian absence is almost always an incidental finding and is detected, at laparoscopy, in approximately 1 in 11 000 women (Sivanesaratum, 1986). In practice it is usually impossible to determine whether the condition represents true agenesis or infarction following torsion prenatally, postnatally or later.

Ovarian Cysts (see also p. 256)

(see also p. 256)

Neonatal ovarian cysts are of germinal or graffian origin and, as such, are follicular, theca lutein or simple cysts in which the cell lining is destroyed. Small follicular cysts, 1 mm or more in diameter, are detectable in approximately one third of the female newborns, often in ovaries which are generally enlarged, and are presumptively due to raised levels of maternal or placental chorionic gonadotrophin (HCG). After birth, HCG level falls and such ovaries revert to normal.

Higher levels of HCG exisiting in maternal diabetes, isoimmunisation and non-immune hydrops have been associated with theca lutein cysts (Ahlvin and Bauer, 1976; Fleming and McCleary, 1981) again with resolution once HCG levels fall following delivery. The same phenomenon has been observed in the fetus delivered prematurely before circulating maternal and fetal hormones produce negative hypothalamic pituitary feedback (Tapanainen *et al.*, 1981). Large cysts in this situation are resolvable by administration of medroxy-progesterone, a synthetic progesterone analogue (Sedin *et al.*, 1985).

The principal complication of larger cysts, 4–5 cm diameter or more, is torsion followed by haemorrhagic infarction and which is reported as occurring in 50% of cases in some series (Widdowson *et al.*, 1988). This event is not necessarily accompanied by any systemic upset and may occur prenatally. Other, occasional, complications include spontaneous rupture, with ascites (Manson *et al.*, 1978), and adhesion intestinal obstruction in associated with ovarian infarction (McClever and Andrews, 1988).

Neonatal ovarian cysts were once considered rare and were detected only if palpable or symptomatic, but the reported incidence has increased considerably with the advent of prenatal ultrasonography (Grapin *et al.*, 1987). They are now recognised as the commonest cause of an intra-abdominal cyst in a female fetus and may be spherical, oval or dumb-bell shaped. Sometimes they are highly mobile (Avni *et al.*, 1993). Differential diagnosis, on fetal ultrasonography, includes urachal cysts, limited to the midline below the umbilicus, hydrocolpos, again limited to the midline and extending deeply into the pelvis, duplication anomalies of the gastrointestinal tract, which tend to be tubular, and distal megaureter (Rizzo *et al.*, 1989). Among other possibilities, renal cysts are readily distinguishable, provided that the organ is not ectopic, but omental and mesenteric cysts are less so and similarly cystic lesions affecting the posterior abdominal wall (Debeugny *et al.*, 1989) or segmental dilatation of small bowel as occurring in cystic fibrosis.

Prenatally or postnatally, presence of a fluid-debris level within the cyst is almost always the result of torsion (Nussbaum *et al.*, 1988).

The low incidence of clinically detectable ovarian cysts neonatally argues that most of these now discovered by ultrasonography resolve spontaneously, as would be expected since the great majority are hormonally driven. There is now ample evidence, by serial ultrasonography postnatally, that this is the case although the process, with larger lesions, may take many months (Widdowson *et al.*, 1988; Croitoru *et al.*, 1991) Torsion followed by infarction represents an alternative fate, but the extremely low level of ovarian absence found at laparoscopy suggests that this is most uncommon.

These considerations bear upon management and there is now general agreement that cysts which are simple, anechoic, with a wall invisible on ultrasound, and which are less than 4–5 cm diameter, can be expectantly managed with serial ultrasound examinations confirming resolution. Cysts so massive so as to cause symptoms undoubtedly call for active intervention and the same can be advocated for smaller lesions still exceeding 5 cm diameter, especially if bilateral, or for the occasional cyst found to enlarge during follow-up or failing to resolve over a prolonged period. Isolated case reports or small series report successful percutaneous cyst aspiration (Grapin *et al.*, 1987; Widdowson *et al.*, 1988; Brandt *et al.*, 1991). Open surgical intervention should be limited to cystectomy or marsupialisation of the cyst since functional ovarian tissue may exist in the remainder of the gonad (Brandt *et al.*, 1991).

Operative intervention, in the form of oophorectomy, is advisable where the presence of a fluid-debris level on ultrasonography indicates that torsion has occurred (Nussbaum *et al.*, 1988).

Solid Ovarian Tumours

These are exceptional neonatally and the handful of recorded examples includes one of granulosa cell carcinoma (Ziegler, 1945) and one of cystadenoma (Bulfamonte, 1942).

Other Ovarian Anomalies

Streak ovaries co-exist with Turner's syndrome (45X karyotype) (see p. 130 Chapter 8) and are also encountered in mixed gonadal dysgenesis, often asymmetrically, with a dysgenetic testis contralaterally or, sometimes, bilaterally. Occasionally one or other gonad is absent.

Dysgenetic gonads are liable to malignant change and gonadoblastoma has been recorded neonatally. Absence of a gonad unilaterally may well represent prenatal torsion and infarction of such a tumour. Accordingly, these gonads should be removed within the first few months of life. As a rule, infants with mixed gonadal dysgenesis are raised as females and excision of the gonads can be combined with suitable genital reconstruction.

True hermaphrodites have both ovarian and testicular tissue which may exist as testis on one side and an ovary on the other, or may be combined as an ovotestis. As a rule, and especially if recognised early, affected patients are better raised as females in which event genital reconstruction is combined with excision of a testis, if present, or, with ovotestis, ideally excision of testicular but not ovarian tissue. In these gonads ovarian tissue is usually polar and testicular tissue central. The completeness of testicular excision can be monitored by serum levels of MIF. If any doubt occurs as to the presence of residual testicular tissue the entire gonad should be excised.

MISCELLANEOUS ANOMALIES

Clitoral Hypertrophy

In preterm females, the clitoris is apt to appear prominent due to immature development of the labia majora, whilst on occasion there is true hypertrophy from persistence of a fetal pattern of steroid production by the adrenal glands. In the mature neonate, clitoral hypertrophy should prompt suspicion of an enzyme deficiency or an intersexual state, even in the absence of urethralization of the urogenital sinus or of 'scrotal' development. Among the former to be considered are partial forms of 3β-hydroxysteroid dehydrogenase deficiency in genetic females and 17β-hydroxysteroid dehydrogenase and 5α-reductase deficiency in genetic males, all of which tend to be associated with minimal virilization neonatally but marked virilization through puberty.

Clitoral hypertrophy may also occur as a feature of neurofibromatosis.

Congenital Short Urethra

The urethra is wide and abnormally short, less than 2 cm in a neonate. Its orifice is unusually evident and capacious (Fig. 5.19). The sphincteric mechanism,

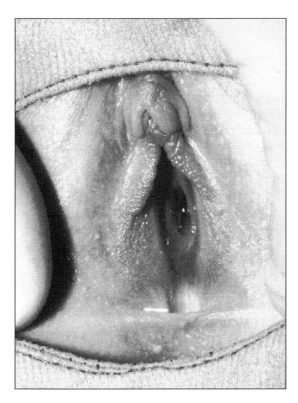

Fig. 5.19 Congenital short urethra. In this case there is co-existing distal vaginal atresia with the introitus represented by a shallow pit. The single wide vulval orifice is of the short patulous urethra.

including the bladder neck, is incompetent and urine dribbles more or less continuously from an empty bladder. The bladder itself is structurally and functionally normal.

Despite the obvious appearance, this anomaly is very rarely detected neonatally, largely by virtue of its extreme rarity, and presents instead in older girls as primary, severe, diurnal enuresis. Treatment requires a combination of urethral lengthening and bladder neck reconstruction.

Urethral Prolapse (Fig. 5.20)

Urethral prolapse, only rarely occurring neonatally, is a complaint largely confined to infants of Afro-Caribbean descent (Jenkins *et al.*, 1984) and supposedly results from poor attachment between the smooth muscle layers of the urethra (Owens and Morse, 1968).

The lesion may either come to light simply by virtue of its appearance or, more often, because of blood-stained discharge resulting from ulceration of its surface. It is distinguishable from prolapsed duplex-system ectopic ureterocele and paraurethral cyst in being entirely circumferential.

Resolution may follow conservative measures in the form of antibiotic therapy and locally applied oestrogen cream (Richardson *et al.*, 1982). Persistent

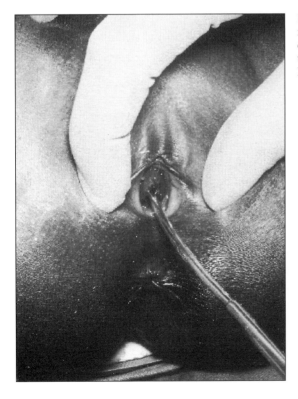

Fig. 5.20 Urethral prolapse in a neonate. The prolapsed urethra extends around the circumference of the urethral orifice. (Patient of Mr Patrick Duffy).

lesions are treatable by excision of the prolapsed segment with primary suture (Jenkins *et al.*, 1984).

Prolapsed Ectopic Ureterocele (Fig. 5.21)

This uncommon complication is confined to ureteroceles occurring as part of a complete duplication anomaly of the upper urinary tract. The ureterocele itself comprises the cystically dilated, intravesical termination of the upper polar ureter with the orifice upon it located distally. The lower polar ureteric orifice is found superiorly on the anterior surface of the lesion. Only unusually large and mobile ureteroceles prolapse. Nevertheless prolapsed ureterocele is probably the commonest cause of an interlabial mass neonatally.

Until recently, presentation occurred either simply because of the appearance of the lesion or because the prolapse caused some degree of bladder outflow obstruction with urinary retention. Nowadays most duplex-system ureteroceles are detected by prenatal ultrasonography and any complicating prolapse is detected upon consequential examination neonatally.

Differential diagnosis includes urethral prolapse and paraurethral cyst. Sometimes the ectopic orifice is visible with urine spurting from it intermittently

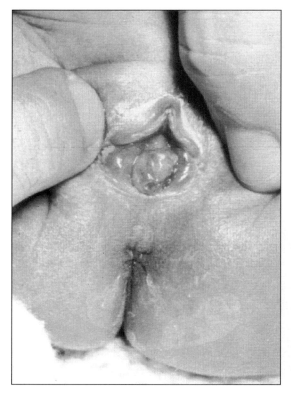

Fig. 5.21 Prolapsed ectopic utererocele in a female neonate. (Patient of Mr Patrick Duffy).

(Thompson and Kelalis, 1964). An abdominal ultrasound examination will always reveal the appearances of the upper renal tracts and bladder typical of duplex-system ureterocele. Immediate treatment is necessary only if the lesion is complicated by bladder outflow obstruction or by urinary sepsis. Reduction, under general anaesthetic, may be facilitated by initial needle aspiration of the ureterocele and completed by cystoscopy. Occasionally open, transvesical, reduction is necessary. Definitive treatment follows, usually in the form of excision of the poorly functioning upper renal pole and decompression of the ureterocele by aspiration of the upper polar ureteric stump (Rickwood *et al.*, 1992).

Paraurethral Cyst

A retention cyst of a paraurethral gland may be present at birth and takes the form of a swelling below the urethral meatus (Fig. 5.22) or one protruding through the meatus simulating a prolapsed ureterocele. Most cysts resolve spontaneously during the first few months of life and active treatment, by way of incision and drainage or marsupialization, is necessary only for infected or persistent lesions.

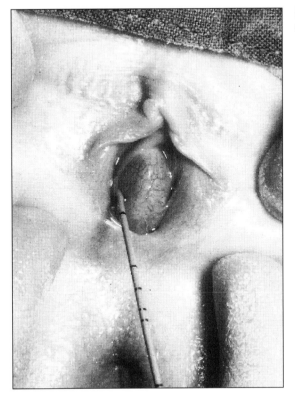

Fig. 5.22 Paraurethral cyst. The catheter is inserted into the urethra.

Hymenal Polyps

Because of the influence of maternal oestrogen, the hymen at birth and for the first few days of life is thickened and oedematous and, on occasion, the posterior portion forms a round or elongated polyp. Berglan and Selander (1962) found that 6% of 1000 newborn girls examined had this abnormality. No treatment is required.

Botryoid Rhabdomyosarcoma

Occasional examples of vaginal sarcoma botryoides have been recorded neonatally (Hays *et al.*, 1985). Treatment is described on p. 253 and the problems peculiar to management neonatally are discussed by Spicer (1995).

Vaginal Cyst

A vaginal cyst resulting from fluid distension of the epoophoron (Gartner's duct) may occasinally be noted neonatally projecting into the lumen of the vagina (Klein *et al.*, 1986). Tense cysts, compressing the urethra and causing obstructed micturition, require excision.

Labial Hypertrophy

Modest degrees of hypertrophy of the labia minora, usually bilaterally, are quite common and require no treatment.

Vascular Lesions

Haemangiomata or lymphangiomata occasionally affect the vulva. Treatment is never indicated neonatally and the majority resolve spontaneously during infancy.

Procidentia

Genital prolapse in the newborn is exceptionally rare and is largely confined to those with paralysis of the pelvic floor, usually from myelomeningocele. It has also been described following impacted breech presentation (Cottom and Williams, 1965). The condition is treated by manual reduction, following which the legs are bound together for a few weeks while the bladder is drained via a catheter. Temporary support with a rubber nipple or pessary restores the uterus to its normal position (Carpenter and Rock, 1988).

Adherent Labia Minora

Although commonly termed 'congenital labial adhesions', this minor complaint is almost certainly acquired, not congenital, as would be expected given that application of oestrogen cream often separates the labia (see p. 118).

FUNCTIONAL COMPLAINTS

Vaginal Bleeding

Vaginal bleeding is occasionally observed neonatally, either directly or as blood-staining of a napkin, and is almost always a transient phenomenon consequent upon circulatory maternal oestrogens (Gillian and Gundy, 1992).

Persistent bleeding demands attention and the principal differential diagnoses comprise ulceration of a urethral prolapse or sarcoma botryoides, the former discernible on vulval inspection, the latter on vaginoscopy.

Vaginal Discharge

Many female newborns have a noticeable and rather thick vaginal discharge for the first few days of life, a phenomenon also ascribable to the effect of circulating maternal hormones.

Trichomonas vaginalis infection can be acquired during passage through an infected birth canal. The discharge is greyish-white and frothy and the diagnosis is confirmed when numerous leucocytes and trichomonads are observed on wet-film microscopy. Metronidazole, 15 mg/kg per day, given for 10 days is curative.

Neonates with diabetes mellitus or immunodeficiency states are susceptible to candidal infection. Here, there is diffuse vulval inflammation with white plaques on the vaginal wall and the diagnosis is confirmable by observing mycelia in a potassium hydroxide preparation or by culture. Treatment comprises 100 mg miconazole or clotrimazole intravaginally for 7 days or 1 ml 0.5% gentian violet solution instilled intra-vaginally for a similar period (Huffman, 1987).

Occasionally there is an underlying structural problem. With some urogenital sinus anomalies, bacterial infection of a urinary hydrocolpos can present as 'vaginal' discharge. Vulval inspection reveals the likely cause of this. With complete duplication of a renal tract, the upper polar ureter may terminate ectopically in the vagina. Where function of the upper renal pole is unusually poor, the small quantity of urine produced pools within the vagina, becomes infected, and appears as vaginal discharge. This form of presentation is exceptional in the neonate.

AMBIGUOUS GENITALIA

General

The birth of a child of indeterminate sex represents a self-evident psychological burden to its parents and, as such, constitutes a paediatric emergency. Nonetheless, it is fundamental to the subsequent well-being of the child that there is correct and appropriate assignment of gender, a process which may necessarily occupy a few days and which requires the collaboration of paediatric endocrinologist, genetecist, urological surgeon and radiologist.

The term ambiguous genitalia implies the presence of a phallus too small for penis, too large for clitoris and almost always exhibiting some degree of hypospadias, typically severe, combined, in the great majority of cases, with gonads which are unilaterally or bilaterally impalpable, maldescended or of indeterminate nature. Additionally, some degree of 'scrotal' development is the rule, with rugosity of the skin, and which tends to be proportionate to extent of virilisation of the phallus.

Fortunately the problem is rare and, with the various forms of congenital adrenal hyperplasia (incidence 1 in 14 000 live births (Pang *et al.*, 1988)) representing 30–40% of cases, can be estimated as occurring in 1 in 4200–1 in 5600 live births.

Various classifications of intersexual disorders exist, most broadly those with ambiguous genitalia and those without (e.g. complete androgen insensitivity syndrome (CAIS) in those with female phenotypes), and, more specifically, those based upon the pathophysiology of sexual development (disorders of chromosomal, gonadal or phenotypic sex) or upon gonadal histology. For neonates with ambiguous genitalia the last proves to be the most helpful classification and comprises female and male pseudohermaphroditism, true hermaphroditism and conditions with dysgenetic gonads. The essential features of these conditions are summarised in Table 5.2.

Table 5.2   Disorders of sexual differentiation

Disorder	Gonads	Mullerian derivatives	Chromosomes
Female pseudohermaphroditism	Ovaries	Present	XX
Male pseudohermaphroditism	Testes	Absent	XY
Gonadal dysgenesis and XY agenesis	Testis + streak/ Bilateral streak	Variable	XO/XY
True hermaphroditism	Testis + ovary	Present	46 XX + mosaics/ 46 XY with Y line

Female Pseudohermaphroditism

The various endogenous forms of this condition (congenital adrenal hyperplasia) are fully described on p. 274; exogenous occurrences, from maternal virilising tumours or from intake of progesterone, are exceptionally rare.

The degree of phallic development varies from little more than mild clitoral enlargement to an organ of normal penile dimensions (Fig 5.23). As a rule, the hypospadiac orifice of the common urogenital sinus is perineal, except in those with more extreme virilization where it may be located more distally or, very rarely, may open terminally on the glans. It remains a truism that any 'boy' with hypospadias and impalpable gonads is best regarded as a 'girl' until proved otherwise. With few exceptions, the degree of 'scrotal' development parallels that of the phallus (Fig. 5.23) and so also the level of urethro-vaginal confluence, with high, suprasphincteric, confluence occurring in only some 5% of cases, almost all of them severely virilised. The ovaries, fallopian tubes, uterus and cervix are normal and even minor vaginal malformations, such as septation, are rare.

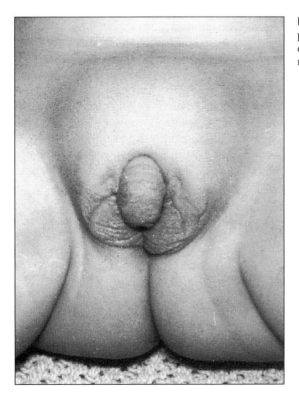

Fig. 5.23 Congenital adrenal hyperplasia showing marked clitoral enlargement and 'scrotal' development.

Male Pseudohermaphroditism

Subcategories within this group associated with ambiguous genitalia (as opposed to micropenis) comprise anomalies causing impaired testosterone production, abnormal testosterone metabolism or end-organ insensitivity to androgens. They are all characterised by absence of structures of Mullerian origin although a distal 'vaginal' remnant, of separate embryological derivation, may be present with the urethral channel distally representing a common urogenital sinus.

The phallus is pathologically underdeveloped, sometimes to the extent of appearing no more than minor 'clitoral' enlargement, with associated perineal hypospadias. The scrotum is typically bifid and the gonads are often incompletely descended or may lie intra-abdominally.

Among conditions associated with impaired testosterone production are various enzyme deficiencies, most of which are inherited as an autosomal recessive trait, and in these individuals serum testosterone does not rise appropriately following HCG stimulation. Some (e.g. 20–22 desmolase deficiency) are also associated with adrenal insufficiency. Deficiency of 17β-hydroxysteroid impairs conversion of androstenedione to testosterone and it is a curiosity of this defect that affected individuals, while severely under-virilized neonatally, even to the extent of being thought normal girls, nonetheless virilize vigorously through puberty, with clitoral enlargement, hirsutism and masculinisation of the voice.

Abnormal testosterone metabolism is largely confined to deficiency of 5α-reductase, necessary in the conversion of testosterone to dehydrotestosterone, and, as with deficiency of 17β-hydroxysteroid, is characteristically associated with marked virilisation at puberty.

The syndrome of complete androgen insensitivity, with a normal femal phenotype, is described elsewhere (p. 142); the incomplete forms have to a variable degree of feminisation of the external genitalia, usually severely so, in an XY male with normal testes (Fig. 5.24). Analysis of the androgen receptor-gene in these patients reveals various mutations explaining the lack of response to endogenous or exogenous androgens.

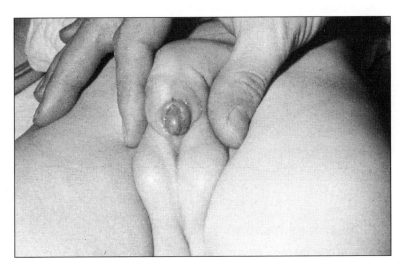

Fig. 5.24 Incomplete androgen insensitivity. There is modest 'clitoral' enlargement and normal testes lie in the scrotum on each side.

True Hermaphroditism

This, the rarest intersexual state, is characterised by the presence of both ovarian and testicular tissue, either as separate gonads or as one or two ovotestes, the commonest combinations being bilateral ovotestes or ovary–ovotestis.

Ovotestes, which may descend fully into the scrotum, characteristically have testicular tissue located centrally and ovarian tissue at either pole. The predominant karyotype is XX, although XY and mosaics have been recorded. The testicular development occurs from translocation of the short arm of the Y chromosome with a retained testis-determining factor gene.

Central to internal genital development in these cases, as also those with gonadal dysgenesis, is that MIF acts not by a circulating endocrine effect but by local diffusion, so that a normally functioning testis will inhibit development of Mullerian structures ipsilaterally, whereas one which is poorly functioning, or dysgenetic, will allow these structures to develop. Thus in true hermaphroditism the anatomy of the internal genitalia is very variable, with the uterus being normal or hypoplastic and the fallopian tubes being present unilaterally or bilaterally depending on the local levels of androgens, oestrogens and MIF. Phallic development is usually poor although, because of the presence of testicular tissue and Wolffian duct structures, paternity has been recorded in large series of Bantu Africans among whom true hermaphroditism is relatively common.

Gonadal Dysgenesis

Some 40% of these patients have a 46 XY karyotype and the bulk of the remainder 45X/46XY mosaicism. In pure gonadal dysgenesis, both gonads are dysfunctional with a female phenotype as with complete androgen insensitivity syndrome. In mixed types, with ambiguous genitalia, a normal testis is associated with an abnormal or streak gonad contralaterally (Fig. 5.25). As to be

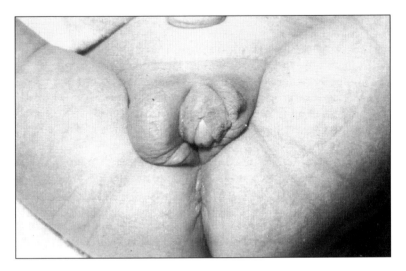

Fig. 5.25 Mixed gonadal dysgenesis. Moderate phallic enlargement is associated with a normal scrotal right testis. A streak gonad was present on the left.

expected in this situation, the anatomy of internal genitalia varies, with most having at least a rudimentary uterus while a fallopian tube is usually present on the side of the streak gonad. Phallic development is usually poor.

Investigation

Clinical

Occasionally the diagnosis is determinable from a relevant family history and very rarely from a history of maternal hormone ingestion or virilising tumour.

On physical examination, presence of any palpable gonad excludes congenital adrenal hyperplasia and other forms of female pseudohermaphroditism, although not the converse, whilst presence of two normal-feeling testes points strongly to a form of male pseudohermaphroditism. Gonads palpable only unilaterally, or which feel abnormal, hint, no more, at true hermaphroditism or gonadal dysgenesis.

A uterus may be felt on rectal examination. Finally, ambiguous genitalia should be distinguished from urethralisation of the female phallus, not an interesexual state, and which is recognisable by the presence of both phallic and perineal orifices combined with anterior anal ectopia.

Laboratory investigations

Useful hormonal investigations in these patients, and their interpretation, are to be found in Chapter 15. Determination of genetic sex is essential and the provisional result on the peripheral karyotype is usually available within three days of sample collection.

Imaging studies

Ultrasound represents the most useful early study and is best undertaken neonatally when the uterus and ovaries are rendered prominent by the physiological effects of circulating maternal oestrogens. Demonstration of a hydrocolpos confirms the presence of a urogenital sinus anomaly occurring from virilisation of the fetus. Demonstration of a uterus and two ovaries reinforces the diagnosis of female pseudohermaphroditism on an XX infant although it should be noted that in 40% of quite normal female neonates only one ovary is identifiable by pelvic ultrasound and in 16% neither (Cohen *et al.*, 1993). Ultrasound may similarly be employed to search for testicular tissue within the pelvis. With ovotestes, the normal uniform structure of the testes is replaced by a heterogenous appearance secondary to the presence of follicles within the ovarian portion of the gonad.

Where no gonadal tissue is seen in the pelvis, inguino-perineal ultrasound, using a high frequency transducer, may identify testicular tissue and thereby exclude female pseudohermaphroditism.

The adrenal glands can also be assessed for evidence of hyperplasia, suggested by normal cortico-medullary differentiation and lengths and widths exceeding 20 mm and 4 mm respectively. Normal sized glands, however, do not exclude congenital adrenal hyperplasia, although a cerebriform appearance is said to be specific (Avni *et al.*, 1993).

Contrast radiography via the orifice of the common urogenital sinus (genitogram) finds use in demonstrating the presence of separate urethral and vaginal canals and their level of confluence (Fig. 5.26).

MRI has become increasingly employed in the investigation of intersexual states with its advantages lying in ability to image in multiple planes and to perform tissue characterisation. Detailed anatomy of Mullerian and Wolffian structures is obtainable and so too of gonads, orthotopic or ectopic, although streak gonads remain difficult to identify. It is also able to differentiate between a penis and an hypertrophied clitoris since with the latter the bulbo-spongeous and transverse perinei muscles are poorly developed or absent (Secat *et al.*, 1994).

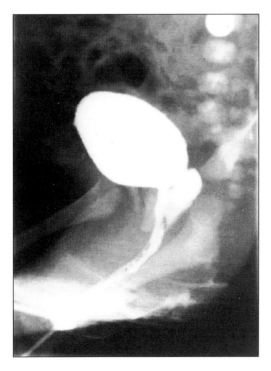

Fig. 5.26 Genitogram. Contrast enters the urethra and bladder anteriorly and the vagina posteriorly. The urethro-vaginal confluence is low.

Endoscopy

Endoscopy of the common urogenital sinus represents an alternative means of demonstrating the urethral and vaginal channels and their level of confluence, also the presence or absence of a cervix uteri or of vaginal septation. This investigation can be omitted as part of the initial investigations provided a satisfactory genitogram has been obtained.

Laparoscopy

With modern equipment, laparoscopy is technically feasible in neonates and has the potential to exactly define intrapelvic anatomy and to obtain gonadal biopsies. In practice, development of newer imaging techniques, notably ultrasonography and MRI, has lessened the need for early laparoscopy although it still finds use at a later stage, particularly for demonstrating the presence or absence of Mullerian-derived structures and in seeking gonads, streak gonads especially.

Management

General

What follows assumes that the intersexual state has been identified neonatally, or shortly thereafter, as is nowadays almost always the case in those with ambiguous genitalia. An occasional exception lies in infants with congenital adrenal

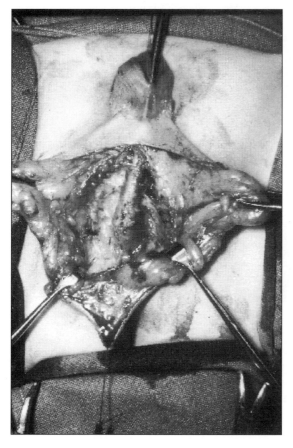

Fig. 5.27 Vaginoplasty for low urethro-vaginal confluence prior to reduction clitoroplasty. A posterior perineal skin flap has been raised to expose the proximal phallic urethra and the site of urethro-vaginal confluence.

hyperplasia, usually non-salt-losing, who are severely virilised, although even here the mistake should not arise where it is discovered that there are no palpable gonads.

On a practical basis, the child's birth should not be registered until a definitive decision has been taken as to gender.

The most straightfoward decision lies in those with female pseudohermaphroditism who should always be raised as girls, no matter how virilized the phallus, since, with appropriate reconstruction, they are potentially able to achieve normal sexual and reproductive function.

In other categories, the decision is apt to be more problematical and, in most cases, hinges upon the size of the phallus and its potential for further growth. The hypospadiac deformity is not, however, a major consideration since this is almost always amenable to full surgical correction. At term, normal stretched penile length is 3.5 ± 0.4 cm, although, in the presence of chordee, measurement of diameter tends to be more helpful, the normal, at term, being $1.0-1.5$ cm. Where length and diameter fall below 1.5 cm and 0.7 cm respectively,

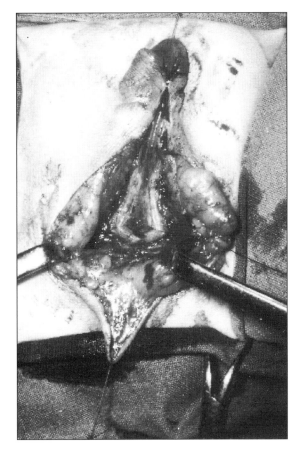

Fig. 5.28 The common urogenital sinus has been opened to expose the vagina posteriorly and the urethral orifice (catheterised) anteriorly. The perineal skin flap will be inset around the vaginal orifice.

construction of a sexually satisfactory penis is not feasible and assignement to the female gender is advisable (Savage, 1982). Between these figures and 2.0 cm and 0.9 cm respectively, a satisfactory correction may or may not be possible, a matter largely dependent upon the judgement of the surgeon concerned. Where doubt exists, a good response to a single injection of testosterone (e.g. Sustanon 100, 25 mg) usefully predicts the effects of androgen stimulation at puberty, while lack of response argues for assignment of the female gender. The latter applies particularly in cases of incomplete androgen insensitivity. In a few finely balanced cases, the decision may ultimately hinge upon the presence or absence of a vagina as demonstrated by genitography or by endoscopy.

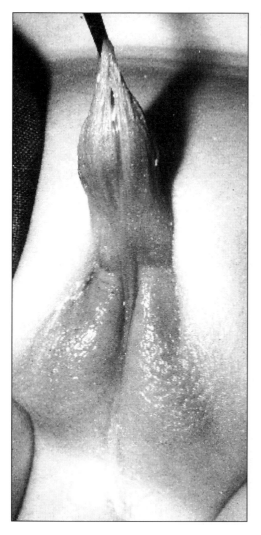

Fig. 5.29   Patient with congenital adrenal hyperplasia prior to clitoral reduction.

Patients with male or true hermaphroditism and gonadal dysgenesis to be reared as girls should have any testicular tissue or streak gonads removed as soon as it is practicable, preferably within the first three months of life.

Female gender surgery

Reduction phalloplasty is undertaken at 3–6 months of age and, where there is low urethro-vaginal confluence, this may be combined with posterior perineal flap vaginoplasty (Figs 5.27, 5.28).

An immediately preoperative view of the phallus is shown in Fig. 5.29. An incision dorsally and laterally around the corona is extended ventrally on each side of the urethral plate back to the urethral meatus, enabling the phallic skin to be mobilised from the underlying corpora (Fig 5.30). The urethral plate is dissected from the corpora ventrally and dorsally the neurovascular bundles are similarly mobilised (Fig. 5.31). Further dissection frees the corpora to their attachment to the pubic bones at which point they are transfixed, ligated and divided, then resected almost to the glans distally. This leaves the glans viable upon the dorsal neurovascular bundles and urethral plate (Fig. 5.32) and it is usually desirable to reduce its bulk by dorsal wedge incision. The trimmed glans is then resutured to the stumps of the corpora. The prepuce is split in the midline vertically (Fig. 5.33) and the resulting flaps sutured around the corona dorsally and laterally then along the urethral strip on either side to form 'labia minora' (Fig. 5.34). The final appearance is shown in Fig. 5.35.

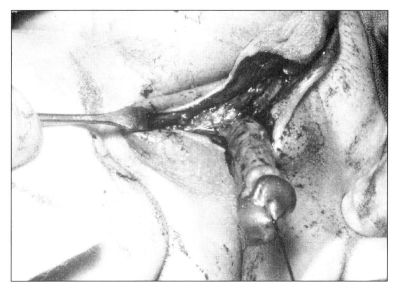

Fig. 5.30 Skin has been mobilised from the phallic shaft and the corpora freed to the pubic bones.

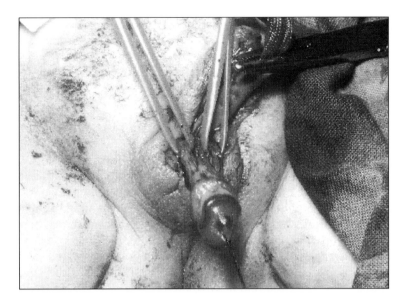

Fig. 5.31 Isolation of the dorsal neurovascular bundles.

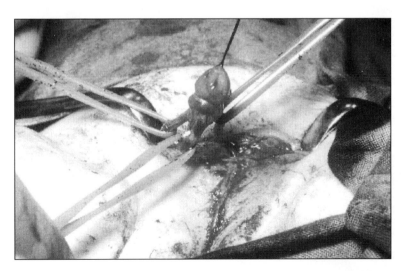

Fig. 5.32 The urethral plate has been freed from the corpora and the latter excised from the glans to close to the pubic bones. Slings hold the urethral plate ventrally and the neurovascular bundles dorsally.

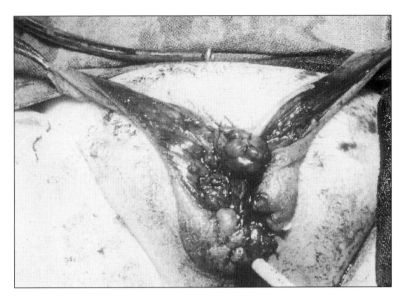

Fig. 5.33 The glans has been reduced in size by dorsal wedge excision and then sutured to the corporal stumps. The prepuce has been split in the midline.

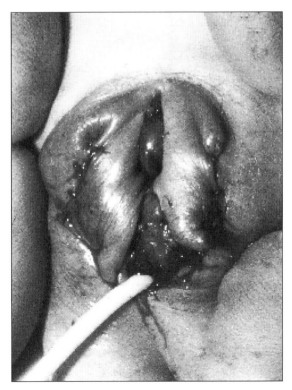

Fig. 5.34 The preputial flaps have been sutured to the urethral plate medially and the skin laterally to represent 'labia minora'.

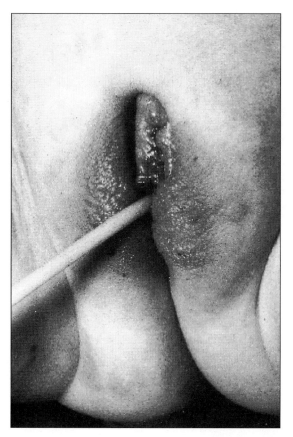

Fig. 5.35 Final appearances at the end of the procedure.

Techniques employed for vaginal reconstruction are outlined in 'urogenital sinus anomalies'.

REFERENCES

Ahlvin RC, Bauer WC, 1976: Luteinized cysts in ovaries of infants born of diabetic mothers. *American Journal of Diseases in Childhood* **93**, 107–109.

Antell L, 1952: Hydrocolpos in infancy and childhood. *Pediatrics* **10**, 306–320.

Avni EF, Godart S, Israel C, Schmitz C, 1983: Ovarian torsion cyst presenting as a wandering tumour in a newborn: antenatal diagnosis and postnatal assessment. *Pediatric Radiology* **13**, 169–171.

Avni EF, Rypens E, Smet MH, Galetty E, 1993: Sonographic demonstration of congenital adrenal hyperplasia in the neonate: the cerebriform pattern. *Pediatric Radiology* **23**, 88–90.

Bailez MM, Gearhart JP, Migeon C, Rock J, 1992: Vaginal reconstruction after initial construction of external genitalia in girls with salt wasting adrenal hyperplasia. *Journal of Urology* **148**, 680–682.

Beazley JM, 1974: Congenital malformations of the genital tract (excluding intersex). *Clinical Obstetrics and Gynaecology* **3**, 571–576.

Bellinger MJ, Duckett JW, 1982: Accessory phallic urethra in a female patient. *Journal of Urology* **127**, 1159–1164.

Beninshka K, 1973: Congenital anomalies of the uterus with emphasis on genetic causes. In Norris HJ, Hertig AJ, Abell MR (eds). *The uterus*. Baltimore: Williams & Wilkins, 68.

Berglen NE, Selander P, 1962: Hymenal polyps in newborn infants. *Acta Paediatrica Scandinavica* Suppl. **135**, 28–30.

Blakely CR, Mills WG, 1981: The obstetric and gynaecological complications of bladder exstrophy and epispadias. *British Journal of Obstetrics and Gynaecology* **88**, 167–173.

Brandt ML, Luks FI, Filitraut D, 1991: Surgical indications in antenatally diagnosed ovarian cysts. *Journal of Pediatric Surgery* **26**, 276–282.

Braren V, 1994: Construction of neovagina. *Dialogues in Pediatric Urology* **20**, 15–16.

Bulfamonte JC, 1942: Large ovarian cyst in a newborn child. *American Journal of Surgery* **55**, 175–176.

Buttran VC, Gibbons WE, 1979: Mullerian anomalies; a proposed classification (an analysis of 144 cases). *Fertility and Sterility* **32**, 40–47.

Canning DA, Gearhart JP, 1993: Exstrophy of the bladder. In Ashcroft KW, Holder TM (eds), *Pediatric surgery*, 2nd edition. Philadelphia: WB Saunders Co., 678–693.

Carpenter SF, Rock JA, 1988: Procidentia in the newborn. *International Journal of Obstetrics and Gynaecology* **25**, 151–152.

Cetallos R, Hicks GM, 1970: Plastic peritonitis due to neonatal hydrometrocolpos; radiologic and pathogenic observations. *Journal of Pediatric Surgery* **5**, 63–68.

Chitayat D, Hahn S, Marion W, *et al.*, 1987: Further delineation of the McKusick – Kaufman hydrometrocolpos-polydactyly syndrome. *American Journal of Diseases of Children* **141**, 1133.

Cohen HL, Shapiro MA, Mandel FS, Shapiro ML, 1993: Normal ovaries in neonates and infants: a sonographic study of 77 patients 1 day to 24 months old. *American Journal of Roentgenology* **160**, 583–586.

Cottom D, Williams E, 1965: Procidentia in the newborn. *Journal of Obstetrics and Gynaecology of the British Commonwealth* **72**, 131–138.

Croitoru DP, Aaron LE, Laberge JM, Neilson IR, Guttman FM, 1991: Management of complex ovarian cysts presenting in the first year of life. *Journal of Pediatric Surgery* **26**, 1366–1368.

Davis GH, Wapner RJ, Kurtz AB, Cihiber G, Fitzsimmons J, Blocklinger AJ, 1984: Antenatal diagnosis of hydrometrocolpos by ultrasound examination. *Journal of Ultrasound in Medicine* **3**, 371–374.

Debeugny P, Huillet P, Cusson L, 1989: Le traitement non-operatoire sytematique de kysites de l'ovaire du nouveau – ne. *Chirurgie Paediatrique* **30**, 30–36.

Dehner LP, 1975: Female reproductive system. In Kassina JM (ed.), *Pathology of infancy and childhood*. St. Louis, CV Mosby, 732.

Donahoe PK, Powell DM, 1993: Treatment of intersex abnormalities. In Ashcroft KW, Holder TM (eds), *Pediatric surgery*, 2nd edn. Philadelphia: WB Saunders Co., 740–765.

Elias S, Simpson JL, Carson SA, *et al.*, 1984: Genetic studies in incomplete Mullerian fusion. *Obstetrics and Gynecology* **63**, 276–278.

Felix W, 1912: The development of the urogenital organs. In *Manual of human embryology*, Volume 2. Philadelphia: JB Lippincott, 436–571.

Fleming P, McCleary RD, 1981: Non-immunological fetal hydrops with theca lutein cysts. *Radiology* **141**, 169–170.

Geary W, Weed JC, 1973: Congenital atresia of the uterine cervix. *Obstetrics and Gynecology* **42**, 217–220.

Gillian M, Gundy MM, 1992: Examination of the neonate including gestational age assessment. In Robertson NRC (ed), *Textbook of neonatology*. Edinburgh: Churchill Livingstone.

Gilsany V, Cleveland RH, 1982: Duplication of the Mullerian ducts and genitourinary malformations. *Radiology* **144**, 793–796.

Grapin C, Montagni JP, Sirinelli D, Silbermann B, Gruner M, Faure CL, 1987: Diagnosis of ovarian cysts in the perinatal period and therapeutic implications (20 cases). *Annals of Radiology* **30**, 497–502.

Grover D, Solanker BR, Banerjee H, 1970: A clinicopathologic study of Mullerian duct aplasia with special reference to cytogenetic studies. *Journal of Obstetrics and Gynaecology* **107**, 133–136.

Grumach MM, Conte FA, 1981: Disorders of sex differentiation. In Williams RH (ed), *Textbook of endocrinology*. Philadelphia: WB Saunders, 423–513.

Hahn-Pederson T, Krist N, Nielson OH, 1984: Hydrometrocolpos: current views on pathogenesis and management. *Journal of Urology* **132**, 537–540.

Hays DM, Shimada H, Raney RB, *et al*, 1985: Sarcomas of the vagina and uterus: the Intergroup Rhabdomyosarcoma Study. *Journal of Pediatric Surgery* **20**, 718–724.

Hendren WH, 1980: Construction of female urethra from vaginal wall and perineal flap. *Journal of Urology* **123**, 657–664.

Hill SJ, Horsch JH, 1989: Sonographic detection of fetal hydrometrocolpos. *Journal of Ultrasound in Medicine* **4**, 323–325.

Howard FS, Hinman F, 1951: Female pseudohermaphroditism with supplementary phallus. *Journal of Urology* **65**, 439–443.

Huffman JW, 1987: Gynecologic infections in childhood and adolescence. In Feigin RD, Cherry JO (eds), *Textbook of Pediatric Infectious Diseases*, Volume I, 2nd edn. Philadelphia: WB Saunders.

Hurwitz RS, Marzoni GM, Ransley PG, Stephens FD, 1987: Cloacal exstrophy: a report of 34 cases. *Journal of Urology* **138**, 1060–1064.

Jenkins GR, Verheeck K, Noe HN, 1984: Treatment of girls with urethral prolapse. *Journal of Urology* **132**, 738–741.

Jost A, 1972: A new look at the mechanism controlling sex differentiation in mammals. *Johns Hopkins Medical Journal* **130**, 28–36.

Kaufman R, Hartman F, McAlister W, 1972: Family studies in congenital heart disease. II. A syndrome of hydrometrocolpos, postaxial polydactyly and congenital heart disease. *Birth Defects* **8**, 85–89.

Klein FA, Vick CW, Broecker BH, 1986: Neonatal vaginal cysts: diagnosis and management. *Journal of Urology* **135**, 371–373.

Koram KS, Salti I, Hajj SN, 1979: Congenital absence of the uterus. Clincopathologic and endocrine findings. *Obstetrics and Gynecology* **50**, 531–533.

Koram S, Mrouch A, 1978: Ovarian biopsy in the evaluation of amenorrhoea. *Acta Obstetrica Gynaecologica Scandinavia* **57**, 301–304.

Krisiloff M, Puchner PJ, Trettor W, *et al.*, 1978: Pregnancy in women with bladder exstrophy. *Journal of Urology* **119**, 478–479.

Lund DP, Hendren WH, 1993: Cloacal exstrophy: experience with 20 cases. *Journal of Pediatric Surgery* **28**, 1360–1369.

Manson R, Rodgers BM, Nelson RM, Young TK, 1978: Ruptured ovarian cyst in a newborn infant. *Journal of Pediatrics* **73**, 324–325.

Marshall FF, 1978: Embryology of the lower urinary tract. *Urological Clinics of North America* **5**, 1–13.

McClever PA, Andrews H, 1988: Fetal ovarian cysts: a report of 5 cases. *Journal of Pediatric Surgery* **23**, 354–355.

McKusick V, Bauer R, Koop C, 1964: Hydrometrocolpos as a simply inherited malformation. *Journal of the American Medical Association* **189**, 813–814.

Mitchell ME, Brito CG, Rink RC, 1990: Cloacal exstrophy reconstruction for continuence. *Journal of Urology* **144**, 554–558.

Mundy AR, 1994: *Urodynamic and reconstructive surgery of the lower urinary tract.* Edinburgh: Churchill Livingstone, 293–341.

Nussbaum AR, Sanders RC, Harman DS, Dudgeon DL, Parmley TH, 1988: Neonatal ovarian cysts: sonographic-pathological correlation. *Radiology* **168**, 817–821.

Owens SB, Morse WM, 1968: Prolapse of the female urethra in children. **100**, 171–176.

Pang S, Wallace MA, Hotman L, *et al.*, 1988: World wide experience in newborn screening for classical congenital adrenal hyperplasia due to 21-hydroxylase deficiency. *Pediatrics* **81**, 866–874.

Pena A, de Vries PA, 1982: Posterior sagittal anorectoplasty: important technical considerations and new application. *Journal of Pediatric Surgery* **17**, 796–811.

Ramenofsky M, Raffensperger J, 1972: An abdominoperineal–vaginal pull-through for definitive treatment of hydrometrocolpos. *Journal of Pediatric Surgery* **6**, 381–387.

Rich MA, Brock WA, Pena A, 1988: Spectrum of genitourinary malformations on patients with imperforate anus. *Pediatric Surgery International* **3**, 110–113.

Richardson DA, Hajj SN, Herbst AL, 1982: Medical treatment of urethral prolapse in children. *Obstetrics and Gynecology* **59**, 69–73.

Rickwood AMK, Reiner I, Jones MO, Pournaras K, 1992: Current management of duplex system ureteroceles: experience with 41 patients. *British Journal of Urology* **70**, 196–200.

Rizzo N, Gabrielli S, Perolo A *et al.*, 1989: Prenatal diagnosis and treatment of fetal ovarian cysts. *Prenatal Diagnosis* **9**, 97–104.

Savage MO, 1982: Ambiguous genitalia, small genitalia and undescended testes. *Clinics in Endocrinology and Metabolism* **11**, 127–158.

Secat E, Hricak H, Godding CH *et al.*, 1994: The role of MRI in the evaluation of ambiguous genitalia. *Pediatric Radiology* **24**, 231–235.

Sedin G, Bergquist C, Lindgren PG, 1985: Ovarian hyperstimulation syndrome in preterm infants. *Pediatric Research* **19**, 548–552.

Shapiro E, Lepor H, Jeffs RD, 1984: The spectrum of the exstrophy-epispadias complex. *Journal of Urology* **132**, 308–310.

Sheldon C, Cormier M, Crone K, Wacksman J, 1981: Occult neurovesical dysfunction in children with imperforate anus and its variants. *Journal of Pediatric Surgery* **26**, 49–54.

Sivanesaratum V, 1986: Unilateral unexplained absence of ovary and fallopian tube. *European Journal of Obstetrics, Gynaecology and Reproductive Biology* **22**, 103–105.

Soper RT, Kilger K, 1964: Vesico-intestinal fissure. *Journal of Urology* **92**, 490–501.

Spicer RD, 1995: Soft tissue tumours. In Freeman NV, Burge DM, Griffiths DM, Malone PSJ (eds), *Surgery of the newborn.* Edinburgh: Churchill Livingstone, 539–545.

Tam PKH, Parikh DH, Rickwood AMK, 1990: Urethralisation of the female phallus with absent urogenital sinus. *British Journal of Urology* **66**, 551–552.

Tapanainen J, Koivisto M, Vihko R, Huhtaniemi I, 1981: Enhanced activity of the pituitary-gonodal axis in premature, human infants. *Journal of Endocrinology and Metabolism* **52**, 235–238.

Thompson GJ, Kelalis PP, 1964: Ureterocele: clinical appraisal in 176 cases. *Journal of Urology* **91**, 488–492.

Tran A, Arensman R, Falterman W, 1987: Diagnosis and management of hydrometrocolpos syndrome. *American Journal of Diseases in Children* **141**, 632–634.

Tridenti G, Armanetti M, Flisi M, Benassi L, 1988: Uterus didelphys with an obstructed hemivagina and unilateral renal agenesis in teenagers: report of three cases. *American Journal of Obstetrics and Gynecology* **159**, 882–883.

Walker B, Krebs D, Lang N, 1988: Pregnancy following repairs of congenital atresia of the uterine cervix and upper vagina. *Archives of Obstetrics and Gynaecology* **51**, 24.

Westerhout C, Hodgman JE, Anderson GV, Slack RA, 1964: Congenital hydrocolpos. *American Journal of Obstetrics and Gynecology* **89**, 957–961.

Widdowson DJ, Pilling DW, Cook RCM, 1988: Neonatal ovarian cysts: therapeutic dilemma. *Archives of Disease in Childhood* **63**, 737–742.

Woodhouse CRJ, 1991: *Adolescent urology*. Blackwell Scientific.

Ziegler EE, 1945: Bilateral ovarian carcinoma in a 13 week fetus. *Archives of Pathology* **40**, 279–282.

CHAPTER 6

Emotional aspects of gynaecological problems at birth

JULIA NELKI AND ADRIAN SUTTON

The detection of any abnormality in a newborn child is an emotionally charged situation. The parents must begin the process of readjustment to the baby who has been born in contrast to the image that had been held, more or less clearly, in mind throughout the pregnancy. Any abnormality can present complex emotional issues but those involving the genitalia particularly intersex disorders, present specific complications. We are primed emotionally, socially and culturally to people being either male or female. To consider a baby who cannot automatically and immediately be thought of as one or the other presents a challenge to the psychological resources of all parties involved but most particularly to the parents. They will be dealing with their grief at the loss of the expected, perfect baby while also needing actively to engage in the unusual and unexpected needs of their actual baby. There may be serious or even life-threatening medical or surgical problems requiring an immediate operative response. The dilemma for professionals is to come to a joint decision with the parents as quickly as possible while supporting them in their shock, grief, anger and uncertainty.

The pain and confusion evoked by uncertainty about how to relate to the baby and how to relate to others about the birth of that baby may make everyone wish to act quickly in order to give certainty back. The recognised advantage of early gender assignment in stabilising gender identity (Stradtman, 1991) can lead to the view that 'gender assignment is an neonatal surgical emergency' (Pinter and Kosztolanyi, 1990). The danger is that this may limit thinking and lead to precipitate action with irreversible consequences. It is as if gender assignment is directly equated with matters of immediate survival.

The sex of a baby is not usually viewed as something over which parents can have direct control although a mythology has grown up around this. The strength of feeling which may occur when this choice is apparently available has become clear through controversies in the arena of *in vitro* fertilisation. The dilemma when there are abnormal or ambiguous genitalia is not only that a decision has to be made but also who it is that should be making this decision and on what basis. Intense conflicting feelings may make clear thinking difficult while advances in surgical techniques may mean that surgeons have continually to question their own established practice and the boundaries of what is possible.

Case Example _____

A baby, chromosomally male, was born with extensive cloacal exstrophy. At birth it appeared that the genitalia could be more readily fashioned as a female. During the first stage of the operation, it was discovered that from a surgical point of view, it would be as easy to construct either female or male genitalia. It was recognised that there would be many other problems – a colostomy, likely incontinence and sterility – but the question of gender became paramount. There were lengthy and heated discussions on the ward with emergency meetings held out of hours: views became polarised between female and male staff. Female staff, primarily the nurses and social worker, expressed the view that, given his genetic make-up and the fact that the parents had been told when the mother was pregnant that they would be having a boy, the boy should 'remain' a boy. Male staff, primarily doctors, felt that even though lifelong hormone treatment would be needed, life as a boy with inadequate external genitalia would be far harder than for a girl for whom the defect would be less obvious. Neither were the parents of a single mind. The final decision was to make the baby a girl on the basis of anatomical considerations and evidence that psychosocial adjustment is easier in females (Moritz *et al.*, 1986).

It did not prove possible to take more time to find out what would be right for this particular family and to help the parents come to a shared view. It was as if there was a rush to reverse or cover up the situation – to make it secret.

The wish to prevent upset and pain is at the heart of the process described. Unfortunately, the wish to act as if the situation has not happened – to remove doubt about gender – may not be fulfilled. Children do know when there are secrets even if they do not know what the secrets are (Kent, 1994; Pincus and Dare, 1980). Often their fantasies are worse than the reality. Support, possibly sophisticated help, may be required but children can usually handle what their parents can handle (Bluebond-Langner, 1978).

For the professionals involved it is of the greatest importance that they realise that the adjustments to be made by the parents involve a process and not a single event or series of isolated events. The ability of parents to absorb information will vary according to a number of different factors which range from tiredness, through the potentially profound effects of the physical presentation to fears for the child's survival. With or without severe medical or surgical complications, to give birth to a child of indeterminate sex evokes powerful feelings in parents. These may be of guilt, blame, 'freakishness' or confusion: along with grief there may be anger. Parents may find themselves trying simultaneously to deal with these experiences whilst also having to make decisions about gender assignment.

Just when they are trying to come to terms with 'not knowing' they are being asked to 'know', to say whether their baby should be a boy or a girl.

Communication from medical and nursing staff to the parents needs to be consistent. Joint conversations involving medical and nursing staff with the parents, particularly if significant decisions about management are being discussed, may guard against some of the potential misunderstandings. The approach needs to be one in which those issues about the child's condition which can be regarded with certainty are made clear while simultaneously those things which are uncertain are delineated and clarified. When the sex of a baby is called into question one realises how much is usually taken for granted in terms of relating to the child as belonging to a particular sex, being given a particular name which is registered on the birth certificate. The sex is assumed to be a fundamental 'given', part of creation, something usually known at birth and occasionally beforehand. The parents will be forced into thinking many years ahead – to school activities and adolescence – and to think of their baby as a potentially sexually active adult or not: they are forced to focus on the genitalia instead of being able to appreciate their baby as it is at that moment.

A lack of certainty may cause considerable anxiety and confusion but the wish to provide an immediate solution in response to this may be less helpful in the medium and long term than the ability of professionals to assist parents in tolerating these feelings.

The relationships and interchanges with parents at this stage will be laying the foundation for future relationships between the child, the family and professionals. This is of particular importance where there is likely to be the need for continuing medical or surgical interventions but will also be important at crucial stages in the child's life, particularly puberty. Establishing a good relationship early on will encourage contact at any times of difficulties, new doubts or questions. The availability of contact over a long period of time will provide some security and support and links with a mental health professional may be helpful.

Many parents find it difficult to talk with their children, or perhaps with adults, about sexual matters (as do many professionals) even when there are no problems. Where there are discrepancies between gender identity and anatomy they are propelled into confronting any ordinary inhibitions they may have, harnessing all their psychological strengths and perhaps developing new ones. The difficulties are greater and the potential for misunderstandings, even with the most respectful approach, is high. Two examples illustrate just how readily they may occur:

1. A parent whose baby was found to have gonads consisting of mixed testicular and ovarian tissue was told that they were 'half and half'. It was only many years later that it was discovered that the mother had thought this meant that ovarian tissue occupied half the gonad and testicular tissue occupied the other half. She had agreed to removal of the gonads. She was left feeling guilty that she may have denied her child the chance to have one or other half and thereby be either male or female rather than the confused

person she was. This underlying guilt was causing considerable distress and contributing to problems which were occurring. When this was understood, it was possible to correct the earlier misunderstanding and to reiterate issues about the possibility of malignant change being of crucial importance in the decision to remove the gonads.

2. The mother of a child with incomplete testicular feminisation syndrome (partial and androgen insensitivity) had been told that her daughter would have 'sexual problems'. She took this to mean that she would be homosexual rather than that male secondary sexual characteristics would develop. This confusion may have contributed to delays in presentation when endocrinological issues arose in the early teens.

The giving of explanations needs to be combined with the process of ensuring that parents report back what they understand has been explained to them. This will also assist in developing truly trusting relationships in which parents can feel that they not only receive explanations but are also listened to. A multi-disciplinary approach to care may ensure better communication and the experience a child and family mental health professional can offer may be particularly helpful. The perspectives of each person will assist in increasing awareness of the different ways in which words can be understood or misunderstood.

It is important to ensure that those issues over which there is no choice are fully appreciated and that parents are not mistakenly left feeling responsible for particular actions where there was no realistic alternative: the 'illusion of choice' may leave parents with a burden of guilt if difficulties arise with gender identity or general emotional development later in life. Decisions may be shared but professionals must feel able to accept responsibility for offering parents a real opportunity to provide informed consent on behalf of their baby.

For some parents, this will not be their first child. Provisional arrangements will have been made for the care of the older child(ren) unless an unanticipated premature birth occurs. These plans may well provide fully for the immediate practicalities but adaptations will rapidly need to be made. The sibling will need to hear in simple terms – using the child's own familiar words – that the new baby is not well and needs to be in hospital: this will also mean that mummy and/or daddy will need to be there as well. The nature of 'not well' should be explained in terms of functions and activities, e.g. the parts of the body to do with 'weeing and pooing', 'the private parts'. The child's questions will need to be listened to carefully and age-appropriate answers given to the extent that is possible. It will again be important to allow for uncertainty. The child's responses will be the best guide of understanding and of ability to cope with her/his emotions as well as those of the parents. Responses may be clear and overt, or subtle and indicated through nuances of language or alterations in behaviour. The support of family, friends and primary health care professionals can be invaluable, practically and emotionally, in addition to that of the nursing and medical staff. Similar issues have been described in relation to children with surgical feeding problems (Sutton *et al.*, 1991) and the involvement of child mental health professionals may, in some cases, be helpful. This may take the form of consultation to the professionals or direct involvement with the family.

There may be difficulties between the siblings later too, with the child with genital abnormalities resenting the 'normal' siblings and the siblings feeling left out because of the attention the child gets because of the parents' worries and need for frequent hospital visits.

Sexual assignment and parental rearing are the most important indicators of future gender identity: given a strong sense of gender, the identity will be firmly fixed by about 3 years of age (Rutter, 1971). It is vitally important to ensure that the parents are convinced of the correctness of the gender to which they are assigning their child. All tests and investigations need to be done as quickly as possible to ascertain the correct sex and make a diagnosis (Lala and Matarazzo, 1990) and the parent's fantasies and confusions understood. Ahlquist (1994) emphasises the importance of concentrating on the social and emotional aspects of gender rather than on the genotypic, gonadal, phenotypic, hormonal or legal ones: '[most important is the] social, how we see ourselves, how others see us and how we approach sexual relationships'. Someone with a strong gender identity will be able to accept chromosomal gonadal and even phenotypic discrepancies even though it may be hard to accept and counselling may be required (see Anonymous, 1994). In some cases, formal psychotherapy may be required.

An effective liaison and/or consultation service between paediatrics and mental health would mean that such problems could be discussed as they arise. Direct referrals are sometimes made because of the anxiety that a particular child or condition evokes, together with the stigma and reluctance to attend that is common (Woodhouse and Pengelly, 1991). Regular liaison where both professionals offer their particular expertise to a child or family, or consultation where the professionals can talk about their dilemmas in relation to a particular child or family, may avoid the need for referral and help develop trusting relationships early on in case they are needed later thus offering a better service to the child and family.

SUMMARY

The starting point for the psychological management of genital abnormality or intersex disorder is full diagnosis of the child and ascertaining whether it is clear to which sex the child belongs or could most successfully be assigned. Parents will need to be given support in their emotional turmoil. A proper balance is required between the wish to avoid unnecessary delay while also recognising that a period of uncertainty is unavoidable. This will also allow time for the important psychological work of assimilating the reality of the new baby. By doing this, decisions can be made jointly by professionals and parents on the basis of understanding current difficulties and future issues which may arise. With sensitive handling of these at birth, a family can be assisted in dealing with their anxieties and worries as they arise and the child and their parents will be able to develop in a way which will better equip them to contend with the emotional challenges which their condition may present as they grow up.

REFERENCES

Ahlquist 1994: Gender identity in testicular feminisation. *British Medical Journal* (Letters) **308**, 1047.

Anonymous, 1994: Once a dark secret. Personal view. *British Medical Journal* **308**, 542.

Bluebond-Langner M, 1978: Knowing and concealing. In *The private worlds of dying children*. Princeton.

Kent A, 1994: *Health Story, Take A Break.*

Lala R, Matarazzo P, 1990: Sex determination in ambiguous genitalia. *Archivio Italiano di Urologia Nefrologica e di Andrologica* **62**, 161–164.

Moritz M, Zigler M, Duckett J, Howell C, 1986: Cloacal exstrophy. In Welch KJ, Judson GR, Ravitch M, O'Neill J (eds), *Pediatric surgery,* Vol. 2, 4th edn. Chicago: Year Book Medical Publishers.

Pincus L, Dare C, 1980: Loss, separation and death. In *Secrets in the family*. Faber & Faber, 135–144.

Pinter A, Kosztolanyi G, 1990: Surgical management of neonates and children with ambiguous genitalia. *Acta Paediatrica Hungaria* **30**(1), 111–121.

Rutter M, 1971: Normal psychosexual development. *Journal of Child Psychology and Psychiatry and Allied Disciplines* **11**, 259–283.

Stradtman EW, 1991: Female gender reconstruction surgery for ambiguous genitalia in children and adolescents. *Current Opinion in Obstetrics and Gynecology* **3**(6), 805–812.

Sutton A, Morton M, Dyer E, 1991: Developing relationships: the value of research in child psychiatric liaison with a neonatal intensive care unit (Unpubl.). Presented at the conference Paediatrics and Psychotherapy, Leuven University Belgium.

Woodhouse D, Pengelly P, 1991: *Anxiety and the dynamics of collaboration.* Aberdeen University Press, 71–100.

CHAPTER 7

Problems in childhood

ANNE S GARDEN

While talking to colleagues about writing this book, one comment I received was, 'If you write it in proportion to the problems seen, 99% of the book will be about vaginal discharge'.

Vaginal discharge is certainly the commonest paediatric gynaecological problem presenting to general practitioners, paediatricians and gynaecologists. It is a very worrying symptom for parents and may significantly disrupt family life. It is difficult to eradicate, even with optimal management and is, in general, very badly managed.

Other gynaecological problems commonly presenting in this age group are vulvar irritation without discharge, labial adhesions and, less commonly, but potentially most serious, vaginal bleeding.

VAGINAL DISCHARGE

At birth, the structure and physiology of the vagina and vulva of the neonate are influenced by levels of circulating maternal hormones, particularly oestrogen. The labia are thick and rounded, the vagina lined with squamous epithelium which is several layers thick and the pH of the vagina is acidic. The newborn female frequently has a physiological vaginal discharge which is white and odourless, similar to that which occurs in adult life and which is also produced by the effect of maternal hormones. Much less commonly, in this immediate neonatal period, the discharge may be bloodstained due to the breakdown of the endometrium which has been stimulated by maternal oestrogen levels.

The level of maternal oestrogen in the neonate starts to fall immediately following delivery and is unrecordable within a few weeks. The genital tract then becomes hypo-oestrogenic – the state in which it will remain until puberty. The labia majora lose their fat; the labia minora become thin and attenuated and do not meet in the midline to close over the vaginal orifice (Fig. 7.1); the vaginal epithelium becomes thin and atrophic and the pH of the vagina rises. All these factors promote the development of infection which physical and hormonal factors would overcome in a post-pubertal girl. Additional factors which promote the occurrence of infection, are the close proximity of the vagina and rectum

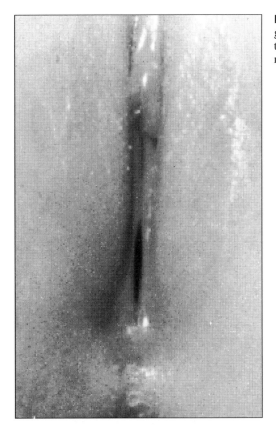

Fig. 7.1 Normal vulva of a prepubertal girl. Note the flattened labia majora and the thin attenuated labia minora which do not meet in the midline.

allowing faecal contamination and the spread of bacteria and the predilection for young girls to sit on the floor or in sandpits preferably without their underwear! The result is recurrent bacterial infections of the vaginal introitus, commonly referred to as vulvovaginitis.

The presenting symptoms are of vaginal discharge and vulvar soreness. The discharge is usually green in colour but may also be yellow or brown. It is usually offensive. It is accompanied by extreme soreness or irritation which is frequently sufficiently severe to prevent the girl from sleeping or even to wake her up at night. The scratching and rubbing precipitated by this irritation causes skin excoriation. The skin irritation and excoriation may cause dysuria and lead to a false diagnosis of recurrent urinary tract infection. Prepubertal girls of any age may be affected but vaginal discharge is most common in girls aged between two and six years, particularly in those who are overweight. When taking a history from these girls and their parents, it is important to find out what treatment has been given in the past and what the response was. Often creams such as Canesten have been used extensively and may in themselves be contributing to the irritation.

A study performed at the Royal Liverpool Children's Hospital (Pearce and Hart, 1992) in which 200 consecutive girls, presenting with genital discharge, irritation, pain or redness to the Accident and Emergency Department, were investigated by having swabs taken from the introitus. The commonest single organism identified was *H. influenzae*. Staphylococci, Streptococci, Coliforms, Gonococci, Gardnerella and Candida were also isolated. Other studies have found different organisms to be more common (Hammerschlag, 1978). The important thing, however, is not so much which specific organism is involved but that the infections are almost exclusively bacterial in origin and not, as is widely believed by mothers and doctors alike, due to Candida. In the Liverpool study, only seven of the 200 girls studied had Candida isolated. Of these, four were pubertal and at least one was sexually active. Anticandidal treatment is a particularly common treatment given to these girls being referred to a paediatric gynaecologist. It is essential that it is realised that Candida infections are rarely found in prepubertal girls and their presence is likely only if the girl is diabetic. The bacterial nature of the discharge can often be confirmed by eliciting a history of improvement in the discharge when antibiotics were given for some coincidental infection, e.g. tonsillitis.

There were no cases of Gonococcus or Gardnerella in the Liverpool study. Gonococcal infection in prepubertal girls usually presents with a copious purulent discharge and is discussed further in Chapter 10. It is due to sexual contact with an infected person and sexual abuse must be considered. Gardnerella infection is also suggestive, but not diagnostic, of a girl being sexually active or being sexually abused. One study reported a higher incidence of Gardnerella infection in a group of girls who had been sexually abused than in the controls. Within the group who had been abused there was a higher incidence of infection in those girls who had been abused on multiple occasions (Bartley *et al.*, 1987).

Poor hygiene is often cited as a cause of vaginal discharge in young girls. While this is certainly an aetiological factor in some girls, vulvovaginitis is also seen in girls in whom there is no doubt about their cleanliness. Care must be taken not to antagonise a mother by the blanket assumption that all girls presenting with this problem are not being washed properly. Indeed I have seen severe vulvovaginitis in one of twin sisters, the other having no symptoms.

Investigation includes examination of the underwear to confirm the presence of discharge (also often giving a clue to the level of hygiene) and of the vulva for the presence of inflammation (Fig. 7.2) and to exclude a dermatological cause for the irritation. Gentle separation of the labia will allow inspection of the hymen and allow a swab to be taken from the introitus. While there will obviously be contaminants from a swab taken in this way, it is my strongly held opinion that to attempt to carry out any other form of bacteriological investigation in a girl of this age, particularly one whose presenting complaint has been of vaginal soreness, is unjustified. Various suggestions have been made as to how a non-contaminated vaginal swab may be obtained, including the insertion of a catheter, the use of a wire loop and the more standard bacteriological swab inserted beyond the hymen. In most cases, identification of the specific bacteria

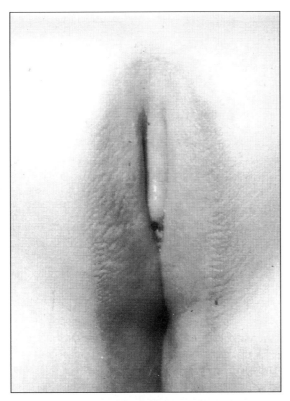

Fig. 7.2 Inflamed appearance of the vulva in a girl with vulvovaginitis.

is of academic interest. If it is considered essential that accurate bacteriological information is obtained, for instance where there are allegations of abuse or where a sexually transmitted infection is suspected, then it is my opinion that this must be done under a general anaesthetic. To persist in a prepubertal, unanaesthetised girl to insert any type of instrument beyond the hymen, at best, will probably inhibit the girl from allowing gynaecological examination again for the rest of her life, with the consequences that may have, and at worst may be considered a form of abuse.

It is not necessary to perform an examination under anaesthesia on all girls presenting with a problem of vaginal discharge. Such a procedure should be restricted to those in whom it is considered essential to obtain accurate bacteriology, those in whom the condition does not respond to the management outlined below and those in whom there is a history of the discharge having been bloodstained. It is mandatory to perform an examination under anaesthesia in all girls from whom a history of vaginal bleeding is obtained.

Examination under anaesthesia is usually performed using an infant laryngoscope. Other instruments that may be used include a paediatric cystoscope or a hysteroscope. It is important, whatever instrument is used, that all the vagina and cervix is visualised. It is easy to miss a lesion or a foreign body which is obscured by the blades of the laryngoscope. Prior to examining the vagina, a high vaginal swab, and if necessary, an endocervical swab should be taken. The vagina, including the posterior fornix is then examined, the appearance of the epithelium noted and a foreign body or tumour carefully looked for.

Having excluded a foreign body or tumour, the management of recurrent vaginal discharge is a mixture of reassurance, advice and persistence. Reassurance is required that the condition is common (most mothers are convinced that her daughter is the only one to have this problem); that it does not mean she has been sexually abused (provided that you can be reasonably sure about this); that it does not mean that she is going to have problems with persistent vaginal discharge in her adult years and that while a cure cannot be promised at present the condition is self-limiting and will improve after puberty. It may also be wise to mention that while the discharge is due to recurrent bacterial infection, the consequences are not those of genital tract infections in adults which may result in pelvic inflammatory disease and tubal damage.

The advice given is mainly to prevent and minimise recurrences and includes instructions on hygiene, if necessary. If there is no evidence of poor hygiene contributing to the problem it is important to say so, otherwise the girl and her parents become obsessed with cleanliness which may cause further short-term and long-term problems. In addition, it is important that this information is given in such a way as does not produce guilt feelings in the mother.

The girl should be advised to wipe her perineum after defaecation from front to back to decrease the risk of vulvar contamination from faecal flora. It may also be advisable to encourage her to wash her bottom after having had a bowel movement. As vulvovaginitis seems to be more common among girls who are constipated, advice about diet and fibre should be given. Similarly, girls who are overweight should be encouraged to lose weight. The girl should wear cotton underwear which should be changed daily and discouraged from wearing trousers, tights and leggings, particularly if made of synthetic fibres. There is no evidence that the use of bubble bath causes vaginal discharge, in contrast to vulvar irritation without discharge (see below) and so they do not need to be proscribed – particularly if their use encourages good hygiene.

If the discharge is particularly troublesome, the best and simplest treatment is the use of salt baths. Two large tablespoonfuls of salt are added to about 16 pints of warm water in a suitable basin. The girl is then encouraged to sit in it for about ten minutes. After drying thoroughly, a bland cream should then be applied to the area. Creams such as E45, Sudacrem, Zinc and Castor Oil or even Vaseline may be used. They have an emollient action on the affected skin and provide a barrier against further irritation from the discharge. Some mothers have reported an improvement with antibacterial creams such as Sultrin. The girl and her parents should be warned about the ineffectiveness of such treatments as Canesten, unless Candida has been proven to be the infecting organism. They should also be advised to re-attend should the discharge become particularly offensive and especially if it should become bloodstained. Because of the chronic nature of the condition and because it is well recognised that patients (and their parents) only retain about one third of information given at any clinic consultation, we have devised an advice sheet at the Royal Liverpool Children's Hospital, incorporating the above factors, which is given to parents whose daughters present with the problem (see Appendix 1).

Persistence is required as naturally the parents are concerned and will often return in the hope that some magic cure can be offered. They require continual reassurance on the cause and the benign nature of the problem and the fact that it will improve with the rising levels of oestrogen at puberty.

If a specific organism is identified on the swab, appropriate antibiotic treatment may be required. Antibiotic therapy may also be helpful to convince the parents that the cause is recurrent bacterial infections. Treatment with a broad spectrum antibiotic will clear the presenting infection but will not prevent future infections. Treatment with repeated courses of antibiotics is obviously not indicated so the preventative measures as outlined above are also required.

Another suggested form of treatment is the use of local oestrogen cream (usually Dienoestrol 0.01%, Ortho) applied to the vulva. Application of local oestrogen cream should produce the changes which occur at puberty and thus increase the girl's own resistance to infection. While in theory this should be of value, I have not found it of great benefit in my own practice. The reason for its failure may be my stressing the adverse effects of the treatment which may result in the parents using it so sparingly that there is no hope of it working! If used too liberally, oestrogen may be absorbed systemically, causing breast development and even menstruation in extreme cases. If it is used, it should be applied sparingly twice daily for no longer than two weeks. Again this treatment may be helpful in convincing the parents that the discharge can be cleared and that it will improve at puberty.

Very occasionally, an ectopic ureter will be the cause of vaginal discharge in young girls. An ectopic ureter may open onto the perineum or into the uterus, cervix or vagina. The discharge is clear and watery although it may be purulent if the urine becomes infected. Diagnosis is with a intravenous urogram.

VULVAR IRRITATION WITHOUT DISCHARGE

While vaginal discharge in childhood is almost exclusively due to bacterial infection, the causes of vulvar irritation without discharge are more difficult to diagnose. The main causes are, in order of frequency of presentation, threadworm infestation, dermatological conditions and non-specific vulvitis.

Threadworm Infestation

Threadworm infestation is extremely common in young children although not all will present with vulvar itching. The causative organism is *Enterobius vermicularis*. Ova are excreted in the stools and are transferred to the child's hands from scratching the perineum. The ova are then transferred from the hands to articles such as toys and cups thus causing the infestation to be spread to the whole family. Threadworms may also be found in the vagina where they also lay ova. The classic symptoms are perianal and vulvar irritation which is caused by the adult threadworms emerging from the rectum at night to lay their eggs. The most straightforward diagnostic test is the so-called Sellotape test (Fig. 7.3). A piece of Sellotape is applied at night to the perianal region. The Sellotape is removed in the morning and attached to a glass slide. In the laboratory, the Sellotape is removed and the slide treated with toluene which removes the debris but leaves the adult worms and the eggs which can then be visualised under low power magnification. Treatment is with mebendazole 100 mg, given as a single dose to all members of the family over the age of two, with the exception of pregnant women.

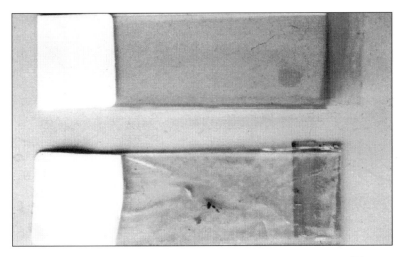

Fig. 7.3   Sellotape test showing the presence of ova in the lower slide.

An alternative means of diagnosis, but one which is less realistic, is to ask the parents to check the perianal region at night with a torch when the worms may be seen moving around. It is a suggestion which in my experience is usually met with incredulous looks!

Dermatological Conditions

The dermatological condition most likely to be seen by the paediatric gynaecologist, as it affects the genital area predominantly, is lichen sclerosus et atrophicus (LSA). The condition occurs at the extremes of life being found in prepubertal girls and postmenopausal women. The girl presents with severe intractable vulvar itching and soreness, occasionally with accompanying bleeding. There is also commonly dysuria from involvement of the skin around the urethra and constipation resulting from pain on defaecation if the perianal area is also affected. Discharge may be a feature due to secondary infection. The aetiology is unknown but it is frequently considered to be auto-immune (Meyrick Thomas *et al.*, 1988). Examination of the vulva shows a specific appearance. The skin is shiny and white (Fig. 7.4) with papules which may coalesce to form plaques. It has a semitranslucent appearance often likened to mother of pearl. In severe

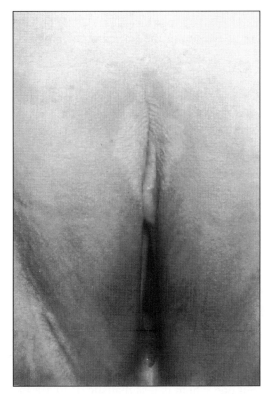

Fig. 7.4 Appearances of mild LSA showing an area of whitened skin on the vulva.

cases, there are areas of purpura, which may give the appearance of bruising, haemorrhagic blisters, excoriation and erosion (Fig. 7.5). These appearances are due directly to the condition and are not secondary to scratching or rubbing. Fissuring may also be present. The appearances are similar to trauma and has resulted in the condition being mistaken for sexual abuse (Handfield-Jones *et al.*, 1987; Bays and Jenny, 1990). This causes additional distress for the parents. The clitoris is often thickened as a result of chronic irritation. In severe cases, atrophic obliterative scarring of the vulva may occur. The appearances are so classical that biopsy is not usually required to confirm the diagnosis. About half the girls affected may also have extragenital manifestations of LSA.

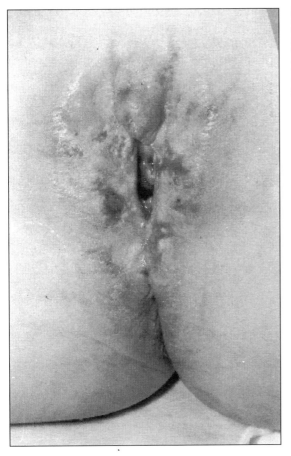

Fig. 7.5 Appearances of severe LSA with thickened white skin with areas of haemorrhage and erosion. There is marked clitoral hypertrophy. Note also the perianal involvement. (with permission from Churchill Livingstone).

If a biopsy is performed, the histological features are of atrophy or hypoplasia of the epidermis with flattening of the rete pegs. There may be hyperkeratosis on the surface of the epidermis. The upper dermis contains an oedematous band of hyalinised collagen and lymphocyte infiltration is present in the deeper dermis.

Treatment is with potent topical steroids such as clobetasol propionate 0.05% (Dermovate, Glaxo) applied twice daily for a maximum of two weeks. In less severe cases, hydrocortisone cream 1% may be used. Steroid creams with additional antibacterial or antifungal activity (Terra-Cortril, Pfizer; Tri-Adcortyl, Squibb) may be helpful as secondary infection is common. Because of this risk of secondary infection, attention to hygiene is imperative. Treatment for constipation may also be necessary. If advice about fibre in the diet is not sufficient, preparations such as Lactulose or Fybogel (Reckitt and Coleman) are helpful.

The condition often improves spontaneously in puberty although this is not the experience of all authors (Berth-Jones *et al.*, 1989). Unlike LSA presenting in the postmenopausal period, there is no risk of malignancy.

Other dermatological conditions which may present with vulvar irritation are eczema, psoriasis (Fig. 7.6) and napkin rash. The latter is commonly the result of poor hygiene, but may also be due to irritation from ammonia, washing powder

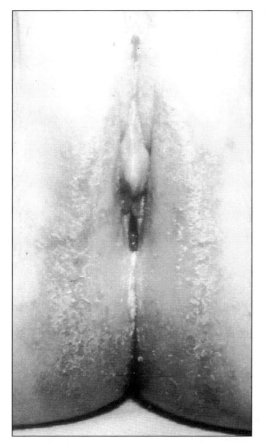

Fig. 7.6   Psoriasis affecting the vulva.

or fabric softener. Super-infection with bacteria or candida (Fig. 7.7) is common. Treatment includes advice about hygiene where appropriate, treatment for any secondary infection and use of such creams as Zinc and Castor Oil to prevent further irritation from ammonia.

Vulvar irritation may also occur from vulvar warts (Fig. 7.8). These are most commonly the result of contact from parents, other family members, baby-sitters or child-minders – anyone with digital warts who may have washed the girl or changed her nappy. Occasionally, perineal warts may be the result of sexual contact, particularly sexual abuse. This will be dealt with further in Chapter 11.

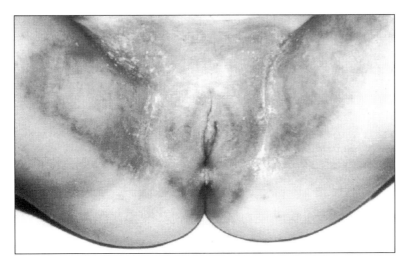

Fig. 7.7 Marked napkin rash. Note the satellite lesions due to added infection with candida.

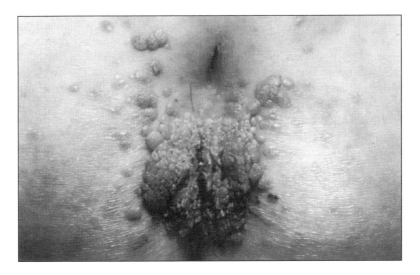

Fig. 7.8 Marked warts affecting the vulva and perianal area.

Non-specific or Allergic Vulvitis

This condition is fairly common but difficult to treat as it is often impossible to identify the precipitating factor. The girl presents with vulvar irritation but no discharge, except in rare cases where there is secondary infection in an area of excoriation. Examination of the vulva shows it to be red and inflamed. Common agents to cause allergies and irritation are washing powders, particularly the biological ones, fabric softeners, bubble bath, perfumed soap, coloured toilet paper, solutions used in the bath such as Dettol and medicated creams which may have been prescribed for treatment of these symptoms. Synthetic fibres, particularly rayon, may also cause irritation. Parents are often of the opinion that factors in the diet, particularly fruit juices are to blame, although there is no objective evidence that irritation specific to the vulva is caused by food items.

Treatment is by elimination of the cause. The girls should wear loose cotton underwear which should be washed separately using mild soap flakes. The girl herself should wash her perineum with a mild soap such as Simple soap and dry herself with a towel which has likewise been washed with soap flakes and without the use of fabric conditioners. Such procedures are tedious for the mother and it is equally important that she is told that if there is no improvement after a few weeks of such measures that she can discontinue them.

Once the most common causes listed above have been eliminated, it then becomes detective work on behalf of the parents to eliminate potential causative factors from the girl's lifestyle.

LABIAL ADHESIONS

Labial adhesions are thought to be the result of chronic vulvar irritation and are found most commonly in young girls aged around 2 or 3. The condition is commonly mistaken for congenital absence of the vagina. The two conditions can be easily differentiated on inspection. In a child with congenital absence of the vagina, inspection of the perineum will show the labia minora, clitoris, urethral meatus and hymenal opening. In a child with labial adhesions, the fused labia prevent visualisation of the clitoris, urethral meatus and hymen and the vulva appears as a flat featureless surface (Fig. 7.9). A thin line running antero-posteriorly marks the area where the labia have fused. The adhesions are usually complete, but if incomplete, the posterior labia is normally the first to fuse and the last to separate.

The condition is due to chronic irritation which traumatises the epithelium of the labia which as they heal causes the two surfaces to adhere. The girl usually presents with her panic-stricken parents who believe that she has a congenital abnormality, or less commonly with a history of chronic irritation, often with discharge. In addition, she may have a problem of dribbling of urine, particularly if the adhesions are almost complete as the urine is excreted behind the adhesion into the vagina and then dribbles out when the angle of the vagina alters when the girl stands up. This may also produce dysuria. Entrapment of urine, in this manner, causes further inflammation and irritation which may worsen the process.

Treatment is by the application of oestrogen cream, usually Dienoestrol 0.01% (Ortho). Application along the line of fusion twice daily for 2 weeks is usually enough to cause separation. Failure of the lesion to separate may mean that the child has resisted the attempts of her mother to apply the cream. If the condition

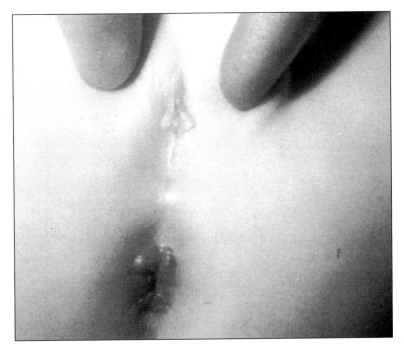

Fig. 7.9   Complete labial adhesions. Note the flat appearance of the vulva and the absence of any features beyond the labia differentiating this from congenital absence of the vagina (with permission from Churchill Livingstone).

does not improve after 2 weeks of using the cream, and it is certain that the cream has been applied, a second course should be given after a break of 2 weeks. Surgical or manual separation of the adhesions should not be carried out as there is a high incidence of refusion and the results of the oestrogen cream application are so good. After separation has occurred, advice should be given about the management of vulvovaginitis (see above) to prevent recurrence.

The finding of labial adhesions often raises the question of sexual abuse. Berkowitz *et al.* (1987) found labial adhesions in 10 girls under the age of 5 from a group of 375 who were referred for assessment of possible abuse. While it would be important to consider abuse as a possible cause in girls who present with recurrent episodes of adhesions, there is certainly no indication to consider it in every girl who presents with the problem.

VAGINAL BLEEDING

Vaginal bleeding is a relatively uncommon presenting symptom in prepubertal girls but is one which causes a great deal of alarm and which is potentially serious.

As has already been said, vaginal bleeding in neonates is likely to be physiological due to the withdrawal of maternal oestrogen stimulation of the
endometrium and no investigation is required. Bleeding in prepubertal girls after
the immediate neonatal period, however, needs careful investigation (Fig. 7.10).
A study of 51 girls under the age of 10 (Heller *et al.*, 1978) who presented to

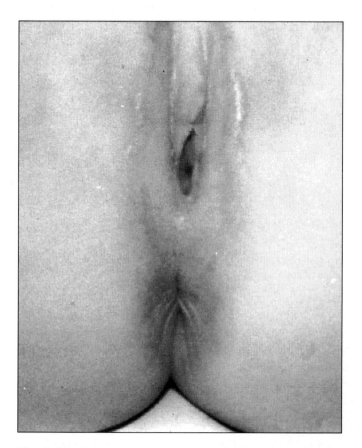

Fig. 7.10 Encrusted bloodstained vaginal discharge due to
foreign body in the vagina.

Great Ormond Street Hospital with vaginal bleeding, found that 37 had some
form of precocious puberty, eight of whom had cyclical vaginal bleeding in the
absence of secondary sexual development or advanced bone age; six had malignant tumours involving the vagina or cervix; four cases were due to trauma;
three were due to vaginitis and one was due to vaginal prolapse. Precocious
puberty is considered in Chapter 15 and genital tract tumours are considered in
Chapter 14 so neither will be considered further here.

Genital Tract Trauma

Genital tract trauma may be due to accidents or to sexual abuse (Chapter 18). The commonest accidents are due to straddle injuries due to falling astride on a fence or the crossbar of a bicycle. The trauma so caused produces a extremely painful haematoma of the labia which is characteristic in appearance (Fig. 7.11). Similar haematomas will be caused by a kick to the perineum. Treatment is by ice-packs and analgesia. If the haematoma continues to enlarge, surgery is necessary to incise the haematoma and evacuate the clot. It is not common to find a specific bleeding point, the haematoma being caused more usually by a general ooze. In these circumstances a drain should be left *in situ* to prevent re-accumulation. Specific bleeding points should, of course, be ligated.

Tearing of the fourchette is never caused by a straddle injury. It is diagnostic of attempted penetration of the vagina.

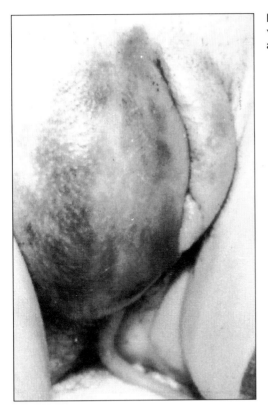

Fig. 7.11 Classical appearance of the vulva in a adolescent girl after falling astride the crossbar of a bicycle.

Vaginitis as a Cause for Vaginal Bleeding

While infection alone may be a cause of vaginal bleeding in childhood, it is more commonly secondary to a foreign body. A foreign body may be inserted inadvertently or deliberately during play, just as they may be inserted into ears and nostrils. Repeated insertion of foreign bodies, however, may require referral to a child psychologist. Foreign body insertion may be accidental such as with toilet paper or a broken off piece of bath sponge. Paradise and Willis (1985) found the prevalence of foreign bodies in girls under 13 years of age, seen as outpatients, to be 4%. Occasionally, the girl will give a history that she has inserted a foreign body, but more commonly she presents with foul smelling vaginal discharge which is bloodstained. The bleeding is commonly slight, no more than spotting, but can be extremely heavy.

The diagnosis usually requires examination under anaesthesia. If the object which has been inserted is radio-opaque, the diagnosis may be made by the use of X-ray or by ultrasound. A negative radiological examination, however, does not rule out the presence of a foreign body. Radiological examination, therefore, is of academic interest as examination under anaesthesia will provide both a diagnosis and cure. It is not uncommon to find multiple objects in the vagina (Fig. 7.12) and examination must be careful to ensure that none are missed. It is particularly important that the examiner continues to study the vagina as the examining instrument is withdrawn to ensure that no foreign bodies are obscured behind the blades of the speculum. Antibiotic treatment may be required after removal of the foreign body to eradicate the infection.

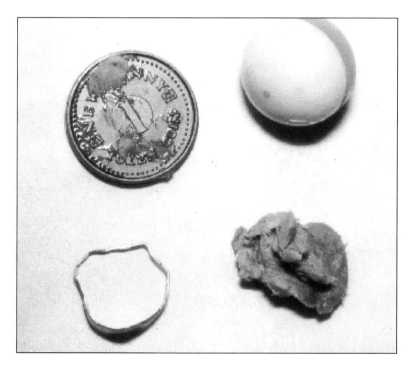

Fig. 7.12 Multiple foreign bodies removed from the vagina (same patient as in Fig. 7.10).

Urethral or Vaginal Prolapse

These are unusual conditions in prepubertal girls which are usually asymptomatic but may present with vaginal bleeding. A urethral prolapse, if large, may also cause urinary symptoms, usually dysuria and, in severe cases, retention of urine. The cause is unknown. It has, however, been reported to respond to treatment with oestrogen cream (Mercer *et al.*, 1988). An alternative treatment is simple excision.

The case of vaginal prolapse reported in the paper by Heller *et al.* (1978) was found in a girl with a meningomyelocoele and presumably was due to poor muscle tone in the pelvic floor secondary to nerve damage.

SUMMARY

In summary, therefore, the commonest presentation of prepubertal girls to a paediatric clinic is with a problem concerning the vulva. Vulvovaginitis due to repeated bacterial infection is by far the most common. Education of the mothers on simple techniques to control the symptom would probably empty the clinic!

REFERENCES

Bartley DL, Morgan L, Rimsza ME, 1987: Gardnerella vaginalis in prepubertal girls. *American Journal of Diseases of Children* **141**, 1014–1017.

Bays J, Jenny C, 1990: Genital and anal conditions confused with child sexual abuse trauma. *American Journal of Diseases of Children* **144**, 1319–1322.

Berkowitz CD, Elvik SL, Logan MK, 1987: Labial fusion in prepubescent girls: a marker for sexual abuse? *American Journal of Obstetrics and Gynecology* **156**, 16–20.

Berth-Jones J, Graham-Brown RAC, Burns DA, 1989: Lichen sclerosus. *Archives of Disease in Childhood* **64**, 1204–1206.

Hammerschlag MR, Alpert S, Rosner I *et al.*, 1978: Microbiology of the vagina in children: normal and potentially pathogenic organisms. *Pediatrics* **62**, 57–62.

Handfield-Jones SE, Hinde FRJ, Kennedy CTC, 1987: Lichen sclerosus et atrophicus misdiagnosed as sexual abuse. *British Medical Journal* **294**, 1404–1405.

Heller ME, Savage MO, Dewhurst J, 1978: Vaginal bleeding in childhood: a review of 51 patients. *British Journal of Obstetrics and Gynaecology* **85**, 721–725.

Mercer IJ, Mueller CM, Hajj SN, 1988: Medical treatment of urethral prolapse in the premenarchial female. *Adolescent Pediatrics and Gynecology* **1**, 181–184.

Meyrick Thomas RH, Ridley CM, McGibbon DH, Black MM, 1988: Lichen sclerosus et atrophicus and auto-immunity – a study of 350 women. *British Journal of Dermatology* **118**, 41–46.

Paradise JE, Willis ED, 1985: Probability of vaginal foreign body in girls with genital complaints. *American Journal of Diseases of Children* **139**, 472–476.

Pearce AM, Hart CA, 1992: Vulvovaginitis: causes and management. *Archives of Disease in Childhood* **67**, 509–512.

APPENDIX 1

Advice Sheet Used at Royal Liverpool Children's Hospital, Alder Hey

Advice to help your daughter

Your daughter has been diagnosed as having vulvovaginitis. This means that she gets recurrent episodes of infection in her private parts (vagina and vulva). This is very common in young girls so you need not think that your daughter is the only girl attending the hospital to have this problem. It happens because young girls, before they start their periods, have less resistance to infection there. This resistance to infection develops automatically as they become older.

There are some things you can do to help, the most important thing is to be particularly careful about keeping the parts of her body around the vulva and vagina very clean. We suggest:

1. She should wear cotton pants and make sure that she changes them at least once a day. It is probably better that she does not wear pants in bed.
2. Try to persuade her to avoid wearing tights and trousers when the soreness is particularly bad.
3. She should (or you should) wash her bottom with soap and water every time her bowels move. Use a non-scented soap (such as Simple Soap), dry her bottom thoroughly afterwards and keep the sponge or cloth that you use for this clean by washing it regularly. You may find that a shower or a shower attachment to the taps is helpful for this.
4. Try to avoid your daughter becoming constipated. Give her plenty of fruit and vegetables in her diet and make sure that she drinks plenty of fluid. If she still has problems with constipation, ask your own general practitioner for help.
5. If the soreness is very bad, you may find that a salt bath before your daughter goes to bed soothes the discomfort. The easiest way to do this is to put 2 large tablespoons of salt to about 16 pints of warm water in a suitable basin and get your daughter to sit in it for about 10 minutes. Do not add disinfectants such as Dettol or TCP.

These things will not cure all cases but should help to control her discomfort. If your daughter's discharge ever becomes bloodstained you must let your doctor know and come back to see us at the clinic. If necessary, you can bring your daughter to the Accident and Emergency Department at Alder Hey.

PART III

GYNAECOLOGY IN ADOLESCENCE

CHAPTER 8

Problems with menstruation

ANNE S GARDEN

INTRODUCTION

The main gynaecological problems in adolescence are related to menstruation – either the absence of periods or, more commonly, periods which are heavy or painful. These constitute the second commonest group of referrals to a paediatric/adolescent gynaecological clinic after children presenting with vulvovaginitis.

An important principle to remember when dealing with gynaecological problems in adolescent girls is that they are just at the beginning of their reproductive life. Careful consideration must be given to the information to be gained from such procedures as vaginal or rectal examination before carrying them out. While, obviously, clinical examination is an important fundamental of good clinical practice, in many instances the information can be obtained by other means, particularly ultrasound. Pelvic examination is not a pleasant procedure for most women and an insensitively performed examination on an adolescent girl may deter her from seeking gynaecological advice, including cervical smears, for the rest of her life with the attendant risks involved.

The average age of menarche has dropped over the last 150 years from 16.5 to 12.8 years. Recently, however, the trend has reversed with a slight rise in the age of menarche. It is suggested that this is more likely to be due to the recent trend for girls to take more exercise in an attempt to stay slim rather than a decrease in the general level of nutrition among adolescents (Rees, 1993). 95% of girls in the United Kingdom will have attained the menarche by the age of 15. The physiology and endocrine changes involved in puberty and the menarche are dealt with more fully in Chapter 1.

AMENORRHOEA

Amenorrhoea is the absence of menstruation. It is classically divided into primary and secondary amenorrhoea – the former being applied when a girl has never had a period, the latter when she has had periods but they have stopped for at least 6 months. Girls presenting with primary amenorrhoea are further divided into those who have normal secondary sexual development and those whose physique is still pre-pubertal. While such distinctions are helpful in planning investigation, they can be misleading. A girl with a chromosome complement 45X/46XX may present with signs and symptoms anywhere in the spectrum from primary amenorrhoea with no sexual development to secondary amenorrhoea with normal secondary sex characteristics or even, in later life, with infertility; the presentation depending on the degree of residual ovarian function. Likewise, girls with ovarian failure may present with either primary or secondary amenorrhoea, with or without secondary sex characteristics, depending on their stage of development at which the ovarian failure occurred. The only thing that can be said with confidence is that if a girl has had a period, she has a uterus and has had some oestrogen production.

Primary Amenorrhoea With No Secondary Sex Characteristics

Primary amenorrhoea in a girl with no secondary sexual development should be fully investigated by the age of 14. The common causes are constitutional delay, chronic systemic disease, absence of ovarian function or hypothalamic/pituitary dysfunction.

Investigation of a girl with primary amenorrhoea and normal secondary sexual characteristics can be delayed until the age of 16. It is important to remember, however, that pubertal development is a continuum and that it is more important to identify breaks in the continuum than to be too strict about a girl's age – a girl who has pubic hair and breast development by the age of ten needs investigation if she has not attained the menarche by the age of 15. Likely causes of amenorrhoea with normal sexual development are commonly anatomical anomalies such as imperforate or absent vagina or an absent uterus.

Reindollar and McDonough (1981, 1983) reviewed 252 girls presenting with delayed puberty and primary amenorrhoea. Primary ovarian failure was the cause in 43%, of whom 63% had a chromosomal abnormality. Hypogonadotrophic hypogonadism was responsible in 31% of the cases. An anatomical abnormality was present in 18% and a further 7% has polycystic ovarian syndrome. Another study (Toublanc *et al.*, 1991) reporting 38 adolescent girls with delayed puberty showed that ovarian failure was the most common cause, although in this study it was usually associated with a normal karyotype. Gonadotropin insufficiency (hypothalamic/pituitary dysfunction) and constitutional delay were the next most frequent causes and in this study were seen equally commonly.

Constitutional delay

These girls have delayed maturation of the hypothalamic–pituitary–ovarian axis with resultant delay in growth spurt, sexual maturation and bone development. There is no underlying pathological process. The condition is frequently familial with a similar history being obtained from her mother or from sisters. Levels of follicle stimulating hormone (FSH), luteinising hormone (LH) and oestradiol will be low, in the pre-pubertal range, although nocturnal peaks of LH may be seen. Radiological estimation of bone age (Fig. 8.1) will show a discrepancy between the girl's chronological age and her bone age. It is unlikely for menstruation to occur below a bone age of 14.5 years.

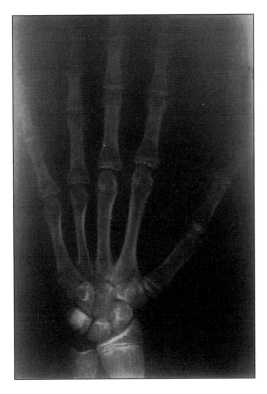

Fig. 8.1 X-ray of wrist from a 16-year-old girl who presented with primary amenorrhoea. The findings are equivalent to a bone age of 14 years.

No treatment is required other than reassurance. Some girls, however, may be extremely embarrassed and upset by their lack of physical development and may be undergoing teasing or even bullying at school as a result of this. In these situations a decision may be made to induce puberty (see p. 136) after discussion with her and her parents. If there are no signs of puberty by the age of 18, induction of puberty ought to be carried out.

Chronic systemic illness

Chronic illnesses due to infection, physical, endocrine or emotional disorders may cause delayed puberty. Tuberculosis infection, though now rare, was traditionally the condition which caused delayed puberty. With the now increasing incidence of this disease, it may be worth considering again particularly in populations where the disease is prevalent. Physical illnesses such as chronic renal or cardiac disease and endocrine disorders, particularly hypothyroidism, may be the cause. Physical illnesses which cause failure to thrive, such as coeliac disease are particularly likely to cause pubertal delay. It may be worth considering screening for coeliac disease in thin girls who present with apparent constitutional delay of puberty but in whom no family history is obtained. With control of the disease process, puberty develops normally.

Absence of ovarian function

The commonest causes for absence of ovarian function are gonadal dysgenesis or ovarian failure. Obviously if the ovaries have been surgically removed in childhood, pubertal development will not occur, but this is rare and is usually elicited in the history. Less commonly, primary amenorrhoea may be due to polycystic ovarian syndrome which will be considered under its more common presentation of secondary amenorrhoea.

Gonadal dysgenesis

The commonest form of gonadal dysgenesis is found in girls with streak ovaries as seen in those with Turner's syndrome.

Turner's syndrome occurs in around 1:2–3000 live female births and is associated with a 45X chromosome complement. Mosaic forms such as 45X/46XX or 45X/46XY are common as are the karyotypes with an abnormal X chromosome such as a partial deletion of one of the arms of the X chromosome (X del [Xp-] or Xdel[Xq-] or an isochromosome X). Girls with deletion of the short arm of the X chromosome (Xdel[Xp-]) have the phenotypic appearance of Turner's syndrome but are fertile while those with deletion of the long arm of the X chromosome (Xdel[Xq-]) are of normal stature but have ovarian failure. About 50% of girls with Turner's syndrome have monosomy X – the remainder have mosaic forms. If two tissues are examined for the presence of mosaicism, the number of girls with the non-mosaic form is decreased to 25% (Held *et al.*, 1992). Recent research has emphasised the need to apply polymerase chain reaction technology in the chromosomal assessment of women and girls with Turner's syndrome in order to detect cryptic mosaicism for part of the Y chromosome. One study obtained positive signals for the SRY gene from 6 of 18 patients tested. The authors suggested that this put these women at risk of virilism and the development of gonadal neoplasms (Kocova *et al.*, 1993). Certainly dysgerminoma and gonadoblastoma have been reported in women with Turner's syndrome (Dominguez *et al.*, 1962; Bonakdar and Peisner, 1980).

Girls with Turner's syndrome are thought to have a normal number of germ cells in their ovaries in utero but to undergo accelerated germ cell atresia leading to the formation of streak ovaries and early loss of ovarian function. In girls with classic signs, the diagnosis is usually made at birth by the presence of lymphoedema of the feet or hands, web neck, coarctation of the aorta, cardiac or renal anomalies. The diagnosis should be suspected in childhood due to short stature and it is worth considering performing a karyotype on all girls whose stature is below the 10th centile. Girls with non-mosaic Turner's syndrome rarely grow above 1.45 m. If the diagnosis is not made at birth or in childhood, girls with Turner's syndrome will present in adolescence with delayed puberty and primary amenorrhoea. While girls with classical features of Turner's syndrome are easy to diagnose (Fig. 8.2), there is difficulty in those individuals who

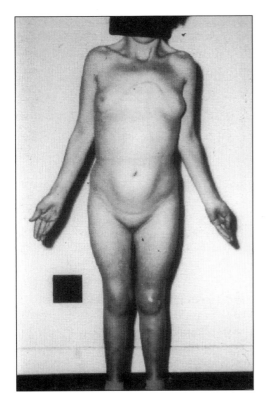

Fig. 8.2 Classic picture of a girl with Turner's syndrome showing a web neck, shield chest with wide spaced nipples and wide carrying angle (with permission from Churchill Livingstone).

have a mosaic form of Turner's syndrome, and in whom there is a high proportion of normal cells, in whom the signs may not be so obvious (Fig. 8.3). It is still regrettable that in many women with Turner's syndrome the diagnosis is not made until adulthood. In the clinic held for adult women with Turner's syndrome in Liverpool, 54% of those who attend were not diagnosed until 12 years of age or older and 21% were not diagnosed until after the age of 16. The signs of Turner's syndrome are listed below:

- short stature
- web neck
- lymphoedema
- shield chest with wide-spaced nipples
- scoliosis

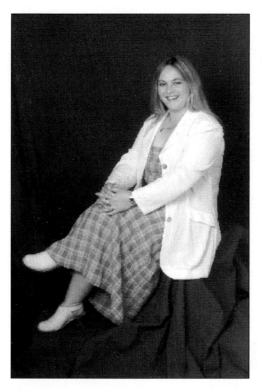

Fig. 8.3 Young woman with Turner's syndrome showing none of the usual obvious features. Picture shown with patient's permission.

- wide carrying angle
- short metacarpals
- soft, curling nails
- low-set ears, low hairline, micrognathia and high arched palate

- coarctation of the aorta
- horseshoe kidney
- strabismus
- ptosis
- multiple naevi

Gonadal dysgenesis may less commonly occur with a 46XY karyotype (Swyer's syndrome and in these circumstances is referred to as pure gonadal dysgenesis as there is no associated short stature and the chromosome complement is normal. These girls are phenotypically female and have a uterus, vagina and fallopian tubes as well as normal female external genitalia. The dysgenetic gonad in utero produces neither androgen, thus allowing the development of female external genitalia, nor Mullerian inhibitory factor (MIF) allowing the Mullerian duct derivatives of tubes, uterus and upper vagina to develop. The presence of a uterus and vagina is the discriminating factor between this syndrome and complete androgen insensitivity syndrome (CAIS).

A familial form of pure gonadal dysgenesis has been described (Simpson *et al.*, 1981). It would appear to have either an autosomal recessive or X-linked pattern.

Occasionally, mixed gonadal dysgenesis may occur. In these girls, one gonad differentiates more than the other resulting in one streak gonad with the other showing varying degrees of testicular differentiation. A degree of masculinisation may be present.

The diagnosis of gonadal dysgenesis is by karyotype and hormone profile which will show elevated FSH and LH levels and low levels of oestradiol. Pelvic ultrasound or diagnostic laparoscopy will determine the presence of a uterus. The uterus will be smaller than normal due to the lack of oestrogen stimulation and careful examination is required. If there is doubt about the presence of a uterus, it may be prudent to repeat the examination after oestrogen therapy when the uterus will be more clearly seen. This is preferable to performing invasive investigations such as laparoscopy, when again because of the small size of the uterus, accurate visualisation may be difficult. Treatment is by induction of puberty and gonadectomy (see below).

Those girls in whom a Y chromosome, or part of a Y chromosome, is present have a 30% lifetime risk of developing either a gonadoblastoma or dysgerminoma (Verp and Simpson, 1987). As these tumours can be very small, it is not sufficient to follow them up with either ultrasound or laparoscopy. Laparotomy and gonadectomy is required. This is probably best performed as soon as the diagnosis is made as the dysgenetic nature of the gonad increases the risk of early malignant transformation which usually occurs within the first two decades of life.

Delayed puberty is also a feature of Noonan's syndrome which has been variously described as 'male Turner's syndrome' or 'chromatin positive females with Turner's syndrome'. This condition, first described in 1963 (Noonan and Ehmke, 1963), is associated with pulmonary stenosis, short stature, pectus deformities, borderline/low intelligence, coarse curly hair, short neck with webbing and typical facial appearance including hypertelorism, down slanting palpebral fissures and ptosis (Noonan, 1968). The karyotype is normal. Hormone profile shows low levels of LH, FSH and oestradiol.

Ovarian failure

Ovarian failure may present with either primary or secondary amenorrhoea depending on the girl's age at the time the failure occurred. The causes of ovarian failure are listed in Table 8.1.

In most girls, it is not possible to identify a cause. In those where a diagnosis is possible, the commonest cause is chromosomal – usually Turner's syndrome. Ovarian failure has also been reported in women who are Fragile X carriers (Schwartz *et al.*, 1994) but this is unusual in girls of adolescent years. Girls with triple X (47XXX) also have a higher incidence of ovarian failure which may be related to a cryptic mosaicism (47XXX/45X) in the ovaries due to non-dysjunction. Although auto-immune ovarian failure has been reported in adults (Alper and Garner, 1985), it is unusual in adolescents. The commonest infection to cause ovarian failure is mumps, the greatest risk of this occurring being in the

Table 8.1 Causes of ovarian failure

Chromosomal	45X/45X mosaic
	Fragile X carrier
	Deletion long arm X
	Familial
Auto-immune	Multiple endocrinopathy
Iatrogenic	Chemotherapy
	Radiotherapy
	Surgery
Infection	Mumps
Metabolic	Galactosaemia
Environmental	
Idiopathic	

fetal or pubertal periods when even a subclinical infection may result in permanent damage (Morrison *et al.*, 1975).

While chemotherapy is a recognised cause of ovarian failure in women in their 30s, it is unusual in young girls although it has been reported (Vergauwen *et al.*, 1994). Radiotherapy, however, does not discriminate between young and old ovaries, but is dose-dependent. Radiation doses up to 500 rads are reported to cause ovarian failure on 60% of patients while doses of 800 rads and over caused ovarian failure in 100% of cases (Baker *et al.*, 1972). While removal of the ovaries in childhood would be an obvious cause of ovarian failure, surgery to the pelvis may disrupt the ovarian blood supply and so cause premature loss of ovarian function even if they are left intact.

80% of girls with galactosaemia experience ovarian failure – although there is controversy as to whether it is the condition itself or the galactose-free diet which causes this. Environmental factors such as smoking do not usually cause ovarian failure in adolescents.

Investigation of girls with ovarian failure will show normal or small ovaries on ultrasound or laparoscopy and raised FSH and LH levels with low or undetectable levels of oestradiol. Treatment is by hormone replacement therapy (HRT) preceded if necessary by the induction of puberty.

Hypothalamus–pituitary dysfunction

The conditions associated with hypothalamic or pituitary dysfunction are many and form a much more heterogeneous and poorly understood group than gonadal failure.

Lesions which cause compression of the pituitary and hypothalamus may cause a decrease in the secretion of FSH and LH. These lesions include tumours of the pituitary, craniopharyngiomas and hydrocephalus. Less common conditions associated with hypogonadotrophic states are the Laurence–Moon-Biedl syndrome, an autosomal recessive disorder characterised by obesity, retinitis pigmentosa, mental retardation, polydactyly and hypogonadism and Prader–Willi syndrome which presents with hypotonia, mental retardation, characteristic facies and obesity. The Kallman syndrome or olfactory–genital dysplasia is characterised by primary amenorrhoea, lack of sexual development and anosmia caused by incomplete agenesis of the olfactory bulbs along with anatomical defects in the hypothalamus. It is thought to be an autosomal dominant condition. In girls with these conditions, however, the diagnosis of the basic condition is usually known so that the amenorrhoea does not present a diagnostic problem.

By far the commonest form of hypogonadotrophic hypogonadism, however, is idiopathic. There are case reports which suggest that some cases are familial. Diagnosis is made by estimation of FSH, LH and oestradiol levels, all of which are low.

Hypothalamic dysfunction resulting in disordered gonadotropin release from the pituitary is also implicated in those girls with delayed puberty and amenorrhoea associated with stress, anorexia nervosa, excessive sports and physical training especially gymnastics and ballet, where it is of advantage to be thin or where the girls have an inadequate dietary intake for the amount of exercise they take. Management of these girls is difficult. In most cases, the condition is reversible when they reach an appropriate weight for their height or when the stress responsible for the amenorrhoea is eliminated. Because of the competitive nature of many sports, however, and the modern fashion for being thin, many girls are unwilling to decrease their training or increase their body weight. Girls with anorexia nervosa, of course, require specialist help to enable them to overcome their problems of disordered body image.

The condition is not a benign one, however, as the hypo-oestrogenic state of these girls predisposes them to loss of bone density and potential osteoporosis. In those who have a high level of physical activity, this places them at risk of sustaining a stress fracture.

Russell (1985) followed up 20 girls who developed anorexia nervosa before puberty. In 6 patients, no breast development occurred even following weight gain and 9 had prolonged primary amenorrhoea, one until the age of 25.

Induction of puberty

Treatment of girls with delayed puberty and primary amenorrhoea is to induce puberty with low dose oestrogen therapy, or, much less commonly, in girls with a hypogonadotrophic state, with pulsatile gonadotrophin releasing hormone (GnRH). It is important to ensure that the girl, her parents and other medical attendants under whose care she may be, realise that the induction of puberty is not an end in itself, purely for cosmetic reasons, but continued treatment is important to prevent the long-term consequences of a hypo-oestrogenic state, namely, osteoporosis and an increased incidence of atherosclerosis and cardiovascular disease. All too often, girls and women on long-term oestrogen replacement have their medication stopped for some spurious reason which indicates that there has been no understanding of the underlying disorder and the need for long-term therapy.

Induction of puberty should as far as possible mimic the normal progress of puberty. Treatment should ideally begin at a age when a girl's ovary would normally begin to secrete oestrogen, around the age of 10 or 11. If the girl has Turner's syndrome, however, induction of puberty may be delayed to allow treatment with growth hormone and maximum skeletal growth to occur before the introduction of oestrogens causing closure of the epiphyses.

Treatment should begin with very small doses of ethinyl oestradiol – 1 µg daily for approximately 6 months, increasing to 2 µg, 5 µg, 10 µg and 20 µg at 6 monthly intervals. Low dose ethinyl oestradiol is not widely available and arrangements need to be made with specialist units for the 2 µg tablets to be made available. The 2 and 10 µg tablets have then to be divided to obtain the 1 and 5 µg dose. Increasing the dose of ethinyl oestradiol at a faster rate than this is said to cause the development of a breast with proportionately too great nipple and areolar development compared to the underlying breast tissue development. On the 20 µg dose, the girl should be warned that she may experience break through bleeding. When that occurs, she should be converted onto a combined oestrogen and progestogen preparation.

An alternative method of inducing puberty using low dose transdermal 17β-oestradiol patches has been reported (Illig *et al.*, 1990). This is probably a better and more physiological method as it avoids the first pass metabolism of oestrogens in the liver and also provides a continuous dose of oestradiol. The patches, however, were made specifically for the study and are not commercially available.

Traditionally, the combined oral contraceptive pill has been the drug of choice for long-term treatment in these girls. With the advent of a large variety of HRT preparations for treatment of post-menopausal women, a greater choice is available. There are reasons to suggest that treatment using HRT may be superior. First, the lower dose of oestrogen contained in HRT preparations is not associated with an increased incidence of hypertension; changes in lipid profiles in women using HRT are theoretically more beneficial than those taking the combined oral contraceptive although no data from long-term studies are available; the hormone regime of oestrogen only followed by combined oestrogen and progestogen more closely mimics the natural cycle than continuous combined oestrogen and progestogen. The final reason, and possibly the most important one, is that 4 week oestrogen regimes are widely available in the various HRT preparations while the combined oral contraceptive pill is only a 3 week regime every 4 weeks. For individuals such as those with Turner's syndrome, who have no endogenous oestrogen production, a 3 week regime reduces their overall oestrogen intake. In girls who may have to take replacement oestrogen for 40 years, it is the equivalent of only receiving 30 years therapy.

There are, however, practical problems. The combined oral contraceptive pill is available free of charge whereas HRT incurs a double prescription charge. Additionally, the combined oral contraceptive pill is acceptable to a girl's peers, whereas HRT may not be – being seen as a drug for older women. It is essential that the girl is happy with the therapy she is receiving so as to ensure maximum compliance.

To ensure adequate doses of oestrogen are being achieved (both in terms of dosage and compliance), levels of oestradiol, FSH and LH should be checked. Adequate dosage of oestrogen will cause suppression of FSH and LH to normal levels. Girls on long-term oestrogen supplementation should also have their bone mineral density checked at regular intervals to ensure that the effects of therapy on their bones is satisfactory. There is currently no means of assessing the effects of therapy on the cardiovascular system, although it may be prudent to check cholesterol levels.

Primary Amenorrhoea with Secondary Sex Characteristics

As has already been said, the differentiation between those girls presenting with amenorrhoea who show signs of sexual development and those who do not is a rather false one. In the group who have signs of sexual development would also have to be considered girls with constitutional delay or some chronic medical condition who have begun to develop but have not yet attained the menarche, girls who are a Turner's mosaic, and those with ovarian failure or hypothalamic–pituitary dysfunction, from whatever cause, where the problem has occurred after the onset of puberty.

There are, however, several causes of primary amenorrhoea which only occur in the presence of normal secondary sexual development. They are usually due to anatomical defects. The fallopian tubes, uterus, cervix and upper two thirds of the vagina develop from the Mullerian ducts between the 8th and 12th weeks of intrauterine life. Failure of the ducts to form or canalise will cause the girl to present with amenorrhoea. As the ovaries have a separate development from the Mullerian duct, oestrogen production is normal and therefore the development of secondary sex characteristics is unaffected.

As 30% of girls with Mullerian duct development abnormalities from whatever cause, will also have renal tract abnormalities, investigation with either renal unltrasound or intravenous urogram is required as part of the management of these girls.

Imperforate or absent vagina

Abnormalities of the vagina are relatively common, occurring in approximately 1:4000 females and varying in degree from the more common imperforate hymen to the relatively rare complete vaginal agenesis.

While these conditions may be diagnosed at birth by routine examination of the genitalia or by diagnosis of hydrocolpos (see p. 51 and p. 246), most cases are not diagnosed until puberty.

An imperforate vagina may be found at any level but is most frequent in the lower third, often just behind the hymen. The abnormality at this level is due to failure of the membrane to break down at the point of fusion between the downgrowth of the Mullerian duct to the upward growth of the urogenital sinus. Failure of canalisation at higher levels of the vagina developing from the Mullerian duct do occur but are usually partial, presenting as strictures rather than complete closures, and cause dyspareunia or problems with inserting tampons.

Less commonly there may be congenital absence of the vagina. As this usually occurs in association with absence of the uterus, it does not cause symptoms of cryptomenorrhoea.

In girls with a functioning uterus and failure of canalisation of the vagina at whatever level, puberty and sexual development proceed normally until menarche when obstruction to the flow of menstrual blood (cryptomenorrhoea) causes lower abdominal pain. The girl presents classically with cyclical lower abdominal pain and a careful history may reveal that cycles occur monthly, although as menstruation is often irregular for the first few cycles after menarche, this may not be the case. There is often a history of admission to a surgical ward with a diagnosis of suspected appendicitis which resolves spontaneously only to recur after one month. If the diagnosis is not made at this stage, an abdominal and pelvic mass may develop due to the accumulation of menstrual blood and the formation of a haematocolpos and haematometra (Fig. 8.4). This in turn may be

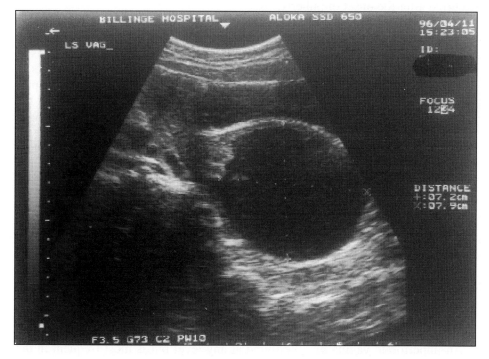

Fig. 8.4 Longitudinal ultrasound image of the vagina showing marked distension in an adolescent girl with haematocolpos (courtesy of Miss Pat Lewis).

sufficiently large to cause retention of urine by compression of the urethra by the expanding vaginal mass.

Examination findings depend on the duration of the cryptomenorrhoea. In advanced stages, a palpable abdominal swelling will be present. In the most common situation where the anatomical defect is in the lower third of the vagina, separation of the labia will reveal the classic bulging blue-coloured membrane (Fig. 8.5). Treatment is by incision and excision of the membrane with release of large amounts of tarry chocolate-coloured fluid – a simple procedure which is

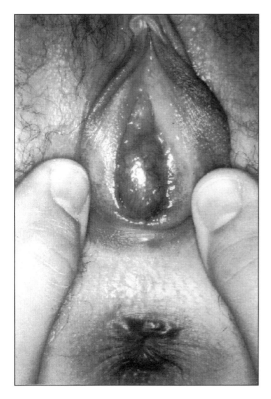

Fig. 8.5   Distended membrane of haematocolpos.

extremely satisfying to both surgeon and patient (Fig. 8.6)! No further treatment is required provided that the redundant membrane is sufficiently excised to prevent recurrence.

In those girls where the obstruction is higher in the vagina, diagnosis and treatment is more complicated. Ultrasound examination of the pelvis will reveal a haematometra and haematocolpos. The length of the haematocolpos, although distended by the accumulated blood, will give some guide to the level of the blockage.

Congenital absence of the vagina in the absence of a uterus will be considered below.

An extremely rare anomaly presenting in the same manner as an imperforate

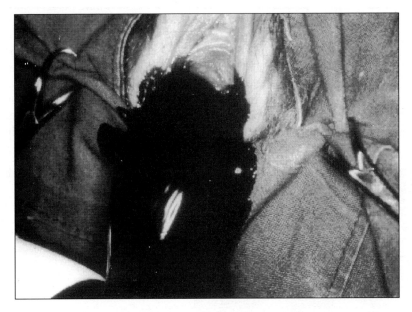

Fig. 8.6   Same patient as in Fig. 8.5. Excision of the membrane with release of copious amounts of tarry material.

or absent vagina is congenital absence of the cervix. Reconstructive surgery in such cases is very difficult and hysterectomy may be required.

Obstruction of menstruation is associated with an increased incidence of endometriosis (San Filippo *et al.*, 1986) the severity of which seems to depend on the duration of symptoms. This may affect future fertility.

Absence of the uterus

The uterus may be absent as a result of surgery, usually for malignant disease of the genital tract, in childhood such as a malignant ovarian tumour or sarcoma boitryoides. If the ovaries are not removed as part of surgery, normal puberty will occur but with failure of menstruation. Obviously, in such girls a history is obtained. More commonly, absence of the uterus is congenital as part of CAIS or of Rokitansky–Kuster–Hauser syndrome.

Rokitansky–Kuster–Hauser syndrome

Rokitansky–Kuster–Hauser syndrome (Griffin *et al.*, 1976) is the congenital absence of the uterus and vagina due to failure of Mullerian duct development. As the ovaries have a different embryological derivation from the uterus, there is normal hormone production and normal development of external genitalia and breasts. The amount of Mullerian duct development varies – the fallopian tubes may be shortened or of normal length; there may be no uterine development, the presence of rudimentary uterine horns (Fig. 8.7a and b) or rarely the presence of

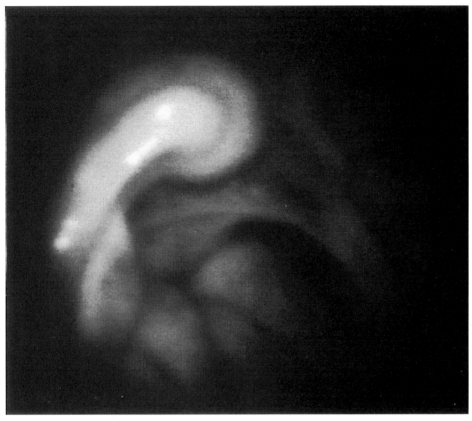

(a)

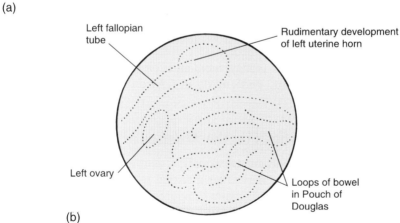

Left fallopian tube

Rudimentary development of left uterine horn

Left ovary

Loops of bowel in Pouch of Douglas

(b)

Fig. 8.7a and 8.7b Laparoscopic view of a teenage girl with a variant of Rokitansky–Kuster–Hauser syndrome showing no development of the right Mullerian duct leading to absence of the right fallopian tube and uterus. On the left, the fallopian tube and rudimentary development of the uterine horn can be seen. The left ovary can also be seen. The Pouch of Douglas can be seen below containing only bowel.

a normal uterus. The upper vagina is almost invariably absent. Examination of the introitus shows normally developed labia and a normal hymen surrounding a central dimple. A varying amount of lower vagina is present as it derives from the urogenital sinus. The diagnosis is confirmed by ultrasound and/or diagnostic laparoscopy. Obviously, in these circumstances, it is not possible to induce menstruation. Treatment is limited to producing a vagina that is of sufficient width and length to allow intercourse.

Complete androgen insensitivity syndrome

Girls with CAIS have a normal 46XY karyotype but are phenotypically female. The genetic basis of CAIS is considered fully in p. 204. They are usually taller than average and are usually described as having good breast development, although the areolae may be underdeveloped. Pubic and axillary hair are sparse. The condition is an X-linked recessive one so the diagnosis may be made at birth if the girl has an affected sibling. More commonly, however, the diagnosis is not made until she presents at puberty with amenorrhoea.

Clinical examination reveals the features already mentioned. Examination of the perineum shows a normal vulva and hymen with a short blind-ending vagina. The hormone profile shows normal male levels of testosterone.

The condition, as the name implies, is due to end-organ insensitivity to androgens. The skin in the genital area, therefore, fails to respond to the androgens and female genitalia develop. The internal organs, however, do respond to MIF resulting in the absence of tubes, uterus and upper vagina. The diagnosis is made by clinical features, 46XY karyotype and absence of a uterus.

The testes are normal and may be found anywhere along the line of testicular descent from the abdomen to the labia. The risk of malignancy is low, around 5%, and is rare before 25–30 years of age (Verp and Simpson, 1987). They may therefore be left *in situ* until after puberty to optimise breast development. They should, however, be removed after puberty.

Girls with CAIS need sensitive management and counselling, preferably from an early age (Goodall, 1991), and particularly in regard to their femininity (see Personal view, 1994).

Treatment of Vaginal Agenesis (in the Absence of a Uterus)

The timing of treatment is important. Obviously, it is important that these girls have a functioning vagina before they enter a sexual relationship, but it is also important that the girl is sufficiently mature to appreciate what the object of the treatment is and that she does not feel pressured into having it by either her parents or the medical staff. Treatment may be either surgical or non-surgical.

Non-surgical methods This technique of producing a functional vagina was first described by Frank in 1938. It can be achieved because of the potential space filled with loose connective tissue between the urethral and anal openings. By teaching the girl to apply a vaginal dilator to the central dimple in the introitus, and so to this potential space, a functional vagina can be produced. If the girl is sexually active, having intercourse will increase the length of the vagina. The advantage of this method, apart from the lack of surgery, is that should the girl cease to be sexually active there is no risk of contracture of the vagina. It does, however, require a great deal of commitment to the technique by the girl. It also requires a reasonable depth to the original vaginal pouch for it to be successful.

Surgical methods Non-surgical methods are not successful in every case, particularly in conditions where there are additional abnormalities of the perineum. In such circumstances a surgical approach will be required.

The simplest of these is probably a Williams' vulvovaginoplasty (Williams, 1964) which involves making a 'U' shaped incision, 4 cm from the midline from the level of the urethra down to the perineum anterior to the anus. The incision is deepened to mobilise the skin edges. The inner skin edges are then sutured together to form a pouch, the deep tissues sutured in front of them and the outer skin edges closed over. A catheter is left *in situ* following the procedure. The disadvantages of the Williams' procedure are that it produces an abnormal looking perineum in adolescents who are already rather sensitive about the fact that they have 'something wrong down there' and a vagina with a plane of axis directly posterior as opposed to axial and slightly anterior. However, once the pouch is made, intercourse will cause dilatation and lengthening of the potential space as with Frank's procedure and satisfactory intercourse can occur. It also has the advantage that dilators are not required to keep the pouch open as when a split skin graft is used.

If the Williams' vulvovaginoplasty is not acceptable to the girl, the options are between a split skin graft or a full thickness graft. The former is often described as a McIndoe's vaginoplasty and involves the removal of a split skin graft, usually from the buttock, sufficiently long to be twice the length of the desired vagina. A vaginal space is created by blunt dissection of the potential space between the bladder and rectum. The skin is then formed into a tube and fitted onto a mould inserted into the dissected space. The mould is held in place by suturing together the labia minora. A urinary catheter is left *in situ*. The mould and catheter are removed after about a week.

A McIndoe's procedure has the advantage of producing a vagina that is of normal position and diameters. It has the disadvantage, however, of producing an unsightly scar at the donor site. A further disadvantage is that to keep it patent the woman has to use vaginal dilators unless she is having intercourse regularly. Failure to use the dilators results in contracture of the graft which can then be very difficult to re-dilate. Rock *et al.* (1983) following up a group of 79 women who had the procedure found 100% functional satisfaction and 91% anatomical satisfaction. The functional satisfaction was higher than in the group who had a non-surgical procedure. Strickland *et al.* (1993) in a much smaller study found a high satisfaction rate with the procedure with none of their patients requiring to use dilators, in contrast with other studies. The main problem experienced by this group was that of vaginal dryness. Other substances used for forming a neo-vagina include colon and amnion. Amnion is no longer used because of the risk of HIV infection.

A more recently described technique involves the use of full-thickness tissue grafts following the use of tissue expansion (Johnson *et al.*, 1991). Tissue expanders are placed in the labia minora and gradually expanded by the addition of normal saline over a 3–5 week period. The potential space between the bladder and rectum is then dissected as before and full-thickness skin flaps created by the tissue expansion inserted to line the neovagina. Care must be taken to ensure that hair bearing skin is not used – hair growth from within the vagina cannot easily be removed. There is no problem with contracture in these patients as the graft is full thickness. The problems are those of infection and a prolonged hospital stay of almost two months.

The most important thing to remember in the management of vaginal agenesis is that the girl is satisfied with the method chosen and the outcome.

Pregnancy is a rare, though not unreported, cause of primary amenorrhoea.

Secondary Amenorrhoea

In contrast, the commonest cause of secondary amenorrhoea is pregnancy and should be tactfully considered in every girl or woman presenting with the symptom. The most frequent pathological cause in this age group is probably hypothalamic–pituitary dysfunction secondary to stress, exercise or weight loss (Morgan and London, 1993). Other common causes are polycystic ovarian syndrome (PCO), resistant ovary and ovarian failure.

Polycystic ovarian syndrome

PCO is a common cause of secondary amenorrhoea or irregular menstruation. It is characterised, endocrinologically, by LH hypersecretion and hyperandrogenism. Polycystic ovaries must be differentiated from the normal multicystic ovary of the pubertal girl. On ultrasound, the multicystic ovary is seen to contain 6 or more cysts of a diameter of 40 mm or more within a normal sized ovary which has a normal stromal appearance. Polycystic ovaries, conversely, are larger than normal with a large number of small cysts arranged circumferentially within the ovary which has increased stromal tissue (Fig. 8.8). This arises from disordered folliculogenesis with failure to produce a dominant follicle. The finding of polycystic ovaries on ultrasound is one which is found in 23% of the population (Polson *et al.*, 1988), however, so that finding alone does not indicate pathology. Periods of remission may occur where normal ovulatory cycles occur and biochemical parameters return to normal.

The use of 'PCO' is limited to those girls or women who, in addition, present with a combination of symptoms which includes amenorrhoea, irregular periods, obesity, acne, hirsutism and, in later life, infertility. In addition to ultrasound imaging of the ovaries, an LH:FSH ratio of greater than 3, with a slightly raised

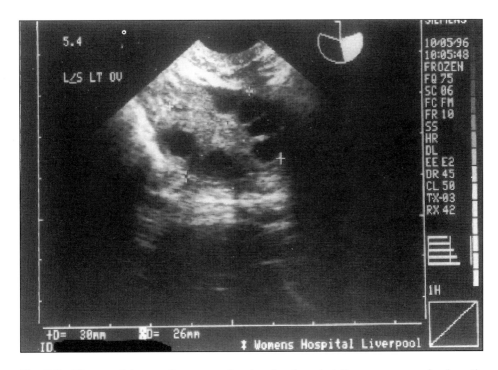

Fig. 8.8 Ultrasound image of an ovary showing the characteristic appearances of polycystic ovary with increased ovarian size and circumferential distribution of the cysts.

testosterone level and low sex hormone binding globulin (SHBG) will confirm the diagnosis.

The cornerstone for treatment for girls with PCO must be to encourage them to lose weight. This reduces the peripheral conversion of oestrone and the circulating levels of LH (Bates and Whitworth, 1982) and has been reported to cause spontaneous onset or return of menstruation. Weight loss of as little as 5% or more is associated with improvements in menstrual cyclicity, hirsutism, rates of ovulation and pregnancy (White and Turner, 1994). Further treatment for those girls whose presenting symptom is amenorrhoea is the combined oral contraceptive pill. This has the beneficial psychological effect for the girl of producing regular withdrawal bleeds. However, there are also good medical reasons for this treatment, too. Most girls with PCO have normal levels of oestrogen but as they are not ovulating they are not producing progesterone. Unopposed oestrogen increases the long-term risk of endometrial carcinoma. This risk is reduced by inducing regular withdrawal bleeds with the pill. Girls and their parents, however, must realise that this treatment is only masking the underlying cause which still exists and that stopping the pill will probably, once again, result in amenorrhoea or scanty, infrequent periods.

Resistant ovary

This is a relatively rare condition which resembles, and is difficult to differentiate from, ovarian failure. The aetiology is unknown. Investigations show raised FSH and LH levels with low oestradiol levels. The differentiation between this condition and ovarian failure may be made by ovarian biopsy which shows the presence of plentiful primordial follicles. Many clinicians, however, do not advocate the use of ovarian biopsy. Even if follicles are identified on histological examination, there is no guarantee that they will develop and that the girl will spontaneously ovulate or menstruate. Conversely, an unrepresentative biopsy may fail to show the presence of follicles when they are actually present in other areas of the ovary. These doubts, in addition to the risks of anaesthesia and laparoscopy, mean that ovarian biopsy is rarely indicated in the clinical management of resistant ovary. As spontaneous ovulation may occur, there is a possible, though extremely rare, chance of pregnancy. Treatment is with HRT as already described to produce withdrawal bleeds and prevent osteoporosis and atherosclerosis. In view of the chance of spontaneous ovulation, although rare, it may be worth considering the use of the combined oral contraceptive pill for HRT in this group if pregnancy is not wished.

Hyperprolactinaemia as a cause of secondary amenorrhoea in this age group is rare. There is some evidence (Teoh *et al.*, 1992), albeit conflicting (Block *et al.*, 1991), that drug use, such as marijuana and cocaine, may raise prolactin levels and thus cause amenorrhoea. It is also important in the assessment of those with period problems to exclude hypo- or hyperthyroidism. The problem of amenorrhoea in association with hirsutism or virilisation is dealt with in Chapter 16.

HEAVY AND/OR IRREGULAR PERIODS

The more common period problem in adolescent girls is heavy periods. The official definition of heavy periods is a menstrual loss greater than 80 ml per cycle. While this is a tidy scientific definition, in practice it is difficult to be objective about menstrual loss. In studies performed in adults with a subjective complaint of menorrhagia, 68% had blood loss less than 80 ml and 42% had a loss less than 50 ml (Cameron, 1989). In dealing with an adolescent girl, there is a further problem that her presentation may be coloured by her mother's experience of menstruation. 'I always had problems with my periods and she is going the same way' is a well-recognised situation and one which requires careful management.

It is extremely important when dealing with girls presenting with this problem that the practitioner does, however, make some attempt to assess the amount of flow. Once treatment has begun, it is impossible to convince the girl (and her mother) that the cycle she presented with was within acceptable limits and did not require treatment. The girl thereafter has a false expectation of menstruation throughout her reproductive life and which may end up with her having unnecessary surgery in later years.

While taking a careful history of cycle length and duration is not always help-ful (Cameron, 1989), questions related to the size and frequency of passing clots, whether she has to get up at night to change her protection or whether she stains her underclothes or sheets may be helpful. Questions related to the amount of sanitary protection required and how often she has to change it may be useful but does depend on the fastidiousness of individual girls. It is also important to assess to what degree her periods affect her lifestyle – her ability to go to school, take part in games, go out in the evenings.

Investigations should include haemoglobin and thyroid function tests. An ultrasound scan of the pelvis may be carried out but is probably not required at this stage of management. An examination under anaesthetic and dilatation and curettage is *not* required. Dilatation and curettage is a diagnostic procedure for the exclusion of serious pathology and there is no serious endometrial pathology related to abnormal menstruation in this age group. The underlying pathophysi-ology is failure of ovulation which is common in the first few months or years following the menarche. A study by Apter and Vihko (1987) showed that while only 15% of cycles were ovulatory in the first year after the menarche, this rose to 75% of cycles by 5 years and 95% by 12 years. Unopposed oestrogen acting on the endometrium causes continued proliferation of the endometrium over a longer than normal period of time and leads to a very thick endometrium. When such an endometrium does break down, understandably, it causes very heavy menstrual loss. Histology of the endometrium, therefore, would show a hyper-proliferative pattern or in extreme cases, a cystic hyperplastic appearance. The pattern in the early years following menarche, therefore, may be that of irregular, infrequent, extremely heavy periods with the passage of large clots. Provided that the loss is not too heavy and that the girl does not become anaemic, assur-ance that the condition is self-limiting may be all that is required, although it is probably wise to put a time limit on the duration of the symptoms before coming back for further management.

If therapy is required, it can be either hormonal or non-hormonal. Non-hormonal therapy is probably only suitable for those with regular heavy periods as it does not affect the duration of the cycle, merely the duration and heaviness of the flow.

The most widely used non-hormonal treatment are the prostaglandin inhibitor group of drugs, the most commonly used being mefanamic acid 500 mg, 3 times daily, taken from the onset of menstruation until the heavy phase of the period has passed (Anderson *et al.*, 1976). A reduction in blood loss of the order of 30% has been reported. The advantage of treatment with mefanamic acid is that treat-ment need only be taken during menstruation, not throughout the cycle as with hormone medication. In addition, dysmenorrhoea, if present, will also be improved. Side effects of mefanamic acid include diarrhoea. They should not be used in those with inflammatory bowel disease and should be used with caution in girls with asthma. The other form of non-hormonal therapy is the fibrinolytic inhibitors. These may be used on their own or in conjunction with the prostaglandin inhibitors. Those most commonly used are tranexamic acid

1–1.5 g, 3 or 4 times daily, or ethamsylate 500 mg 4 times daily. As with mefanamic acid, these preparations only require to be take throughout the days of heavy menstrual flow.

For girls who have irregular periods or in whom non-hormonal treatment has not been successful, hormonal treatment is required. The first line of treatment are the progestogens, either norethisterone 5 mg 2 or 3 times daily, dydrogesterone 5 mg twice daily or medroxyprogesterone 5 mg twice daily. All are taken from day 12 to day 26 of the cycle. All the progestogens cause some water retention and weight gain which may make them unacceptable for weight conscious teenagers. It is often preferred by her mother, however, who may not be happy at the alternative of their daughter going on the combined oral contraceptive pill. Progestogens in high doses may be used to stop an exceptionally long and heavy period.

If progestogen therapy is not tolerated or successful, the treatment of choice is the combined oral contraceptive pill. The choice of which pill to use is left to the individual practitioner but it is rare that doses in excess of 30 µg ethinyl oestradiol are required.

It should be explained to the girl and her parents that such hormonal treatment is only masking her own cycle and producing regular withdrawal bleeds while the girl's ovulation and hormone pattern matures. Stopping the medication therefore may result in the symptoms recurring.

It is advisable that the girl does stop treatment at 6–12 monthly intervals to ascertain what has happened to her own cycle (unless in the meantime she has begun to require the pill for contraception). She should choose a time when her life would not be disrupted too much if her previous period pattern were to recur, e.g. not in the middle of her GCSEs! If there has been no improvement in her periods, she should restart treatment.

A great deal of research has been carried out on the risk of oral contraceptives, particularly in young girls. Pike *et al.* (1983) suggested that oral contraceptive use during the time of breast development might increase the risk of breast cancer. Two studies (Bernstein *et al.*, 1990; Wingo *et al.*, 1991) specifically examined the duration of oral contraceptive use during teenage years in relation to the risk of breast cancer in young women and reported a slightly increased risk. A more recent study from Holland (Rookus and van Leeuwen, 1994) concluded that 4 or more years of oral contraceptive use, especially if partly before the age of 20, is associated with an increased risk of breast cancer developing at an early age. The Collaborative Group on Hormonal Factors in Breast Cancer (1996) defined this risk as being 0.5 excess cancers per 100 000 women for use at the age 16–19 (see *Lancet* report, 1996). While this risk has obviously to be balanced against the risk to the girl of anaemia and loss of schooling, it is equally important that the girl does not take the combined oral contraceptive pill for longer than is necessary.

Failure to respond to the above treatment suggests an underlying pathology. The commonest in this age group is one of the congenital or acquired haematological disorders such as Von Willebrand's disease or idiopathic thrombocytopenia. One study has suggested that of adolescents presenting with severe menorrhagia up to 50% may have an underlying bleeding disorder (Classens and Cowell, 1982).

DYSMENORRHOEA

Dysmenorrhoea or painful menstruation is a frequent symptom in teenagers, about 50% having symptoms severe enough to cause some disruption of their school or social life. It occurs in ovulatory cycles. As already discussed, the first few cycles after the menarche are usually anovulatory and are therefore usually painless. The history, therefore, is usually of the onset of painful cycles several months after the menarche. The pain usually starts on the first day of menstruation although it may occur a day or two premenstrually and lasts until the second or third day of the cycle. The pain is colicky in nature and is suprapubic often radiating to the back and the inner aspect of the thighs. It is often accompanied by nausea, vomiting and diarrhoea. Some girls have symptoms so severe as to cause them to faint or to miss several days schooling each month. It is caused by contractions of the myometrium associated with excessive prostaglandin production (Dawood, 1990). Treatment is with the prostaglandin inhibitors or with the combined oral contraceptive pill as already mentioned.

While dysmenorrhoea in the adolescent is rarely associated with pathology, two conditions merit mention and should be considered in those girls who fail to respond to the treatment outlined above.

Endometriosis

Endometriosis is a condition where tissue identical to the endometrium of the uterus is found outside the uterus, usually in the pelvis around the uterosacral ligaments or ovaries. It causes chronic pelvic pain and dysmenorrhoea, which unlike that already described, lasts throughout the menstrual flow. It has usually been considered a disease of women later in their reproductive life, but with the more widespread use of laparoscopy making the diagnosis easier, it has been realised that it also affects adolescents. Vercellini *et al.* (1989) in a study of 47 adolescent girls with chronic pelvic pain diagnosed endometriosis in 38%.

The treatment of endometriosis in adolescents is aimed at reducing the pain and preserving future fertility. This can be achieved by using a variety of hormonal medications which produce a hypo-oestrogenic state thus causing the endometriotic deposits to atrophy. Drugs used include progestogens, danazol and GnRH analogues.

Progestogens cause a hypo-oestrogenic state and amenorrhoea by suppressing gonadotrophin release. The most widely used progestogens are norethisterone 10 mg daily increasing if necessary to 25 mg daily, dydrogesterone 10–15 mg daily and medroxyprogesterone acetate 30 mg daily and should be used continuously. Danazol acts by suppressing the hypothalamic–pituitary axis and reducing the frequency of GnRH pulses (Maouris *et al.*, 1991) thus reducing oestrogen production. It also directly inhibits ovarian hormone production. Unfortunately, it also has an androgenic effect both by its action of decreasing SHBG levels thus displacing testosterone from SHBG and by binding to intracellular androgen receptors. The side effects of danazol are mainly related to the androgenic effects – weight gain, decreased breast size, acne and oily skin. More rarely but more seriously, virilising effects may occur including cliteromegaly, hirsutism and deepening of the voice. These side effects may be irreversible. Treatment must be stopped immediately if any virilising side effects occur. Muscle cramps and headaches have also been reported. Gestrinone has a similar mode of action and side effects as danazol. GnRH analogues act by causing down regulation of the pituitary thus causing hypogonadotrophic hypogonadism. They can be given either as a nasal snuff (Buserelin, Nafarelin) or as slow release depot preparations (Goserelin, Leuprorelin). There is some evidence to suggest that the depot preparations are more effective that the nasal sprays (Shaw, 1988). The side effects are similar to the symptoms of the climacteric – hot flushes, night sweats, depression and a reduction in breast size. Vaginal dryness and loss of libido are also common but may not be mentioned by teenagers without specific prompting. The GnRH analogues also cause bone loss – a reduction in bone density of the distal forearm of between 2% and 4.6% being reported and between 2% and 6% in the spine (Fogelman, 1992). This is of particular importance in young women as the risk of osteoporosis in later life is related to the peak bone mass attained in early life. The effect, however, does appear to be reversible with nor-

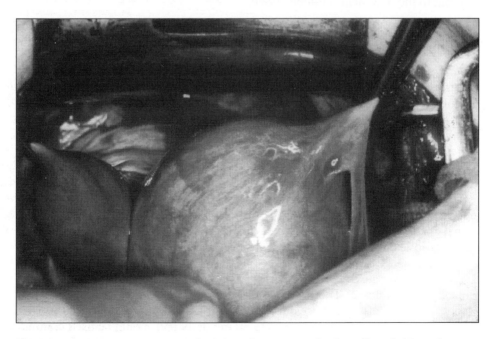

Fig. 8.9 Laparotomy appearances of a right rudimentary uterine horn distended from the accumulation of menstrual blood in a teenager who presented with dysmenorrhoea.

mal levels reported 6 months post-treatment. Treatment with GnRH analogues, however, is limited to 6 months therapy because of this. The use of 'add-back' regimes where oestrogen or progestogen are given in doses which prevent side effects or bone loss but are not sufficient to cause endometrial stimulation are being assessed. Whatever treatment option is used, it is prescribed at a dose sufficient to cause amenorrhoea for 6 months. There is a risk of recurrence with all regimes.

Rudimentary Blind Horn

A second rare but important cause of refractory dysmenorrhoea is a *rudimentary blind horn* of the uterus (Fig. 8.9). This occurs due to incomplete fusion of the Mullerian duct. Unlike cryptomenorrhoea due to an imperforate or absent vagina, the diagnosis may be delayed as there is normal menstrual flow from the normal uterine horn. The diagnosis may be suspected when severe dysmenorrhoea, lasting throughout the duration of the menstrual flow, occurs immediately from the menarche. Diagnosis may be confirmed by ultrasound (Fig. 8.10) or by laparoscopy. Treatment is by excision of the blind horn with preservation of the normal uterine horn. As with other Mullerian duct abnormalities, investigation of the renal tract must be carried out. Both these conditions, although rare,

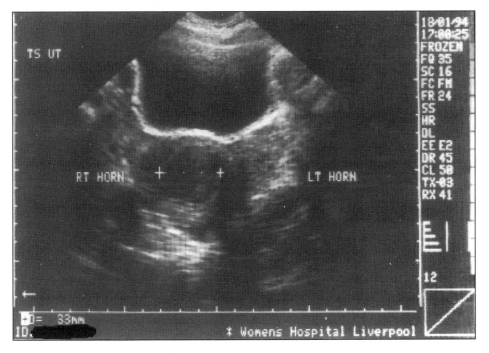

Fig. 8.10 Transvaginal ultrasound appearance of the same patient showing the distended uterine horn initially diagnosed on these appearances as being an ovarian cyst.

should be considered when dysmenorrhoea lasts throughout menstruation or fails to respond to therapy outlined above.

REFERENCES

Alper MM, Garner PR, 1985: Premature ovarian failure: its relationship to auto-immune disease. *Obstetrics and Gynecology* **66**, 27–30.

Anderson ABM, Haynes PJ, Guillebaud J, Turnbull AC, 1976: Reduction of menstrual blood loss by prostaglandin synthetase inhibitors. *Lancet* **i**, 774–776.

Apter D, Vihko R, 1978: Hormonal patterns of adolescent cycles. *Journal of Clinical Endocrinology and Metabolism* **47**, 944–954.

Baker WJ, Morgan RL, Pickham MJ, Smithers DW, 1972: Preservation of ovarian function in patients requiring radiotherapy for paraortic and pelvic Hodgkins disease. *Lancet* **ii**, 1307.

Bates GW, Whitworth NS, 1982: Effect of body weight reduction on plasma androgens in obese infertile women. *Fertility and Sterility* **38**, 406–409.

Bernstein L, Pike MC, Krailo M, Henderson BE, 1990: Update of the Los Angeles Study of oral contraceptives and breast cancer: 1981 and 1983. In Mann RD, (ed.), *Oral Contraceptives and Breast Cancer*. London: Royal Society of Medicine, 169–180.

Block RI, Farinpour R, Schlechte JA, 1991: Effects of chronic marijuana use on testosterone, luteinizing hormone, prolactin and cortisol in men and women. *Drug and Alcohol Dependence* **28**, 121–128.

Bonakdar MI, Peisner DB, 1980: Gonadoblastoma with a 45, XO karyotype. *Obstetrics and Gynecology* **56**, 748–750.

Cameron IT, 1989: Dysfunctional uterine bleeding. *Balliere's Clinical Obstetrics and Gynaecology* **3**, 315–327.

Classens EA, Cowell CA, 1982: Acute adolescent menorrhagia. *American Journal of Obstetrics and Gynecology* **139**, 277–280.

Collaborative Group on Hormonal Factors in Breast Cancer. Breast cancer and hormonal contraceptives: collaborative re-analysis of individual data on 53 297 women with breast cancer and 100 239 women without breast cancer from 54 epidemiological studies, 1996. *Lancet* **347**, 1713–1727.

Dawood MY, 1990: Dysmenorrhoea. *Clinical Obstetrics and Gynecology* **33**, 168–178.

Dominguez CJ, Greenblatt RG, 1962: Dysgerminoma of the ovary in a patient with Turner's syndrome. *American Journal of Obstetrics and Gynecology* **83**, 674–677.

Fogelman I, 1992: Gonadotropin-releasing hormone agonists and the skeleton. *Fertility and Sterility* **57**, 715–724.

Frank RT, 1938: The formation of an artificial vagina without operation. *American Journal of Obstetrics and Gynecology* **35**, 1053–1055.

Goodall J, 1991: Helping a child understand her own testicular feminisation. *Lancet* **337**, 33–35.

Griffin JE, Edwards C, Madden JD, Harrod MJ, Wilson JD, 1976: Congenital absence of the vagina. The Mayer–Kuster–Hauser syndrome. *Annals of Internal Medicine* **85**, 224–236.

Held KR, Kerber S, Kaminsky E *et al.*, 1992: Mosaicism in 45, X Turner Syndrome: does survival in early pregnancy depend on the presence of two sex chromosomes? *Human Genetics* **88**, 288–294.

Illig R, DeCampo C, Lang-Muritano MR *et al.*, 1990: A physiological mode of puberty induction in hypogonadal girls by low dose transdermal 17β-oestradiol. *European Journal of Pediatrics* **150**, 86–91.

Johnson N, Batchelor A, Lilford RJ, 1991: Experience with tissue expansion vaginoplasty. *British Journal of Obstetrics and Gynaecology* **98**, 564–568.

Kocova M, Siegel SF, Wenger SL, Lee PA, Trucco M, 1993: Detection of Y chromosome sequences in Turner's syndrome by Southern blot analysis of amplified DNA. *Lancet* **342**, 140–143.

Maouris P, Dowsett M, Edmonds DK, Sullivan D, 1991: The effect of Danazol on pulsatile gonadotropin secretion in women with endometriosis. *Fertility and Sterility* **55**, 890–894.

Morgan A, London S, 1993: Effects of excessive exercise and weight loss on adolescent menstrual cyclicity. *Adolescent Pediatrics and Gynecology* **6**, 63–70.

Morrison JC, Gimes JR, Wiser LW, Fish SA, 1975: Mumps oophoritis: a cause of premature menopause. *Fertility and Sterility* **26**, 655–659.

Noonan JA, 1968: Hypertelorism with Turner phenotype. *American Journal of Diseases of Children* **116**, 373–380.

Noonan JA, Ehmke DA, 1963: Associated non-cardiac malformations in children with congenital heart disease. *Journal of Pediatrics* **63**, 468–470.

Personal view, 1994: Once a dark secret. *British Medical Journal* **308**, 542.

Pike MC, Henderson BE, Krailo MD, Duke A, Roy S, 1983: Breast cancer in young women and use of oral contraceptives: possible modifying effect of formulation and age at use. *Lancet* **ii**, 926–930.

Polson DW, Wasdworth J, Adams J, Franks J, 1988: Polycystic ovaries – a common finding in normal women. *Lancet* **i**, 870–872.

Rees M, 1993: Menarche when and why. *Lancet* **342**, 1375–1376.

Reindollar RH, McDonough PG, 1981: Etiology and evaluation of delayed sexual development. *Pediatric Clinics of North America* **28**, 267–286.

Reindollar RH, McDonough PG, 1983: Adolescent menstrual disorders. *Clinical Obstetrics and Gynecology* **26**, 690–701.

Rock J, Reeves L, Retto H *et al.*, 1983: Success following vaginal creation for mullerian agenesis. *Fertility and Sterility* **39**, 809–813.

Rookus MA, van Leeuwen FE, 1994: Oral contraceptives and risk of breast cancer in women aged 20–54 years. *Lancet* **344**, 844–851.

Russell GFM, 1985: Premenarchial anorexia nervosa and its sequelae. *Journal of Psychiatric Research* **19**, 363–369.

San Filippo JS, Wakim NG, Schikler KN, Yussman MA, 1986: Endometriosis in association with uterine anomaly. *American Journal of Obstetrics and Gynecology* **154**, 39–43.

Schwartz C, Dean J, Howard Peebles P *et al.*, 1994: Obstetric and gynaecological complications in fragile X carriers. *American Journal of Medical Genetics* **51**, 400–402.

Shaw RW, 1988: LHRH analogues in the treatment of endometriosis – comparative results with other treatments. *Clinics in Obstetrics and Gynaecology* **2**, 659–675.

Simpson JL, Blagowidow N, Martin AO, 1981: XY gonadal dysgenesis. Genetic heterogeneity based upon clinical observations, H–Y antigen status and segregation analysis. *Human Genetics* **58**, 91–97.

Strickland JL, Cameron WJ, Krantz KE, 1993: Long-term satisfaction of adults undergoing McIndoe vaginoplasty as adolescents. *Adolescent Pediatrics and Gynecology* **6**, 135–137.

Teoh SK, Lex BW, Mendelson JH, Mello NK, Cochin J, 1992: Hyperprolactinaemia and macrocytosis in women with alcohol and polysubstance abuse. *Journal of Studies on Alcohol* **53**, 176–182.

Toublanc JE, Roger M, Chaussain JL, 1991: Etiologies of late puberty. *Hormone Research* **36**, 136–140.

Vercellini P, Fedele L, Arcaini LJ *et al.*, 1989: Laparoscopy in the diagnosis of chronic pelvic pain in adolescent women. *Journal of Reproductive Medicine* **34**, 827–830.

Vergauwen P, Ferster A, Valsamis J, Chanione JP, 1994: Primary ovarian failure after prepubertal marrow transplant in a girl. *Lancet* **343**, 125–126.

Verp MS, Simpson JL, 1987: Abnormal sexual differentiation and neoplasia. *Cancer Genetics and Cytogenetics* **25**, 191–218.

White MC, Turner EI, 1994: Polycystic ovarian syndrome: 2. Diagnosis and management. *British Journal of Hospital Medicine* **51**, 349–352.

Williams EA, 1964: Congenital absence of the vagina. A simple operation for its relief. *Journal of Obstetrics and Gynaecology of the British Commonwealth* **4**, 511–512.

Wingo PA, Lee NC, Ory HW, Beral V, Peterson HB, Rhodes P, 1991: Age-specific differences in the relationship between oral contraceptive use and breast cancer. *Obstetrics and Gynecology* **78**, 161–170.

CHAPTER 9

Colposcopy in teenagers

JENNIFER HOPWOOD

Worldwide, cancer of the cervix is the most common female cancer. In the United Kingdom it is the fifth most frequently occurring cancer in women. The aim of the National Health Service (NHS) Cervical Screening Programme is to reduce the mortality from squamous carcinoma of the cervix. Reduction in the incidence of cervical cancer could be achieved by regular screening of women between 20 and 65 years in order to detect and treat conditions which could have a significant risk of progressing to cancer. After treatment and eradication of such abnormalities, women are returned to the screening programme (Duncan, 1992).

The range of activities in a cervical screening programme are closely inter-related and comprise:

- identifying and inviting eligible women for cervical smears
- smear taking
- cytological examination of smears
- giving the results
- colposcopy and treatment
- follow-up and failsafe devices
- education and information

The same principles apply to all women throughout the cervical screening programme, but there are some special considerations for the young. These involve:

- the age at which testing should start
- preservation of fertility
- choice of treatment of cervical intraepithelial neoplasia (CIN)
- primary prevention measures – information and education

CERVICAL SMEARS IN ADOLESCENTS

Traditional teaching suggests that there is disease progression from normal epithelium through grades of CIN finally becoming invasive cancer in some women after 10 to 15 years. Occasionally, probably due to extremes in the range, cervical cancer will occur in the very young. In 1988 in England and Wales, there were 4 registered cases between the ages of 10 and 19 years, and in the years 1988–92 none of the women who died from cervical cancer was a teenager (Office of Population and Census Studies data).

This epidemiological data may not provide justification for screening teenagers, provided there is good compliance in the 20–25 age group. However, for those health carers who have seen even one woman undergo a hysterectomy for an invasive lesion before she has had the chance to have children, the epidemiological theory may be hard to put into practice. Many clinicians offer an opportunistic smear test soon after the start of sexual activity, regardless of age.

Some women of 20 years, when due for their first call for a smear may have had sexual partners for as long as 8 years and even in adolescents, risk factors for cervical cancer could have been present for many years.

The offering and taking of a smear may in itself have an educative and encouraging role, facilitating discussion not only about prevention of cervical cancer and HIV infection but also about fertility preservation. Although adolescents may not often have or die from cancer of the cervix, it may be that what they do at this time of their lives contributes to their developing precancer and cancer in later years.

A proportion of teenagers will have CIN, including the higher grades. The important issue is whether invasive cancer is likely to develop before the CIN is detected (Martinez *et al.*, 1989).

Although women under 20 years are not *called* by the community programme for a smear, they will enter the *recall* system once a smear has been registered, at whatever age.

Women have the option of having their smears taken by their general practitioners or in community family planning and well woman clinics. Some prefer having the examination by someone they know; others prefer relative anonymity. In all situations they can request that a woman doctor or nurse takes the smear.

It is particularly important in young women to make the examination as comfortable as possible and that an optimal smear is obtained so that neither pain nor worry about an 'inadequate' results are reasons for not having smears in the future.

The thought of a cervical smear is daunting to many women. Information should be given so that the decision to have one is freely given. Never should there be such bribes as 'you must have a smear or I will not give you any more pills'.

There are some practical difficulties which may arise in offering cervical smears to young women. Young people may change address often, so that letters of invitation do not reach them and for the same reasons it may be difficult to ensure notification of an abnormal result.

Adolescents may not want letters about smears sent to their home, because they do not want family to know they are having sex. Their wish should be respected by marking the smear form with the instruction 'no correspondence home'.

Young women attending a department of genito-urinary medicine may be offered a smear test there, and in this situation, the result will not be sent either to their home or to their general practioner unless permission is specifically given.

It is essential, however, in *any* situation before taking a smear, to establish sufficient confidence to negotiate an alternative contact point; perhaps a friend's address or a telephone number so that the young woman can be reached in the event of an abnormality being found.

Case Study

When Susan was 19 years old she had her first smear, having been on the contraceptive pill for 3 years. She smoked 20 cigarettes per day. Occasional dyskaryotic cells were noted and a repeat smear advised in 6 months time. She had forbidden correspondence to her home and left no other means of contact. Despite being told verbally after 3 months that a further smear should be taken, she 'disappeared' for over a year. By this time she had invasive carcinoma, obvious clinically as well as cytologically. At the age of 21, and with no children, she underwent a Wertheims hysterectomy.

In addition to the problem of the request for 'no correspondence home' it is not uncommon for young people meeting health carers in family planning, termination or genito-urinary medicine services to give false names, addresses or dates of birth (even all three) so that tracing them and correlating previous results is difficult.

The Adolescent Cervix in Smear Taking

At the time of puberty and during adolescence, the female genital tract enlarges in response to increasing levels of ovarian hormones and then continuing stimulation by the physiological levels attained. This increase in size is most apparent in the body of the uterus, but the cervix also enlarges and changes in shape, resulting in the columnar epithelium, initially lining the lower part of the cervical canal, now being situated on the vaginal portion of the cervix. This columnar epithelium is exposed to the acidic environment of the vagina and this may encourage the process of metaplasia whereby it is to a varying degree replaced by squamous epithelium. The term 'transformation zone' is used to describe where this is occurring.

The colour of the normal cervix is caused by the thickness of the cell layer overlying the connective tissue, together with the degree of vascularity of the area. A thin covering of columnar cells results in a red appearance, whereas the thicker filter of multilayered squamous epithelium produces a pink appearance. The junction of the red and pink is the squamocolumnar junction or transformation zone and is from where a smear should be taken as this is where intraepithelial neoplasia usually arises. (The red area used to be termed an 'erosion'. This is sometimes misheard by young people as 'corrosion'! Ectopy is a better term.)

PRESERVATION OF FERTILITY

Preservation of fertility in the context of cervical screening in young women relates to awareness and accurate management of infection and pelvic inflammatory disease. At colposcopy, it is important that the treatment modality used should not affect future fertility or pregnancy outcome.

Case Study

Anne was 33 years old and infertile. 'I had always thought that as I had had regular smears from the age of 18, any abnormalities or infection would show up.' She did have abnormal cells and underwent cone biopsy at 25 years, but her recurrent abdominal pain and 'cystitis' were investigated only after her partner was treated for urethritis some years later. She was chlamydia-positive and was treated, but the tubal damage, sustained over the years is severe and could have been prevented.

There are women who attend for investigation of infertility who ask if previous treatment to their cervix for abnormal cells could have been the cause. This is unlikely. However, infection present at the same time as the CIN may well have damaged the reproductive tract.

It is vital that cervical cytology results are not extrapolated to the health of the reproductive tract as a whole. A negative smear does not indicate pelvic health. Inaccurate use of cervical cytology results to evaluate infection can cause iatrogenic infertility. A cervical smear may show trichomonads, yeasts, bacteria suggestive of bacterial vaginosis, evidence of herpes simplex virus (HSV) and of human papilloma virus (HPV) infection. It is *not* efficient at detecting *Chlamydia trachomatis* or *Neisseria gonorrhoea*, both of which can cause pelvic inflammatory disease. Thus, treatment for example of cytologically reported trichomonas may leave unseen co-existent chlamydia to damage the fallopian tubes. Testing for chlamydial infection (the most common sexually transmitted disease apart from HPV) by taking an endocervical swab, could be offered at the time of cervical cytology as a screening measure

(Hopwood and Mallinson, 1995). Many colposcopists test for the infection at the colposcopic assessment. The justification for this is four-fold:

- Chlamydial infection may be associated with low grade cytological abnormalities which may resolve after its treatment.
- Contact bleeding when a smear is taken may result in an unreadable smear. This can be caused by chlamydial infection. Repeated bloodstained smears may lead to 'colposcopy to clarify'.
- Chlamydial cervicitis and endometritis can cause discharge and bleeding which may be incorrectly attributed to the cytological abnormality (though 60% of women with the infection have no symptoms).
- Chlamydial infection may result in morbidity after treatment for CIN.

A confirmed positive chlamydia result should lead to correct treatment together with partner notification. This is best done in a department of genitourinary medicine. (See Chapter 10).

COLPOSCOPY AND TREATMENT

The colposcope is a binocular microscope with a focal length of 150–200 mm. It is provided with bright illumination and a magnification which varies from ×10 to ×60. It enables simple outpatient examination and treatment of the cervix.

If cervical smears *are* taken in adolescents then abnormal reports will result in referral for colposcopy, with the potential for overtreatment of conditions which could revert to normal without intervention (Sivakamar *et al.*, 1990; Walker *et al.*, 1990). Although a simple procedure in medical terms, colposcopy can be frightening both in anticipation and experience, so every attempt should be made to give as much information as possible (e.g. an information leaflet sent with the appointment card), to be friendly, and to cause minimal pain, indignity and discomfort. It is usually carried out in a hospital setting, but there are a few general practices and community clinics offering the service and some young women find these venues less daunting. It may be helpful to have an accompanying relative or friend throughout the visit to the colposcopy department. Pictures and music may be helpful distractions (Vaughn *et al.*, 1994). In some centres, the patient can (if she wishes) watch the procedure on a closed circuit television screen. It is extremely important that this meeting with health care does not make her (and the friends to whom she recounts the experience) reluctant to attend in the future.

Indications for Colposcopy

Referral for colposcopy may be for *cytological* or for *clinical* reasons.

Cytological

Dyskaryotic smear

There is a case for managing women with mildly dyskaryotic smears by cyto-logical review, because many cases will revert to normal without intervention. If they persist, however, then colposcopic assessment is advisable in order to exclude a more serious lesion (Flannelly *et al.*, 1994). However, as mentioned previously, the problem with cytological surveillance in the young is that there may be poor response to invitations for a repeat smear, especially if there is a change of address. It may be that future development of HPV typing will enable adolescents and young women with high risk types (such as 16 and 18) to be selectively monitored and treated (Bavin *et al.*, 1993). Women with severe dyskaryosis should always be referred for colposcopy and most would refer those with moderate dyskaryosis.

For clarification

Cytology is used for clarification when there are recurrent, inadequate or border-line smears. Some will be from a worse lesion, others may have an infective cause, but sometimes no abnormality is found. Whatever the outcome, colposcopy will have clarified the issue rather than repeating smears over a long period.

Blanket antibiotics should never be given for this group of smear results, in case pelvic inflammatory disease should result from inadequate therapy as mentioned above.

Clinical reasons

When signs and/or symptoms such as contact bleeding or post-coital bleeding or a suspicious appearance of the cervix are present. These reasons for colposcopy always override a previous negative smear report, no matter how recent.

Colposcopic examination of the vagina and vulva can be carried out to look for co-existent pathology, for example in the follow up of vaginal adenosis (see p. 249) and colposcopy may be a useful tool in the evaluation of a child with sus-pected sexual abuse (see Chapter 19).

Colposcopic Appearances

Dysplastic epithelium is thicker than normal epithelium and thrown into folds into which blood vessels enter. The resultant patterns on the cervix can be more clearly evaluated with the colposcope than by naked eye. Saline may be applied to enhance these appearances.

Acetic acid (5%) is applied to demonstrate these changes as acetowhite areas. The time taken for the acetowhite to develop and to fade, together with the den-sity of the whiteness, the character of demarcation of white from normal appear-ances, plus vascular patterns (described as punctation and mosaicism) all help to grade the extent and degree of abnormality. It is a subjective evaluation and may be expected to correlate with histological findings in 70% of cases. (Not all acetowhite change is dysplastic. It can be caused for example by immature meta-plasia. Misinterpretation of this appearance could lead to overtreatment which is an especially important consideration in young women.)

Lugol's Iodine may be applied to carry out Schiller's test. Normal squamous epithelium stains black because of the glycogen content, in contrast to non-stain-ing dysplastic epithelium which does not contain glycogen. This often allows clear visualisation of the extent (though not the degree) of abnormality, but it is not a specific test.

Management

Diagnosis is made by considering the colposcopic appearances, together with the cytology and the histology reports. One or more biopsies are taken from an area of suspected abnormality. It is not true that the cervix is insensitive. Pain, no matter how transient by taking a biopsy and often covered with such advice as 'just cough, dear' may result in the young woman not returning for future appointments. Local anaesthetic should be considered when biopsies are taken as well as for treatment.

If the diagnosis seems certain then treatment after taking the biopsy may be offered at the first visit ('see and treat'), but if there is doubt about the diagnosis then management will be deferred for a few weeks until the histology report is obtained. Diagnosis and treatment at one visit is a great advantage for those who find it difficult to attend either because of commitments or because of fear. The disadvantage is that there may be overtreatment which should be avoided espe-cially in very young women. Diathermy loop excision (DLE) provides treatment and diagnostic procedure in one process, and is increasingly popular, though there is an awareness of the potential for overtreatment.

Treatment Modalities

Treatment for CIN may be *ablative* or *excisional* and is usually carried out under local anaesthesia.

Ablation

This destroys the tissue and may be carried out: (a) by 'cold coagulation' which in fact is hot (!) – probes are applied to the cervix at a temperature of $100°C$ destroying the affected area of cervix; (b) by laser (light amplification by stimu-lated emission of radiation) operating at $1000°C$, or (c) by cryocautery.

Excision

Excision removes the abnormal area and preserves it for histological diagnosis (enabling microinvasion to be excluded). In the past this involved formal knife conisation, but currently, use of either the laser in cutting mode or a diathermy loop enables a cone of cervix to be removed as an outpatient procedure. (Laser equipment is very expensive and treatment with it usually takes longer than DLE, with no added benefits so that its use is becoming less popular).

The choice and timing of treatment is determined by the severity of lesion, whether the upper limit can be seen within the endocervical canal, by local facilities and preferences, and whether the adolescent woman is likely to return.

Each treatment modality has advantages and disadvantages. All are capable of restoring the cervix to normal, cytologically and histologically in approximately 95% of high grade CIN without affecting cervical function. The appearance of the cervix after healing is usually entirely normal. An adolescent's perception of the whole experience of the procedure and care she receives are, equally, if not more important, in the success of her treatment and follow up, than are medical preferences.

As the age of women referred for colposcopy has decreased, so it has become important for the less radical methods of treatment to be developed to replace formal conisation which can affect child bearing. This is especially important in caring for adolescents. There is no convincing evidence that DLE has a detrimental effect on pregnancy. When other relevant factors such as smoking are taken into consideration there is no evidence of increased fetal loss, preterm labour, cervical incompetence or stenosis (Cruikshank *et al.*, 1995). This may in part reflect the smaller size and depth of tissue removed as compared to knife conisation.

In treating adolescents there is an awareness that the factors causing the cervical abnormality are likely to persist (e.g. contact with HPV) so that treatment may need to be repeated on several occasions.

After Treatment

Adequate information after treatment is as important as pretreatment counselling. It should be in both verbal and written form, stating the type of treatment used and what to expect afterwards. It should be explained that there is likely to be discharge as part of the healing process and that there should not be penetrative sex for a month or use of tampons for a similar time. (*Before* treatment is carried out, it is a kindness to ask if there are imminent holidays, examinations, etc. which would make a discharge a real embarrassment or inconvenience).

Follow Up

Local guidelines do vary, but there could be a persistent or recurrent abnormality so that follow up policies should be made which can be modified in the light of audit of outcomes. The immediate outcome measures are a negative smear and colposcopy. The long-term outcome is that the woman should not develop a recurrence or invasive disease.

After follow up (one or more) in the colposcopy clinic the woman is transferred back to the local call–recall system for her cervical smears. Development of a formal system for ensuring this transfer is important. Annual smears may be advised for several years but until there is accurate epidemiological data, it is not possible to say categorically for how long.

Practical Issues

Every effort should be made to encourage effective contraception to be continued prior to the colposcopy appointment. Many people associate an abnormal smear with the contraceptive pill and think they should stop taking it, but an unwanted pregnancy only compounds the worry. The referring doctor should give positive counselling to ensure that contraception is *not* stopped prior to the appointment and that useful advice is given about taking consecutive pill packets with no break, in order to prevent a withdrawal bleed if due at the time of the appointment. (This is a common reason for non-attendance.)

Following treatment, taking consecutive packets of pills with no break removes the inconvenience of a bleed in addition to the discharge.

EDUCATION AND INFORMATION

Practical information about what a smear involves, how the result is obtained, what an 'inadequate' smear is and what happens if an abnormality is detected are vitally important. It should be explained to women that a cervical smear is not a diagnostic measure for discharge or possibility of infection. It should be stressed that cervical smears are to find 'early warning cells'; not to detect cancer.

For there to be accurate, effective and non-judgemental information to give to young people about cervical cancer and its prevention, there must be knowledge about its aetiology. However, this is incomplete at present. Knowledge about the natural history of the disease is also incomplete, especially the factors influencing the progression of CIN, despite a huge amount of research into the subject. There is general consensus that some types of HPV play an important causal role in the development of cervical cancer, but that cofactors are necessary to transform HPV-infected tissue into intraepithelial or invasive disease.

Coitus is the major prerequisite for the development of cervical carcinoma. Several epidemiological studies show that women with cervical cancer are more likely to have become sexually active during adolescence than matched controls without the disease.

Previously reported associations with age of marriage and of pregnancy, increased parity, racial factors and low socioeconomic groups may all reflect early age of intercourse and this is the common denominator with all other variables dependent upon it (Fitzpatrick *et al.*, 1992).

Although promiscuity is viewed as having several partners at the same time, serial monogamy may have the same deleterious effect even though it is currently socially more acceptable. It is important that men and women understand that what the male does is vitally important to his partner's cervical health.

There is correlation between cigarette smoking and risk of developing CIN and cervical cancer (Berggren and Sjostedt, 1983; Lyon *et al.*, 1983). Although at first this was thought to be due to associated early coitarche and multiple partners, careful controlled studies show that the risk is maintained even after controlling for other factors. This information should be given so that young people can make their own informed choice about smoking. The effect may result from impaired immune mechanisms (Barton *et al.*, 1988) or to a local carcinogenic or co-carcinogenic mechanisms.

CIN and invasive cancer are more common in women who are immunosuppressed. Adolescent women in this category include those with leukaemia, renal transplant recipients and those with HIV infection, so that regular cervical smears may be indicated.

The choice of contraceptive may be associated with other factors influencing the development of cervical cancer. The duration of use of the combined oral contraceptive pill increases the risk of developing cervical cancer but it may not be causal but by association of other factors, such as change in sexual behaviour in society over the same time.

The use of barrier methods of contraception ought to protect the cervical epithelium from any causative agent transmitted through intercourse. As the squamocolumnar junction is often on the ectocervix after sexual maturity is attained this vulnerable region will be exposed to any agents responsible for the chain of events leading to cervical carcinoma. Young women are encouraged to use the 'double dutch' method i.e. the pill for contraception together with use of the condom to protect the cervix. Consistent condom use for young people is especially difficult to achieve despite their own knowledge about the benefits. Spermicides are virucidal.

Early education of young *men* and women about the risks of early intercourse and multiple partners (of either partner) may be of value, even as early as in the school setting. It is difficult to achieve a satisfactory balance so that fear does not prevail over romance! However, when adolescents are already sexually active, a sexual history compounds any guilt feelings, and is of no scientific value in the clinical situation. Skilled listening for clues about abuse, relationships and fear is more important than adding to the commonly held belief that there is some blame to be apportioned if a smear result is abnormal.

We should help the young by giving accurate advice at an early age so that they can make choices about behaviour. But we should diagnose, treat and follow up with as little intrusion as possible.

Terminology (Evans *et al.*, 1986)

Cervical intraepithelial neoplasia (graded CIN 1, 2 and 3)

This is histological terminology and allows distinction from invasive disease when changes extend through the basement membrane. Dysplasia is a term loosely used in this context.

Dyskaryosis

A cytological term meaning abnormal nucleus. Mild, moderate and severe dyskaryosis as detected on a cervical smear can be expected to reflect CIN 1, 2 and 3 respectively.

Colposcopy

This word is derived from the Greek κολπσσ – a bay or hollow – and σκοπεν – to inspect.

REFERENCES

Barton SE, *et al.,* 1988: Effect of cigarette smoking on cervical epithelial immunity; a mechanism for neoplastic change? *Lancet* **ii**, 652–654.

Bavin PJ, Giles JA, Deery A *et al.*, 1993: Use of semiquantitative PCR for human papillomavirus DNA type 16 to identify women with high grade cervical disease in a population presenting with a mildly dyskaryotic smear report. *British Journal of Cancer* **67**, 602–605.

Berggren G, Sjostedt S, 1983: Preinvasive carcinoma of the cervix uteri and smoking. *Acta Obstetrica et Gynecologica Scandinavia* **62**, 593–598.

Cruikshank ME, Flannery G, Campbell DM, Kitchener HC, 1995: Fertility and pregnancy outcome following large loop excision of the cervical transformation zone. *British Journal of Obstetrics and Gynaecology* **102**, 467–470.

Duncan D, 1992: *NHS Screening programme. Guidelines for clinical practice and programme management* March.

Evans DMD, Hudson EA, Brown CL *et al.,* 1986: Terminology in gynaecological cytopathology. Report of the working party of the British Society for Clinical Cytology. *Journal of Clinical Pathology* **39**, 933–944.

Fitzpatrick C, McKenna P, Hone R, 1992: Teenage girls attending a Dublin sexually transmitted disease clinic: a sociosexual and diagnostic profile. *Irish Journal of Medical Science* **161**, 460–462.

Flannelly G, Anderson D, Kitchener HC *et al.,* 1994: Management of women with mild and moderate dyskaryosis. *British Medical Journal* **308**, 1399–1403.

Hopwood J, Mallinson H, 1995: Chlamydia testing in community clinics – a focus for accurate sexual health care. *British Journal of Family Planning* **21**, 87–90.

Lyon JL, Gardner JW, West DW *et al.,* 1983: Smoking and carcinoma in situ of the uterine cervix. *American Journal of Public Health* **373**, 558–562.

Martinez J, Smith R, Farmer M *et al.*, 1989: High prevalence of genital tract papillomavirus infection in female adolescents. *Pediatrics* **82**, 604–608.

Sivakumar K, Silva AD, Roy RB, 1990: Colposcopy in teenagers [letter]. *Genitourinary Medicine* **66**, 228.

Vaughn I, Richert VI, Kozlowski KJ, Warren A, *et al.*, 1994: Adolescents and colposcopy: the use of different procedures to reduce anxiety. *American Journal of Obstetrics and Gynecology* **170**, 504–508.

Walker EM, Dodgson J, Duncan ID, 1990: Is colposcopy of teenage women worthwhile? An eleven year review of teenage referrals in Dundee. *Journal of Gynecology and Surgery* **5**, 391–394.

CHAPTER 10

Sexually transmitted diseases

OLWEN E WILLIAMS ───────────────────────────────────

Sexually transmitted diseases (STD) contribute a major health risk to all sexually active individuals. Adolescents are no exception to this rule. Their sexual experience, risk-taking behaviour and immature reproductive system put them at a greater risk, not only of acquiring a sexually transmitted infection, but also of suffering the consequent morbidity complicating such diseases.

BACKGROUND

In both the United Kingdom and United States, female adolescents account for 25% of all reported sexually transmitted infections in women. Studies on the epidemiology of STD in adolescent women in the United Kingdom show a vast range in the incidence of the specific infections as shown in Table 10.1. The variation is multifactorial in origin; certain behavioural parameters and context of study should be considered when evaluating results. The sexual behaviour of adolescents will affect the prevalence of STDs and human immuno deficiency virus (HIV) in this age group.

Having the first sexual encounter at an early age is associated with an increased number of lifetime partners (Dunan *et al.*, 1990) and an increased risk of acquiring an STD (Greenberg *et al.*, 1992). Curtis *et al.* (1988) reported that 25% of British females were sexually active by the age of 16 years. One American study (Orn *et al.*, 1989), reported 21% of girls had had at least one coital experience by the age of 12 years. Most studies indicate that adolescents are more sexually active than their peers of 10 years ago. There is also a gender difference, females appear to be more sexually active, and at an earlier age, than their male contemporaries. This is reflected in the STD figures in the United Kingdom (see Summary Information form KC60, 1992).

Adolescent condom use varies from between 9.3 to 37.5%. A study from Norway highlights the fact that adolescents who use condoms, do so for protection against unintended pregnancy, not protection against STD or HIV (Tracen *et al.*, 1992) in contrast to a study from Sweden (Persson and Jarlbro, 1992). Active educational intervention raising this age group's awareness of STDs and HIV,

Table 10.1 Summary of literature

Author	Location	No. of patients	Sex	Age (Years)	% with STD	Specific infection (expressed as % of total)				
						GC	CT	TV	HPV	HSV
Robinson et al., 1983	London 1972	1372	F	16–19	80	8	–	21	9	3
	London 1982	1799	F	16–19	56	6	–	14	8	3
Mulcalchy and Lacey, 1987	Leeds	210	F	12–16	57	14	16	16	4	1
Thin et al., 1989	London	121	M+F	11–18	100	19	6	6	7	2
Thin et al., 1989	Swansea	95	M+F	11–18	100	12	12	0	19	1
Clarke et al., 1990	Leeds	56	F	12–16	19	11	7	9	5	0
Opaneye and Willmott, 1991	Birmingham	159	F	13–16	75	10	12	9	13	4
Fitzpatrick et al., 1992	Dublin	32	F	15–19	71.9	3	6	0	18.8	0
Young and Keane, 1992	Leicester	183	M+F	<16	36	4	20	–	12	4
Williams, 1992	Clwyd	88	M+F	16–19	100	9	35	–	50	6

GC, = N. gonorrhoea; CT, = C. trachomatis; TV, = T. vaginalis; HPV, = human papilloma virus (anogenital warts); HSV, = herpes simplex virus (genital herpes).

may influence behaviour and condom use (Weisman *et al.*, 1991; Mellanby *et al.*, 1992).

From a biological perspective, the cervix in the physically mature woman provides defence mechanisms against ascending infection and subsequent pelvic inflammatory disease (PID). Cervical mucus production and humoral-immunity are absent until ovulation begins, thus potentiating the risk of such complications in the adolescent. The columnar epithelium generally extends from the endo-cervical canal onto the porto-vaginalis of the cervix in early puberty. Exposure to oncogenic pathogens such as HPV, enhances the risk of dyskaryosis and carcinoma at an early age (Mosciki *et al.*, 1989).

Combination of all these factors enhances the vulnerability of the young females' reproductive tract and sexual health.

PRESENTATION OF SEXUALLY TRANSMITTED INFECTIONS IN ADOLESCENTS

In the majority of cases, the presentation of an STD is similar to that seen in the adult. Asymptomatic infection and the co-existence of several sexually transmitted infections is common. Hence, comprehensive screening facilities should be available to the physicians involved in the reproductive and sexual health of the young woman. The ability to contact trace partners and offer health education is essential. If such facilities are unavailable, referral to a Department of Genito-urinary Medicine (GUM) is recommended. The following sections will outline specific aspects of each STD. For more comprehensive information, reference to a major text is recommended (Holmes *et al.*, 1990).

Gonorrhoea

Despite the recent decline in reported cases of *Neisseria gonorrhoea* in the United Kingdom, it remains an important pathogen (Catchpole, 1992). One third of all female cases of post-pubertal gonorrhoea occurred in those under the age of 20 years, between 1988–92 (see Summary Information form KC60, 1992). The incidence amongst female adolescent STD clinic attenders is around 20% (Thin *et al.*, 1989). Females in residential care are particularly at risk of infection (Mulcalchy and Lacey, 1987).

Asymptomatic carriage is particularly common in adolescents. Failure to recognise and treat appropriately leads to PID in 15% of infected teenagers, others will progress to disseminated disease (Hedberg and Anberg, 1965).

Acquisition of *N. gonorrhoea* may be secondary to voluntary sexual activity, sexual assault or abuse. Fomite spread has been reported in children (Blackwell and Eykyn, 1986), but not in adolescents.

N. gonorrhoea is identified by the presence of Gram negative intracellular diplococci on Gram staining, and by culture. The organism infects columnar epithelium, so the immature cervix of the adolescent is readily colonised. The urethra, rectum and oropharynx may also be involved.

Once infected, the majority – an estimated 85% of females – will be asymptomatic. Vulvar itching, a minor vaginal discharge, urethritis and proctitis have been reported after an incubation period of between 2–5 days. In pre-pubescent girls, a purulent vulvovaginitis may occur. Symptoms suggestive of salpingitis/PID occur when the organism has ascended the genital tract. PID in the adolescent, is particularly likely to cause tubal occlusion and resultant infertility (Hedberg and Anberg, 1965). A combination of the following signs and symptoms – lower abdominal pain and tenderness, cervical motion pain 'excitation' and adnexal tenderness all support a clinical diagnosis of PID. Fever, a raised white cell count, elevated (ESR) and an adnexal mass at ultrasonography support the diagnosis. Laparoscopy and screening for pathogens should be considered before laparotomy (Kalm *et al.*, 1991).

Therapeutic intervention depends on the age, pregnancy status and presence of complications. In uncomplicated adult orogenital infection, Ciprofloxacin 500 mg as a single oral dose is recommended. It is contra-indicated during pregnancy and is not yet recommended in children by the manufacturer. Ceftriaxone 250 mg im, or Spectinomycin 2 g im, both as a single dose, may be used. As a large proportion of gonococcal isolates worldwide are now resistant to penicillin and tetracycline, these are no longer recommended for the treatment of gonorrhoea.

As co-infection with *Chlamydia trachomatis* occurs in 45% of individuals infected with gonorrhoea, it is prudent to screen for it and treat with doxycycline 100 mg bd for 7 days, or erythromycin 250 mg qid also for 7 days (Fraser *et al.*, 1983).

In complicated cases, where salpingitis has developed, hospitalisation is recommended as compliance is notoriously low in this age group. There are several recommended drug regimens, and these should cover for *N. gonorrhoea*, *Chlamydia trachomatis* and anaerobes, e.g. ciproxin 500 mg bd for 2 days or spectinomycin 1 g im qid for 2 days, plus doxycycline 100 mg orally or iv bd for 14 days, plus metronidazole 400 mg qid orally for 1 week.

Management of gonococcal infection is not complete without screening and treating sexual partners, an area often neglected when individuals are diagnosed outside the genito-urinary medicine department.

Chlamydia

Chlamydia trachomatis is more common in adolescence than *N. gonorrhoea* (Fraser *et al.*, 1983). The prevalence is high among sexually active adolescents with reports of between 10–34% of those screened (Chacko and Lorchik, 1984; Robinson *et al.*, 1985; Mulcalchy and Lacey, 1987; Thin *et al.*, 1989; Clarke *et al.*, 1990; Opaneye and Willmott, 1991; Fitzpatrick *et al.*, 1992; Young and Keene, 1992; Williams, unpublished data). This is similar to gonorrhoea in that the majority of females infected are asymptomatic, and also that there is a high risk of developing PID (Fraser *et al.*, 1983). Chlamydia is a major factor in infertility by virtue of being a common STD. It is thought to be responsible for a condition known as silent PID, where resultant infertility occurs without any signs or symptoms of PID (Moore and Cates, 1990).

It is usually sexually acquired, but vertically acquired chlamydial disease – ophthalmia neonatorum, infant pneumonia and vulvar vaginitis are well documented in infants. The organism has been isolated from the vagina for up to 1 year following birth (Bell *et al.*, 1986) but one must strongly suspect sexual abuse or voluntary sexual activity in adolescence.

Symptoms which may alert the physician to chlamydial infection in the adolescent are inter-menstrual bleeding, post-coital bleeding and occasionally an increase in vaginal secretions (Fig. 10.1).

Occasionally, confusion occurs if the young girl is going through her menarche or has started on the oral contraceptive pill. However, the majority of infected women are asymptomatic. Due to the asymptomatic nature of the

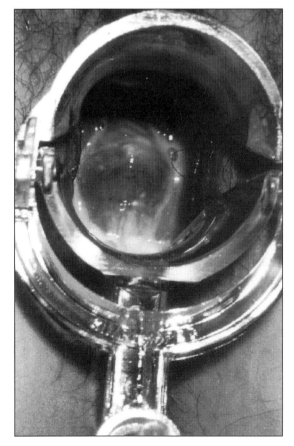

Fig. 10.1   Vaginal discharge in an adolescent girl typical of the appearance of chlamydia infection.

infection, screening all sexually active adolescents may be advisable (Hughes *et al.*, 1989), especially girls who present seeking contraceptive advice, during pregnancy, or are requesting termination of pregnancy.

Termination of pregnancy can promote ascending chlamydial infection with resultant PID. Untreated chlamydia during pregnancy puts the neonate at risk of ophthalmia neonatorum and chlamydial pneumonitis.

There are several diagnostic tests for *Chlamydia trachomatis* (Taylor-Robinson and Thomas, 1991). The 'Gold Standard' is tissue culture and this should always be used if sexual abuse is suspected, as the other tests ELISA, and direct immuno-fluorescent or polymerase chain reaction (PCR), may give false positive results. The most common site from which to isolate chlamydia is from the cervix; however, urethral carriage may occur. Serological tests such as micro immuno-fluorescence can be used, but are of little significance without a positive tissue culture or ELISA test.

The recommended treatment for chlamydial infection is doxycycline 100 mg bd for 7 days. In children and during pregnancy, tetracyclines should be avoided and erythromycin 250 mg qid for 7 days should be used. The penicillins and cephalosporines are ineffective and have no role in the treatment of chlamydial disease. Chlamydial PID should be managed with bed rest and 14 days of oral doxycycline 100 mg bd, plus metronidazole 400 mg qid for 7 days. There is evidence to suggest that, despite adequate treatment, on-going damage to the fallopian tubes can occur secondary to chlamydial PID.

Syphilis

Current statistics for syphilis in the United Kingdom show a dramatic change compared to 20 years ago. In 1992, only 18 female adolescents were reported to be suffering from the infection (see Summary Information form KC60, 1992). Screening for syphilis still remains a vital part of monitoring its prevalence and is done in GUM clinics, the antenatal and blood donation clinics. Discontinuation of antenatal screening in the USA in 1986 saw a 500% rise in congenital syphilis by 1988 (see MMWR, 1989). This has also been associated with a change in epidemiology of the disease; syphilis is now associated with inner-city deprivation, black ethnicity and drug use, especially cocaine, and consequent 'sex for drugs'.

The characteristic presentation of syphilis is seen in the adolescent as in the adult. They present with primary chancre, secondary syphilis, latent syphilis or positive syphilis serology as the only evidence of infection (Rawson *et al.*, 1993).

Management is best left to a specialist/GUM physician, as decisions as to whether the adolescent has congenital or acquired syphilis needs to be made.

Genital Warts

Ano-genital warts are due to sexually transmitted HPV, Types 6, 11, 16, 18, 31 and 35. They are the most common STD in the adolescent age group with over

6000 cases reported in 1992 in England (see Summary Information form KC60, 1992). There has been a huge rise in the incidence of genital warts and a resultant growing awareness of the oncogenic potential of the virus.

Ano-genital warts present as condylomatous, papular or flat (subclinical) lesions (Fig. 10.2). The classical condylomata is soft and fleshy and is found in moist areas such as the vaginal introitus, urethra, perianal and perineal areas. During pregnancy and in immuno-suppressed adolescents, they can become very large. The papular genital warts are flatter and slightly keratinised, whereas flat lesions are those that are only identified with magnification on application of dilute 5% glacio-acetic acid, when the lesions show up as white patches on infected skin. Genital warts must be differentiated from molluscum contagiosum, skin tags, naevae, neurofibromata and other benign tumours. Condylomata lata, seen in secondary syphilis, also resemble warts, and despite being rare, syphilis should be excluded by the appropriate laboratory tests.

Clinical examination is a poor predictor of the HPV type, this requires specific geno-type probe, only available in certain centres (deVilliers, 1992). However, if

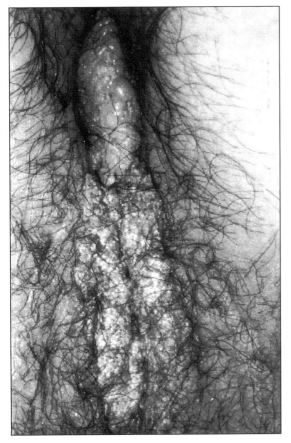

Fig. 10.2   Genital warts in an adolescent girl with a history of sexual abuse.

abuse is suspected and the suspected assailant also has genital warts, viral typing may prove helpful (Oriel, 1992). Screening for other STDs is recommended.

Treatment involves chemical destruction of the warts by a topical cytotoxic agent such as Podophyllin, physical destruction with trichloracetic acid, cryotherapy or CO_2 laser. Follow-up is indicated as warts often recur and condom use should be stressed. Adolescent girls with genital warts should have regular cervical cytology and cytological follow-up at yearly intervals for at least 5 years.

Genital Herpes

Genital herpes is the most common cause of sexually transmitted genital ulcer disease. Over the past 10 years, there has been a 80% rise in new cases reported. With 17% of all female primary HSV infections occurring in women aged under 19 years, this puts this population at a greater risk of HIV infection. Genital ulcer disease can act as a co-factor in the transition of the HIV virus (Piot and Laga, 1989).

Both HSV Types 1 and 2 give rise to genital herpes. Genital herpes usually presents between 5 and 7 days post infection. Symptoms are initially mild; the patient may complain of a tingling sensation on the affected site which is then followed by the appearance of vesicles, which rapidly break down to give rise to painful ulcers (Fig. 10.3). Dysuria, vaginal discharge, vulvar oedema and painful swollen inguinal lymph nodes, and a flu-like illness with meningism may be features of the attack. Urinary retention occurs secondary to sacral radiculopathy in severe cases. Symptoms may take up to 2 weeks to subside.

Management should include accurate diagnosis; swabs from the lesion should be taken as early as possible during an attack to maximise virus isolation; culture and typing for both HSV1 and HSV2 is preferable. Other sexually transmitted infections should be excluded. Antiviral therapy should be commenced as early as possible with acyclovir 200 mg × 5 times daily for 5 days. Adequate analgesia should be prescribed and practical advice as regards micturating in a warm bath of water, wearing loose clothing and bed rest should be given. Retention of urine should be managed by suprapubic catheterisation. Unless co-existence of other pathogens is evident, antibiotics are not usually necessary.

Recurrent genital herpes occurs more frequently with HSV type 2. Predicting who will progress to recurrent disease is impossible. Certain trigger factors have been found, namely, sexual intercourse, stress, immuno-suppression and illness. Management of recurrent genital herpes involves assessing frequency and severity of attacks and the psychological impact of the disease. Disease suppression by use of antiviral products should be considered on an individual basis. Currently, acyclovir 400 mg daily for a period of up to 1 year, has been used successfully (Mindel *et al.*, 1984).

The incidence of psychological problems secondary to genital herpes, is very high (Carney *et al.*, 1994). Therefore in the adolescent girl who acquires herpes, it is important that she is given adequate counselling and correct information

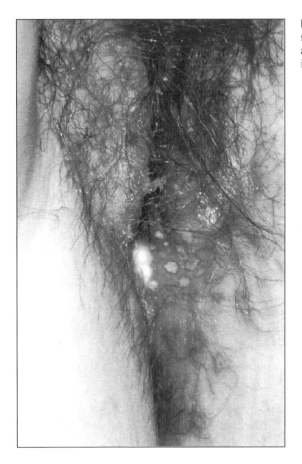

Fig. 10.3 Typical appearance of shallow ulcers on the vulva of an adolescent with Herpes simplex infection.

about the disease. It is important to inform her that she is only infectious to a sexual partner when she is actively shedding the virus i.e. when she has an acute attack. As regards pregnancy, the risk of vertical transmission is around 3% and only occurs in women who, at the time of delivery, are actually shedding the herpes virus.

Vaginal Infections

It is essential for a systematic approach to be used in the management of the adolescent complaining of vaginal discharge (Adler, 1992).

Use of a flow chart may be of value (Fig. 10.4). It is also prudent to screen for sexually transmitted pathogens if the adolescent has had a change of sexual partner recently.

Trichomonas vaginalis, candidiasis and bacterial vaginosis are the 3 usual pathological causes of vaginal discharge. Other causes include retained tampons,

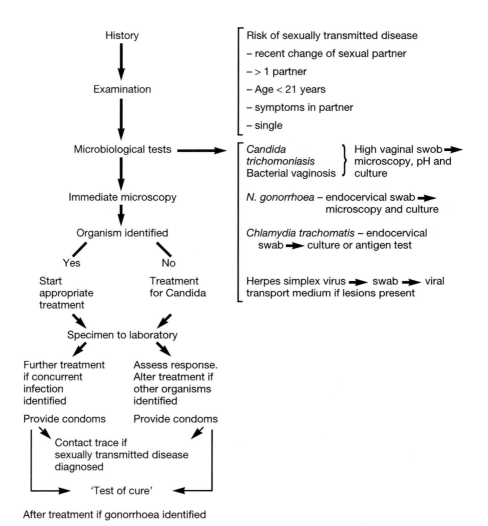

Fig. 10.4   Management of vaginal discharge.

other foreign bodies, cervical ectopy, secondary to cervical infections such as gonorrhoea or chlamydia and physiological discharges. An adolescent girl may have anxieties regarding the presence of vaginal discharge or staining of underwear, which is worse at mid-cycle and during sexual arousal. Reassurance that this is probably a physiological discharge is essential, otherwise anxieties may persist into adult life and psychosexual problems could develop. However, if the individual is at risk of a STD, screening should be carried out. Occasionally, adolescent girls complain of post-coital vaginal discharge, only to be embarrassed to discover that ejaculate is fluid in nature!

Trichomonas

Trichomonas vaginalis is a sexually transmitted pathogen. This protozoan causes an offensive malodorous vaginal discharge with vulvar soreness and irritation. On examination, there is usually marked vulvovaginitis; the cervix may exhibit red punctations. Although the discharge is classically described as being 'frothy' it is not always so.

Diagnosis is made on examining a wet preparation of the discharge under a light microscopy and by culture (high vaginal swab). Occasionally the pathogen can be identified at cervical cytology. As it is an STD, screening for other STD pathogens is essential. Metronidazole 200 mg tds orally for 7 days is the standard treatment, however, a single oral dose of 2 g metronidazole is also effective. It is also important that alcohol is avoided while taking this medication. An alternative, but less effective method of treatment which is safe in pregnancy, is clotrimazole pessaries. Sexual partners must be treated concurrently. Recurrence of symptoms may be due to poor compliance, failure to treat the partner or resistance to metronidazole.

Candida

Candida albicans, a yeast, is a common vaginal pathogen. It is not sexually transmitted, but the sexual partner may develop symptoms. It is uncommon in adolescent girls prior to puberty.

Classically the adolescent girl presents with vulvitis and an associated 'cottage cheese-like' discharge. She may also complain of dyspareunia, a perianal soreness and fissuring at the introitus. Itching is also a common symptom. Infection may be precipitated by antibiotic therapy, pregnancy, diabetes and immuno-suppression. Attacks of candida/vulvitis may be cyclical in nature and correspond to menstruation.

Diagnosis is made from microscopy of vaginal discharge which will show pseudohyphae and spores. Gram staining will demonstrate the hyphae spores as Gram positive structures. These occasionally are apparent on cervical cytology. Culture of the discharge on Sabouraud's medium will also aid diagnosis. Treatment may be local using nystatin, clotrimazole, miconazole or econazole, in the form of pessaries, vaginal cream or local application cream in either multiple or single doses. Oral therapy using fluconazole 150 mg stat dose is probably worth considering in adolescent girls who have recurrent proven candidal vulvitis. In all cases, it may be wise to investigate for underlying causes such as diabetes.

It is important that adolescent girls who complain of symptoms suggestive of candidal vulvitis, are examined, as often the symptoms of itching and discharge could also be attributed to genital herpes, *Trichomonas vaginalis* or a chemical vulvitis. Occasionally, women who have candidal vulvitis also have episodes of bacterial vaginosis sequentially and it is important to recognise this, as the bacterial vaginosis will not respond to anticandidal therapy.

Bacterial Vaginosis

Bacterial vaginosis is thought not to be a STD although it tends to be found in women who have been sexually active. It has been reported in adolescent girls without any evidence of sexual activity.

Our increasing awareness of this condition, has highlighted that it may be implicated in premature rupture of membranes in a pregnant woman and endometritis. Essentially, it is a polymicrobial condition where the predominant lactobacilli found in the vagina, are replaced by mixed flora to include *Gardnerella vaginalis*, Bacteroides SPP, Mobiluncus and occasionally Mycoplasma. Symptoms if present, are of a thin, grey, malodorous vaginal discharge which, after sexual intercourse, may be particularly fishy in odour. There is no associated vulvitis therefore the patient will not complain of itching or soreness.

Diagnosis is made on microscopy. Gram stain smears show clue cells. These are normal epithelial cells coated with small Gram variable rods. Lactobacilli are rare. The pH of the vagina is usually raised and is greater than 4.5. The amine test is usually positive. Culture is not necessary to confirm the diagnosis. Treatment is usually indicated in girls who have symptoms. Metronidazole in a single dose of 2 g or as a 1-week therapy at 200 mg tds may be used. Clindamycin 2% vaginal cream nightly for 7 nights may also be used. There is no evidence that treating the sexual partner will have an effect on patient's recurrences.

Foreign Bodies

The retained tampon causes an offensive mucopurulent vaginal discharge with associated vulvitis. Quite often the young girl will have forgotten to remove the last tampon used and symptoms will appear around 1–2 weeks post-menstruation. Examination and removal of the tampon is essential. Metronidazole 200 mg tds for 7 days will cover the anaerobic colonisation that will have occurred in the vagina. Other foreign bodies are not uncommon, either placed there as part of the sexual act or as part of self-harm (Figs 10.5 and 10.6). Again, removal of these foreign bodies will relieve symptoms.

HIV Infection

In the United Kingdom to date, the incidence of acquired immuno deficiency syndrome (AIDS) and HIV in female adolescents is very low. In 1991 and 1992 the percentage of asymptomatic HIV positive girls aged 16–19 years presenting to GUM clinics for the first time, was 0.7 and 0.5% respectively. They, however, represented 4.3% and 2.8% of the total number of positive women presenting in those years. By the end of March 1992, only 0.4% of the 2 183 018 positive patients in the United States were teenagers. However, 19.5% AIDS patients were aged between 20 and 29 years (Bowler *et al.*, 1992; see Centres for Disease Control, 1991a).

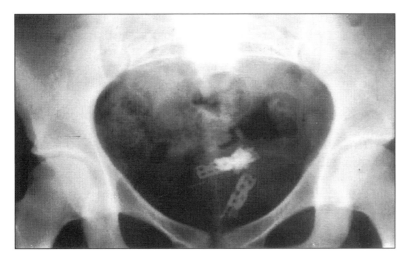

Fig. 10.5 X-Ray of the pelvis showing razor blades placed there as an act of self-harm. (Courtesy of Dr Sheila Moss).

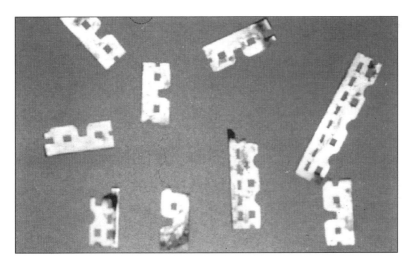

Fig. 10.6 The razor blades after removal under general anaesthetic. (Courtesy of Dr Sheila Moss).

As the average incubation period of HIV infection is 8 years and it is likely that many of these young adults became infected as adolescents. In the United States, it appears that adolescents are more likely to have acquired their infection heterosexually than adults (9% vs 4%). More HIV positive adolescents are female than male (14% vs 7%) as they are physiologically more vulnerable. They are usually black or Hispanic. Barriers to HIV/AIDS prevention and treatment exist. The risk of acquiring HIV is higher in those adolescents who engage in unprotected sex, have multiple sexual partners, share injecting drug equipment and have sex with a 'high risk' person. Poverty, social and cultural barriers and the lack of, or inadequate, health care services for adolescents, potentiate the problems. Denial, 'it happens to others' and other coping mechanisms occur.

The implications of teenage girls being infected with HIV are serious (Williams, 1992), as these individuals become the mothers of tomorrow and may infect their babies via vertical transmission. In New York, 0.7% of teenage women delivering live births are HIV positive. The probability of these babies being infected varies between 13 and 30%.

No significant gynaecological, menstrual, endocrine or reproductive problems arise in females who are HIV positive (Shah *et al.*, 1994). However, there are reports of increased progression rate of CIN in immuno-suppressed women, but the incidence of cervical cancer is rare, as death secondary to the manifestations of AIDS occurs before advanced cervical disease. Annual cytology, however, is advisable.

As there is no effective cure of HIV infection, prevention strategies are imperative. All adolescents should be aware of the mechanism of transmission of HIV and be able to negotiate safer sexual practices such as condom use for penetrative sexual intercourse, and to avoid drugs (Ford, 1992).

Sexually Transmitted Diseases and Rape

The risk of acquiring an STD as a result of rape is unknown due to a multiplicity of factors. The prevalence of rate of STDs in women having been raped has been reported as being between 3.5 and 56% (Murphy, 1990; Jenny *et al.*, 1990). As the age of the majority of rape victims is between 15 and 35 years, corresponding to the same age as the population at highest risk of acquiring a STD, it is important to differentiate between infections existing prior to the assault and those acquired during it. Consequently, documentation of the type of assault, whether or not ejaculation occurred and a sexual history both prior to and subsequent to the incident, is important. The risk of HIV infection should also be assessed as, in many cases, the assailant is known.

All victims should be offered comprehensive STD screening including screening and counselling for HIV infection. Timing of the STD screen must take into account the incubation time of pathogens. It is, therefore, prudent to screen near the time of the assault, 1 week later and again at 3 months, for HIV testing. Some authorities believe that an STD present for up to 72 hours following rape (Murphy, 1990), is a pre-existing infection and this should be borne in mind.

Treatment is directed at whether an infection is isolated as per current guidelines. Prophylactic antibiotics may be offered, especially if the assailant has an infection or if there are signs or symptoms in the victim. Ciprofloxacin 500 mg as a stat oral dose to cover gonorrhoea, followed by doxycycline 100 mg bd for 7 days to cover chlamydial infections, has been recommended.

If there is a risk of pregnancy and the person is seen within 72 hours of the attack, post-coital contraception in the form of Shearing PC4 is advisable (see p. 343). The intrauterine contraceptive device (IUCD) is best avoided due to the risk of disseminating lower genital tract infections. Follow up is essential to provide further screening, advice as regards pregnancy, counselling and HIV testing, also psychological support.

Sexually Transmitted Infections and Sexual Abuse

The presence of a sexually transmitted infection in an adolescent who denies voluntary sexual activity may be secondary to sexual abuse and should be managed appropriately. It is also important that adolescents who report sexual abuse, have the opportunity to be screened for STDs and HIV. Not only might the examination provide important forensic evidence but it is also important for its own sake, as the psychological, psychosexual and physical consequences of having an untreated STD are self-evident.

CONCLUSION

It is important that all adolescents are given accurate and clear information about sexual health. There should be open access, well publicised, confidential adolescent medicine clinics run by a multidisciplinary team. These clinics should offer STD screening, HIV counselling and testing, contraception advice, pregnancy testing, abortion counselling, advice on substance misuse, health education and psychological support, tailored to meet the specific needs of adolescents. Currently, the worried adolescent may access numerous services, before obtaining the appropriate health care.

It is of utmost importance that these services offer patient confidentiality, as young people entering into their sexual activity, sometimes as a means of asserting their independence, despise any parental involvement. Therefore, if teenagers suspect that their parents will be informed about any aspect of their sexual behaviour, they will be reluctant to attend these services and subsequently suffer the consequences of delayed diagnosis. Parental involvement should be encouraged but bringing undue pressure is likely to be counter-productive.

As in all aspects of good STD control, partner notification is important. Tracing sexual partners decreases the likelihood of recurrent infection once sex is resumed following treatment. It also prevents further disease transmission. The psychological effects of STD in adolescents should not be dismissed. Despite being in an era where permissiveness is allowed, a certain amount of guilt and shame is still associated with contracting a STD and, if not treated appropriately, may develop into a psychosexual problem later in life.

REFERENCES

Adler M, 1992: *ABC of sexually transmitted diseases*. BMJ publications.

Bell TA, Stamm WE, Kuo CG, *et al.* 1986: Chronic Chlamydia trachomatis infections in Chlamydial infections. In Oriel JD, (ed.), Cambridge: Cambridge University Press, 305–308.

Blackwell AL, Eykyn SJ, 1986: Paediatric gonorrhoea: non-venereal epidemic in a household. *Genito-urinary Medicine* **62**, 228–229.

Bowler S, Sheon AB, D'Angelo LJ, Vermund SI, 1992: HIV and AIDS among adolescents in the United States: increasing risk in the 1990's. *Journal of Adolescence* **15**, 345–371.

Catchpole MA, 1992: Sexually transmitted diseases in England and Wales: 1981–1990. *Communicable Disease Report* **2**, R1–R6.

Carney O, Ross E, Ikkes G, Mundel A, 1994: A parospective study of the psychological impact on patients with first episode genital herpes. *Genito-urinary Medicine* **70**, 40–45.

Centres for Disease Control (1991) HIV/AIDS October 1991, Atlanta GA.

Chacko MR, Lovchik JC, 1984: *Chlamydia trachomatis* infection in sexually active adolescents: prevalence and risk factors. *Pediatrics* **73**, 836–840.

Clarke J, Abram R, Monteiro E, 1990: The sexual behaviour and knowledge about AIDS in a group of young adolescent girls in Leeds. *Genito-urinary Medicine* **66**, 189–192.

Congenital syphilis – New York City 1986–1988. 1989: *MMWR* **38**, 825–982.

Curtis HA, Lawrence CJ, Tripp JH, 1988: Teenage and sexual intercourse and pregnancy. *Archives of Disease in Childhood* **63**, 373–379.

Duncan E, Tibanx A, Pelzer A, *et al.* 1990: First coitus before menarche and risk of sexually transmitted disease. *Lancet* **335**, 338–340.

de Villiers EM, 1992: Laboratory techniques in the investigation of Human papilloma virus infection. *Genito-urinary Medicine* **68**, 50–54.

Fitzpatrick C, McKenna P, Hone R, 1992: Teenage girls attending a Dublin sexually transmitted disease clinic: a socio-sexual and diagnostic profile. *Irish Journal of Medical Science* **161**, 460–462.

Ford N, 1992: The AIDS awareness and sexual behaviour of young people in South West England. *Journal of Adolescence* **15**, 393–413.

Fraser H, Retig PT, Kaplan DW, 1983: Prevalence of cervical *Chlamydia Trachomatis* and *Neisseria gonorrhoea* in female adolescents. *Pediatrics* **71**, 333–336.

Greenberg J, Magder J, Aral S, 1992: Age at first coitus. A marker for risky sexual behaviour in women. *Sexually Transmitted Diseases* **19**, 331–334.

Hedberg E, Anberg A, 1965: Gonococcal salpingitis: views on treatment and prognosis. *Fertility and Sterility* **16**, 125–129.

Holmes KK, Märdh P, Sparling PF, *et al.* 1990: Sexually transmitted disease. New York: McCuran Hill Inc.

Hughes EG, Maratt J, Spence JE, 1989: Endocervical Chlamydia trachomatis in Canadian adolescents. *Canadian Medical Association Journal* **140**, 297–301.

Jenny C, Hooton T, Bowers A, *et al.* 1990: Sexually transmitted disease in victims of rape. *New England Journal of Medicine* **322**, 713–716.

Kalm JG, Walker CK, Washington EA, *et al.* 1991: Diagnosing pelvic inflammatory disease – a comprehensive analysis and consideration for developing a new model. *JAMA* **266**, 2594–2604.

Mellanby A, Phelps F, Lawrence C, Tripp JH, 1992: Teenagers and the risks of sexually transmitted diseases: a need for the provision of balanced information. *Genito-urinary Medicine* **68**, 241–244.

Mindel A, Faherty A, Hindley D, *et al.* 1984: Prophylactic oral acyclovir in recurrent genital herpes. *Lancet* **ii**, 57–59.

Moore DE, Cates W Jr, 1990: Sexually transmitted diseases and infertility. In Holmes KK, Mardh PA, Sparling FP, *et al.* (eds), *Sexually transmitted diseases.* New York: McGraw-Hill.

Mosciki AB, Winkler B, Irwm CE, Jr, Schachter J, 1989: Differences in biologic maturation, sexual behaviour with and sexually transmitted disease between adolescents with and without cervical intra-epithelial neoplasia. *Paediatrics* **115**, 487–493.

Mulcalchy FM, Lacey CJN, 1987: Sexually transmitted infections in adolescent girls. *Genito-urinary Medicine* **63**, 119–121.

Murphy SM, 1990: Rape, sexually transmitted disease and human immuno deficiency virus infection. *International Journal on STD and AIDS* **1**, 79–82.

New cases seen at NHS Genito-urinary Medicine Clinic in England – Summary information from form KC60 1992; DOM 1992.

Opaneye AA, Willmott C, 1991: The role of genito-urinary medicine in adolescent sexuality. *Genito-urinary Medicine* **67**, 44–46

Oriel JD, 1992: Sexually transmitted diseases in children: human papilloma virus infection. *Genito-urinary Medicine* **68**, 80–83.

Orr DP, Wilbrandt ML, Brack CJ, *et al.* 1989: Reported sexual behaviour and self-esteem amongst young adolescents. *American Journal of Diseases of Children* **143**, 86–90.

Persson E, Jarlbro G, 1992: Sexual behaviour amongst your clinic visitors in Sweden: knowledge and experiences in an HIV perspective. *Genito-urinary Medicine* **68**, 26–31.

Piot P, Laga MM, 1989: Genital ulcers, other sexually transmitted diseases and the sexual transmission of HIV. *British Medical Journal* **298**, 623–624.

Rawson SA, Bromberg K, Hammerschlay MR, 1993: STD in children: syphilis and gonorrhoea. *Genito-urinary Medicine* **69**, 66–75.

Robinson AE, Forster GE, Munday PE, 1985: The changing pattern of sexually transmitted disease in adolescent girls. *Genito-urinary Medicine* **61**, 130–132.

Shah PN, Smith JR, Kitchen VS, Barton SE, 1994: HIV infection and the gynaecologist. *British Journal of Obstetrics and Gynaecology* **101**, 187–189.

Taylor-Robinson D, Thomas BJ, 1991: Laboratory techniques for the diagnosis of chlamydial infections. *Genito-urinary Medicine* **67**, 256–266.

Thin RN, Whatley JD, Blackwell AL, 1989: STD and contraception in adolescents. *Genito-urinary Medicine* **65**, 157–160.

Tracen B, Lewin B, Sundet JM, 1992: Use of birth control pill and condoms among 17–19 year old adolescents in Norway: contraceptive versus protective behaviour? *AIDS Care* **4**, 371–380.

Weisman CS, Plichta S, Nathanson C, Ensminger M, Robinson JC, 1991: Consistency of condom use for disease prevention among adolescent users or oral contraceptives. *Family Planning Perspective* **23**(2), 71–74.

Williams OE, 1992: HIV, the consequences in Women Postgraduate Doctors.

Williams OE: Incidence of STD in females and males under 19 years of age in Clwyd. (Unpubl. data).

Young SM, Keane FEA, 1992: Children seen by Leicester genito-urinary medicine physician 1988–1990. *Genito-urinary Medicine* **68**, 423.

CHAPTER 11

Female genital mutilation

SANDRA D'SILVA ────────────────────────────

Female genital mutilation is a complex and painful issue which embraces aspects of sexuality, health, education and human rights – the rights of women and children and the right to development. The continuation of the practice offers a challenge to all who support the safety and well being of women and children.

Paediatricians, general practitioners and gynaecologists who work in areas where the practice is encountered should have an understanding of the physical and psychological consequences of the procedure and of the ways it may affect a girl's gynaecological health.

THE PRACTICE

Female genital mutilation (see definitions following) is practised in 26 African countries from the Atlantic to the Red Sea, and from the Indian Ocean to the eastern Mediterranean. The prevalence in these areas varies from 5 to 99% (Toubia, 1994). Excision is also practised in Oman, South Yemen and in the United Arab Emirates. Circumcision is practised by the Muslim populations of Indonesia, Malaysia and East Africa, and Boar Muslims in India and Pakistan. It is more associated with the ethnic group than with the geographical area. Because of the secrecy associated with the practice, there are few data available on the incidence in the United Kingdom which varies with the numbers of people from ethnic groups within any local population. The common practice in the United Kingdom is for girls from areas where mutilation is practised to return to their country of origin during school holidays and have the operation carried out while they are there. There have been reports of back street practitioners in the United Kingdom but these have not been substantiated. The age at which mutilations are carried out vary from birth to during the first pregnancy depending on the area. The age at which it is encountered in the United Kingdom appears to becoming younger (Dorkenoo and Elworthy, 1992).

TYPES OF MUTILATIONS

The type of procedure performed also varies with the ethnic group. Four main types are encountered.

1. Circumcision or cutting off the prepuce of the hood of the clitoris known in Muslim countries as Sunna (Dorozynski, 1994).
2. Excision, meaning the cutting of the clitoris and all or part of the labia minora.
3. Infibulation – the cutting of the clitoris, labia minora and at least the anterior two thirds if not the whole of the medial part of the labia majora. The two sides of the vulva are then pinned together by sutures or thorns, thus obliterating the vaginal introitus except for a very small opening preserved by the insertion of a piece of wood to allow the passage of urine or menstrual blood (Fig. 11.1).
4. Intermediate, meaning the removal of the clitoris and varying amounts of the labia majora or minora.

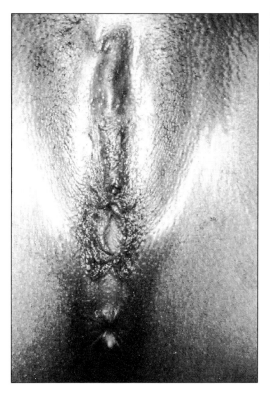

Fig. 11.1   Infibulation performed on an adolescent Somali girl. The clitoris has been removed along with a large part of the labia minora which have been stitched together leaving only a small space for urine and menstrual blood to pass.

MOTIVES FOR FEMALE GENITAL MUTILATION

Customs and beliefs surrounding the various forms of female genital mutilation are widespread and more research needs to be done to understand the motives.

Psychosexual

There is deep-rooted mythological belief in some parts of the world such as Mali, Nigeria, and Kenya that the clitoris is 'the attenuation of sexual desire' (Dorkenoo and Elworthy, 1992). Excision is believed to protect the woman against her oversexed nature, while preserving her chastity.

Religious

While religious arguments are often quoted to justify the practice of female genital mutilation, Dr Taha Ba'asher (1978) in a World Health Organisation (WHO) report clarifies the position that there is no basis in any of the world religions for the practice of female genital mutilation.

Sociological

In many areas (such as Northern Sudan, Kikuyu in Kenya, Banbara in Mali), female genital mutilation is a practice associated with initiation rites and development into adulthood.

In many societies, female virginity is an absolute prerequisite for marriage. A non-infibulated girl, at best, will stand little chance of getting married and, at worst, will be ridiculed and may be forced to leave her community.

Hygiene

In countries towards the east of Africa (Egypt, Sudan, Somalia, Ethiopia), the external genitalia are considered dirty. The uncircumcised girl is therefore considered unclean and rejected by her community.

PHYSICAL CONSEQUENCES

Most frequently, the operations are performed by old women in the village. Except in hospital, anaesthetics are rarely used. The instruments are rarely sterilised. Health risks and complications depend on the degree of the mutilation, hygienic conditions and the skill and eyesight of the operator. The immediate consequences will probably not be seen by medical personnel in the West, but the long-term complications will.

IMMEDIATE COMPLICATIONS

According to recent documentation from the WHO, the most frequent complications that follow female genital mutilation are: severe pain; haemorrhage from the internal pudendal artery or the dorsal artery of the clitoris; urinary retention due to tissue trauma, pain or local oedema; infection of the wound from the procedure being performed in crude, unsterile conditions; and damage to adjacent tissues and organs. Few records of the immediate effects of female genital mutilation are recorded or reported.

LONG-TERM COMPLICATIONS

The most common long-term complications likely to present to a doctor in this country are recurrent urinary tract infections and dysmenorrhoea. It should always be considered that a girl or adolescent might have undergone female genital mutilation if she presents with these symptoms and is from a community where the practice is known to be widespread. The symptoms occur due to the inability of urine or menstrual blood to escape freely due to the infibulation. Pelvic inflammatory disease (PID) may also ensue due to the retention and subsequent infection of menstrual blood. Other long-term complications which may occur are keloid formation and the growth of implantation dermoid cysts along the scar line. The latter may vary in size from a few millimetres to as large as grapefruit.

These adolescents and women, of course, have severe dyspareunia. Very little research has been done on the sexual experiences of mutilated women but one report suggested that some mutilated women had never experienced an orgasm (Ba'asher, 1978). One author with experience of working in the Sudan reported that many infibulated women (and presumably adolescents) have a syndrome of chronic anxiety and depression arising from worry over the state of their genitals, intractable dysmenorrhoea and fear of infertility (Toubia, 1994). Further complications may arise as a result of childbirth which are outside the scope of this book.

HIV TRANSMISSION

There is also a risk of HIV infection particularly in areas with high prevalence of the virus. The use of one instrument in multiple operations conveys a high risk of transmission of infection.

PSYCHOLOGICAL CONSEQUENCES

There are few data on the psychological aspects of female genital mutilation. Ba'asher states:

> It is quite obvious that the mere notion of surgical interference in the highly sensitive genital organs constitutes a serious threat to the child and that painful trauma is a source of major physical as well as psychological trauma (Ba'asher, 1978).

The psychological consequences of female circumcision among immigrants differ from those where the practice is prevalent. Circumcised girls living in societies where the procedure is not performed may have serious problems in developing their sexual identity (Toubia, 1994).

Many girls experience anxiety, fear and terror from being seized in the middle of the night by a trusted adult, the unbearable pain and feeling of betrayal by parents, particularly the mother. There is great deal of confusion in the girl's mind because the ceremony is associated with good food and presents so that she has difficulty in coping with the differing signals of pain and pleasure. In addition, the girls are often separated from their parents, with their feet tied together, until the wound heals which adds to their pain and confusion.

Conversely, however, if community pressure is put on the child to believe that the clitoris is dirty, she will feel relieved to have the procedure performed and to be made like everyone else.

In the United Kingdom, female genital mutilation can be used by families as a powerful weapon to control a girl's sexuality and as a means of deterring them from marrying outside the community. Girls may shun vigorous activities such as physical education in the fear that the scar will split open. Schools are often not aware of the condition. For fear of mockery, girls may be too embarrassed to reveal their condition and therefore live with the pain. This has a detrimental effect on their development and a culture of silence often prevails.

Female genital mutilation can be a constant source of psychological conflict leading to distortion of self-image, suicide and parasuicide. In a helpline organised by Forward (an independent non-government organisation which co-ordinates the work on female excision for the Minority Rights Group), many circumcised girls call to seek help on sexuality issues. Efua Dorkeeno of Forward (Dorkenoo and Elworthy, 1992) states that the ordeal of excision leaves an indelible mark, related to the inflicted psychological trauma. The extent and nature of the immediate and remote psychiatric disturbances depend largely on the girl's inner defences and prevailing social environment.

LEGAL ISSUES

In 1982, the WHO issued a statement that female circumcision should never be carried out by professional medical staff in any setting. In the United Kingdom, the 'Prohibition of Female Circumcision Act' came into force in 1985. Under the Act, it is an offence for any person to:

- excise, infibulate or otherwise mutilate the whole or any part of the labia majora or clitoris of another person; or

- aid, abet, counsel or procure the performance by another person of any of those acts on that other person's own body.

Female genital mutilation has been incorporated into child protection procedures in some local authorities in the United Kingdom.

In France, there are no specific laws against female genital mutilation, but cases have been tried against child abuse laws. In the cases that have been brought to court, most of the parents and professional excisionists have been set free or received light sentences as 'there was no criminal intent' (Dorozynski, 1994).

The Vienna Declaration of the World Conference on Human Rights (1993) held that traditional practices such as female circumcision were violations of human rights. In 1992, the International Federation of Gynaecology and Obstetrics published a joint statement with the WHO condemning the practice and calling for it to be abolished (see International Journal of Gynaecology and Obstetrics, 1992). A press release from the Royal College of Obstetricians and Gynaecologists in 1993 stated that:

> The agreed definition of the word infibulation is that it is 'a stitching together of the labia'. By definition, therefore, when an obstetrician is faced with the repair of the vulva of a woman who has delivered a baby vaginally following a previous infibulation it is illegal then to repair the labia intentionally in such a way that intercourse is difficult or impossible.
>
> Further, although the law states that a surgical operation can be performed on the vulva for the mental health of that person: it states clearly that if a vulval operation is thought necessary for the mental health of that woman, it cannot be performed if only for the purpose of custom or ritual.

Female genital mutilation, then, is a health issue that health workers must be aware of in areas where it is likely to be encountered, so that they can give sensitive help to girls, adolescents (and women) who have had it performed.

REFERENCES

Ba'asher T, 1978: Psychological aspects of female circumcision. Paper presented to the symposium on the changing status of Sudanese women.
Dorkenoo E, Elworthy S, 1992: *Female genital mutilation: Proposals for change*. London: Minority Rights Group.
Dorozynski A, 1994: French court rules in female circumcision case. *British Medical Journal* **309**, 831–832.
International Federation of Gynaecolgy and Obstetrics, 1992: Female circumcision: Female genital mutilation. *International Journal of Gynaecology and Obstetrics* **37**, 149.
Royal College of Obstetricians and Gynaecologists, 1993: Female circumcision (female genital mutilation). Press release. London: Royal College of Obstetricians and Gynaecologists.
Toubia N, 1994: Female circumcision as a public health issue. *New England Journal of Medicine* **331**, 712–716.
World Conference on Human Rights: the Vienna Declaration and Programme of Action, June 1993. New York: United Nations Department of Public Information (United Nations Publication no DPI/1394/39399).

CHAPTER 12

The XY girl

ALAN FRYER

INTRODUCTION

This Chapter is concerned with those individuals who have a Y chromosome but whose external genitalia fail to develop as expected for normal males. Many textbooks describe these patients as male pseudohermaphrodites. Some authors apply this term only to those whose external genitalia are ambiguous while others use the term more liberally. I am going to concentrate in this Chapter on those male pseudohermaphrodites whose external genitalia are frankly female or predominantly female as the diagnosis and management of patients with ambiguous genitalia are discussed in Chapter 5. I will, however, discuss some conditions where the presentation is always, or nearly always, with ambiguous genitalia because they are closely related to other disorders that properly fit within this discussion.

CLINICAL PRESENTATION

The majority of patients in this group remain undetected until adolescence when they present with either primary amenorrhoea and lack of secondary sex characteristics (as in those patients with XY gonadal dysgenesis) or primary amenorrhoea with secondary sex characteristics (as in complete androgen insensitivity syndrome (CAIS)). Some patients do present in early childhood because of the other features of their underlying condition, such as salt-wasting in some defects of androgen biosynthesis. An important early presentation of patients with CAIS is inguinal hernia – 50% of individuals with this syndrome develop inguinal hernias and it is recommended therefore to check the chromosomes in all pre-pubertal girls with inguinal hernias, although the majority will be 46XX.

In some cases the sex reversal comes to light unexpectedly when the child's chromosomes are checked for other reasons. Two of my most recent cases presented in this way. One infant had severe developmental delay and deafness and a 46XY karyotype – the cause of her sex reversal remains obscure. The other girl presented in the newborn period with pedal oedema and a diagnosis of Turner's syndrome was considered. Her chromosomes (blood and skin) revealed a 46XY karyotype in all cells examined. In this latter case, the presence of an undetected 45X cell line remains a strong possibility.

NORMAL SEXUAL DEVELOPMENT

Before considering the possible causes of XY sex reversal, it is necessary to understand the normal process of sexual development. In mammals, sex is determined by the presence or absence of a Y chromosome. Males usually have a Y chromosome and females do not. In the presence of a Y chromosome, the undifferentiated gonad develops into a testis and in its absence an ovary develops. The primary male determining signal (testis determining factor, TDF) is carried by the Y chromosome and in its presence the supporting cells which surround the incoming germ cells become transformed into Sertoli cells. These cells secrete anti-Mullerian hormone which suppresses the formation of the female internal genitalia. They also stimulate the interstitial cells to produce testosterone, which is essential for the differentiation of the Wolffian ducts and male external genitalia. The Sertoli cells form tubular structures around the incoming germ cells, inhibit meiosis and nurture the spermatogonia. Without a Y chromosome the supporting cells become the pre-follicular cells of the ovary and these surround the germ cells which enter meiosis and become primordial follicles. In the absence of anti-Mullerian hormone, the Mullerian ducts develop into uterus, fallopian tubes and upper vagina.

Testosterone is the principle androgen secreted by both the fetal and adult testes. The onset of testosterone secretion occurs just prior to the onset of virilisation in the male embryo, at about 8 weeks of gestation. Testosterone acts directly to stimulate the Wolffian ducts and induce development of the epididymis, vasa deferentia and seminal vesicles. In contrast, the development of the urogenital sinus and the external genitalia is induced by dihydrotestosterone. This acts in the urogenital sinus to produce the male urethra and prostate and in the urogenital tubercle to produce midline fusion, elongation and enlargement of the male external genitalia. Dihydrotestosterone is largely formed by reduction of testosterone, catalysed by the enzyme 5-alpha reductase.

GENETIC CONTROL OF SEXUAL DEVELOPMENT

The first step towards the discovery of the testis determining factor (TDF) was to locate the site of the gene(s) on the Y chromosome. This process was assisted by the observation of patients with abberations of the Y chromosome. First of all, TDF was mapped to the Y short arm (Yp) following the observation that patients with a 46X,i(Yq) karyotype were female. Such patients have Y chromosomes with two long arms (or q arms) instead of a long arm and a short arm. They are in effect deleted for the short arm (p arm). Later the tip of the short arm was excluded because patients with ring Y chromosomes proved to be male. When a ring chromosome forms, the tips of both the short arm and the long arm are deleted and the two 'sticky' ends come together to form a ring. Such observations were consistent with the fact that during male meiosis the X and Y chromosomes pair and exchange genetic material. This obligatory pairing region is known as the pseudoautosomal region and involves the distal part of Yp. One would not expect this area to contain the sex-determining gene(s) as any cross-over event would transfer the TDF to the X chromosome! The boundary between the pairing and the non-pairing region of the Y (pseudoautosomal boundary) therefore marked the distal limit of the male-determining region. Studies of other patients with terminal Yp deletions helped to define the proximal limit, i.e. the most distal breakpoint in the non-pairing region found in patients with a female phenotype. By such means the area of interest was narrowed to band Yp11.2 and one candidate gene, the H-Y antigen, was excluded as the TDF as it mapped to Yq.

The subsequent search required molecular technology and concentrated on those unusual patients who were XX males and XY females. The majority of XX males were found to contain Y-specific sequences in their DNA. How did this arise? Whilst recombination in male meiosis is common in the pseudoautosomal region, it is very unusual in the rest of the Y. However, on rare occasions the point of exchange is displaced proximally and can result in the transfer of TDF to the X chromosome. A sperm carrying such an X will give rise to an XX male and conversely a sperm containing the abnormal Y without TDF will result in an XY female. Studies of the Y-specific sequences present in the XX males and the rare XY females who had lost Y-specific sequences revealed candidate genes for the TDF.

The first plausible candidate gene was described by Page in 1987 (Page *et al.*, 1987) and termed ZFY. This gene coded for a zinc finger transcriptional activator (hence ZF) and was found to have a homologous sequence on the X (known as ZFX). However several pieces of evidence subsequently excluded ZFY as the TDF:

- a Y-positive XX male was found who lacked ZFY
- ZFY proved to be autosomal in marsupial species that have an X-Y sex determining system
- ZFY was found to be expressed only in the germ-cell lineage in the mouse and not in embryonic testes that lacked germ cells. Thus ZFY cannot be involved in testis determination but may have an important role in germ cell maturation.

The search continued with a study of sequences present in XX males that lacked ZFY and in 1990 a gene termed SRY (for sex-determining region Y) was isolated (Sinclair *et al.*, 1990). There was strong evidence that SRY is the testis-determining gene:

- it is conserved and Y-specific amongst a range of mammals
- it was deleted in an XY female mouse

- it is expressed in the gonads of male mouse embryos at the critical stage of testis differentiation
- *de novo* mutations were identified in the SRY gene in human females with XY gonadal dysgenesis (Berta *et al.*, 1990; Jager *et al.*, 1990)
- injecting the gene into XX mouse embryos resulted in XX male mice.

SRY is thus the sex-determining gene and currently it appears that mutations in this gene are an important cause of XY sex reversal. McElreavy *et al.* (1992) studied 25 patients with XY gonadal dysgenesis and found point mutations in the SRY gene in four cases. In one other case, they identified a Yp deletion which did not interrupt the SRY gene and a similar observation has been made by Capel *et al.* (1993) who observed three XY female mice with different Yp deletions but with the SRY locus remaining intact in each case. In one of these mice SRY expression was studied and found to be undetectable at the critical stage of testis development. They postulate that the deletion caused a failure of SRY expression by position effect i.e. the deletion could have brought SRY under the influence of the Y centromeric heterochromatin and thereby silenced SRY expression.

The cause of XY gonadal dysgenesis in those patients without SRY mutations or Yp abnormalities is unknown but there are several strands of evidence to suggest that SRY is not the only gene involved in testicular differentiation. One family reported by Vilain *et al.* (1992) is fascinating because a mutation in the SRY gene is identified which results in XY females in 3 family members but two others carry the mutation and are fertile XY males. One hypothesis considered by the authors is that the SRY allele could generate two different phenotypes by interacting with two independently segregating alleles of a second gene. They cite evidence from mouse genetics reviewed by Eicher and Washburn (1986) who comment on 3 XY female mice where autosomal mutations are responsible. Homologous autosomal genes in the human could exist which may interact with the product of SRY. Indeed, studies in *Drosophila* and the nematode *C. elegans* (Hodgkin, 1990) indicate that the genetic control of sexual differentiation in these species results from a cascade of genes, each gene switching on the next gene in the series. In *C. elegans*, the regulatory cascade consists of seven interacting autosomal genes controlled by three X-linked genes (Hunter and Wood, 1992). It may be that a similar process occurs in the human.

SRY codes for a putative transcription factor and so presumably controls the transcription of at least one secondary gene. Indeed SRY seems not only to bind to DNA but to bend it, suggesting that it might switch on its downstream target(s) by bringing it close to essential regulatory sequences.

The presence of downstream targets might also account for those XX males who lack SRY and yet develop a complete male phenotype (Vilain *et al.*, 1994) and similarly there are some XX true hermaphrodites who have both testicular and ovarian tissue yet lack SRY. Presumably in these groups of patients, there must be a 'gain of function' mutation later in the pathway of testicular differentiation. McElreavy *et al.* (1993) postulate that a second gene exists, which they term Z, that acts as a negative regulator of male sex determination. They hypothesise that SRY suppresses Z to allow testicular development. Recessive mutations in Z would result in an XX male in the absence of SRY and a mutation in Z which makes it insensitive to the action of SRY could result in XY females. i.e. Hypothetical cascade:

(a) Normal male:	SRY– – – – – – I	Z ⟶	Male genes	ON
(b) Normal female:		Z– – – – – I	Male genes	OFF
(c) XX male:	*mutation in*	Z ⟶	Male genes	ON
(d) XY female:	SRY– – $\frac{\text{fails to}}{\text{inhibit}}$ – I	Z– – – – – I	Male genes	OFF

(a) Normal male: SRY with *inhibition* to Z

If a gene with a function like Z exists or genes with other functions within the sex determination pathway exist, what are they and what is their chromosome location? There is evidence for an X-linked gene from both family studies and isolated reports. There are rare families in which there are sibships containing Y-negative true hermaphrodites, Y-negative XX males and normal males and females where the pattern of inheritance is consistent with X-linkage – the mutation being transmitted by normal males or non-manifesting females where the mutation is subject to X-inactivation. There are also families reported with XY gonadal dysgenesis which appear to follow X-linked inheritance (Sternberg *et al.*, 1968; German *et al.*, 1978; Mann *et al.*, 1983) although another possibility in these families is autosomal dominant inheritance with sex-limitation to males.

Further support for the presence of an X-linked gene comes from the observation of cases of sex reversal in XY patients who have X-chromosome duplications (Bernstein *et al.*, 1980; Scherer *et al.*, 1989; Stern *et al.*, 1990). These cases have all shown duplications of the same region, Xp21/p22. Furthermore Ogata *et al.* (1992) reported a sex-reversed child with a 46X,Yp+ karyotype and the Yp+ was derived by a translocation of an Xp fragment (Xp21–22.3) to Yp resulting in duplication of this Xp region. There are other XY cases with Xp duplications where the patients are phenotypically male i.e. Xp22.1–Xp22.32 (Coles *et al.*, 1992), Xp22.1–22.3 (Narahara *et al.*, 1979) and Xp11.2–21.2 (Brondum-Neilson and Langkjaier, 1982), suggesting that the relevant sex-determining gene is located at Xp21.3 – the only segment present in the phenotypic females but not in the males. Ogata and Matsuo (1994) indicate that from molecular studies the relevant gene (which they term TDF-X) may be situated between the anonymous DNA segment DXS28 and the Ornithine carbamyl transferase gene, OTC. Bardoni *et al.* (1994) mapped this locus to a 160 Kb region of Xp21, which includes the adrenal hypoplasia congenita locus (AHC). Such a gene might act by inhibiting male differentiation – when duplicated, it might exceed the threshold for inhibition by SRY and so some authors have given this locus the alternative name of DSS (dosage-sensitive sex-reversal). Swain *et al.* (1996) have suggested that a gene termed DAX1 could be responsible, at least in part, for the DSS phenotype. Functional deficiency of this gene, due to deletions or point mutations, is responsible for AHC and hypogonadotrophic hypogonadism in a male. Studies in mice show that DAX1 is expressed in the developing gonad as well as the adrenals, hypothalamus and anterior pituitary gland. Indeed, the onset of its expression in the genital ridge occurs at the same time as SRY and at the time that SRY expression disappears, DAX1 expression in the testis decreases dramatically, whilst it persists in the ovary. One possible explanation is that SRY may initiate differentiation into a testis which in turn results in repression of DAX1. Possibly a high level of DAX1 as in the DSS phenotype could overcome this repression. In XX individuals, DAX1 may be important in ovarian development.

Some autosomal loci may also be involved in the gene cascade. Simpson *et al.* (1981) ascertained from the literature at the time all cases of XY gonadal dysgenesis for genetic analysis. In 18 families there was more than one affected child and in three further families the pattern suggested either X-linked or male-limited autosomal dominant inheritance. The authors performed a segregation analysis in those 18 families whereby they counted the numbers of recurrences in males born subsequent to the ascertained case. The result of this study was not statistically different from the 25% expected in autosomal recessive inheritance compared to the 50% expected in X-linked recessive inheritance. There have also been reports of XY gonadal dysgenesis from consanguineous unions which adds support to the existence of an autosomal recessive form. Possible locations for these autosomal genes have been suggested by the observation of sex-reversal in both patients with anomalies of the autosomes and patients with syndromes due to single gene mutations that follow autosomal inheritance (see below).

MULTIPLE ANOMALY SYNDROMES INVOLVING XY SEX REVERSAL

Chromosomal Anomalies

Defects of 9p, 10p and 11p13 have been associated with multiple anomaly syndromes including XY sex reversal, although lesser defects such as undescended testes have been reported in a wide range of aneuploidies. Hoo *et al.* (1989) reviewed 4 cases of XY sex reversal associated with 9p anomalies. All four cases showed female external genitalia and a uterus. The gonads in 2 cases revealed immature testicular tissue containing Sertoli cells but no germ cells. They argue that since most 9p deletions do not show sex reversal there may be a recessive gene at 9p24 that is important in early testis development (i.e. these 4 cases might carry a recessive allele on the normal 9 which was unmasked by the deletion on the other).

Wilkie *et al.* (1993) reported two cases of XY sex reversal with 10q terminal deletions – case 1 had female external genitalia with a uterus and cervix but no ovaries visualised and would fit with XY gonadal dysgenesis. In case 2, the genitalia were ambiguous and there was testicular tissue present.

Deletions of 11p13 can result in XY sex reversal. Such cases involve the

Wilms tumour gene WT-1 which is expressed at high levels in the gonadal ridge of the developing gonad and Sertoli cells of the testis as well as the developing kidney. Point mutations in this gene have also been identified in the Denys–Drash syndrome (see below).

Deletions at Xq28 in two boys with myotubular myopathy and abnormal genital development have recently been reported and may indicate a gene at this location that is implicated in male sexual development (Hu *et al.*, 1996)

It is not known whether any of the genes affected by the above deletions are involved in testicular differentiation or whether they are involved in testis development post-differentiation. Indeed it has been argued that the effects of chromosome deletions may be non-specific, i.e. deletion of certain genes may result in inhibition of cell division during testis differentiation and hence result in a partially formed testis.

Single Gene Disorders

Table 12.1 lists a number of reported syndromes which may involve complete XY sex reversal and hence result in female or predominantly female external genitalia. In some of these syndromes, the defective gene may be involved in testis differentiation or development but in other cases the aetiology may lie in androgen biosynthesis etc. One of the most interesting syndromes is campomelic dysplasia, a rare and often lethal skeletal dysplasia which is frequently associated with XY sex reversal. Mutations in the gene SOX9 on chromosome 17q have been identified in a number of patients with this syndrome (Foster *et al.*, 1994; Wagner *et al.*, 1994). SOX9 is a member of a group of SRY-type genes and would seem to have a role in sex determination. An up-to-date review is given by Sinclair (1995). Another gene that lies close to but is distinct from SOX9 has also been discovered and appears to be expressed specifically in the testis – its role is yet to be elucidated (Ninomiya *et al.*, 1996).

There are many syndromes that can result in ambiguous/incompletely masculinised external genitalia and some which result in normal male external genitalia but female internal genitalia (e.g. persistent Mullerian duct syndrome). A complete review of these syndromes is not possible here and the interested reader should consult textbooks of dysmorphology or a computerised database.

CAUSES OF NON-SYNDROMAL XY SEX REVERSAL

Failure of Testis Differentiation

The above discussion on the genetic control of sexual differentiation highlights a number of possible causes of XY sex reversal and these may be summarised thus:

- Chromosome anomalies, i.e. abnormal Y with deletion of male determining region; Xp21 duplications.

Table 12.1 Multiple anomaly syndromes featuring XY sex reversal

Name	Inheritance	Genitalia	Other features	References
Brosnan	AR	Female Gonadal dysgenesis	Short stature, low IQ scalp defects, cleft palate facial dysmorphism, VSD	Brosnan, 1980
Campomelic Dysplasia	AD ?AR	Female/male/ambiguous Internal genitalia are very variable (from normal male to normal female)	Short-limbed dwarfism, usually lethal in newborn. Facial dysmorphism, cleft palate, cardiac and renal anomalies	Foster et al., 1994 Wagner et al., 1994 Houston et al., 1983
Denys–Drash	? 11p15	Female or ambiguous Streak gonads Gonadoblastoma	Wilms tumour, nephritis	Drash et al., 1970 Friedman and Finlay, 1987 Hastie, 1992 Baird et al., 1992 Ogawa et al., 1993 Mueller, 1994
Frasier	?	Female Streak gonads	Nephritis (Wilms not reported)	Frasier et al., 1964 Haning et al., 1985
Gardner–Silengo–Wachtal	AR/XLR	Female or ambiguous	Cardiac defect, cleft palate (? overlap with Smith–Lemli–Opitz)	Greenberg et al., 1987
Double vagina Cardiac, Pulmonary Genital syndrome	?	Female with evidence of testicular tissue	Cardiac, pulmonary and diaphragmatic defects	Maaswinkel-Mooij et al., 1992 Toriello and Higgins, 1992
Nivelon	AR	Female with female internal genitalia	Unusual facies, bone dysplasia	Nivelon et al., 1992
Smith–lemli–Opitz type 2	AR	Female or ambiguous	Unusual facies, syndactyly, polydactyly, neonatal death, cleft palate, cardiac, renal anomalies, Hirschprung's disease, defect in cholesterol synthesis	Irons et al., 1993 Tint et al., 1994
Verloes	AR	Female or ambiguous Mullerian structures are present	Mental retardation, unusual facies, obesity, anal anomaly, spina bifida	Verloes et al., 1990 Schipper et al., 1991

- Loss of SRY as a result of abnormal meiotic recombination during male meiosis (or in a spermatogonial mitosis preceding meiosis). It is however only a minority of XY females who have lost SRY by abnormal X–Y interchange (Ferguson-Smith, 1992).
- Mutations in genes responsible for testicular differentiation. As previously stated mutations in SRY may cause XY gonadal dysgenesis. Genes elsewhere including the X (DSS) may be responsible for several more cases.

These problems will all lead to XY gonadal dysgenesis and will present similarly. The same phenotype can also be produced by sex chromosome mosaicism, i.e. the presence of a 45X or 46XX cell line which has remained undetected on the chromosome analysis. The most common mosaic karyotype in this context is 45X/46XY and these patients usually have normal male genitalia though some can present with normal female or ambiguous genitalia (Chang *et al.*, 1990). These patients can have dysgenetic gonads even in the presence of normal male genitalia and are at risk of developing gonadoblastoma as in 46XY gonadal dysgenesis.

Some patients with true hermaphroditism can have predominantly female external genitalia. Most cases of true hermaphroditism are 46XX and Simpson (1990) has suggested that most 46XY cases are unrecognised 46XX/46XY chimaeras.

Failure of Androgen Production or Action

Even if the gonad differentiates into a testis, there are other possible reasons for the failure of the development of normal male external genitalia:

- abnormal testes, e.g. Leydig cell agenesis/testicular regression
- defect in androgen biosynthesis
- androgen receptor defect
- 5-alpha reductase deficiency

Some of these conditions will result in normal female external genitalia and others in incompletely masculinized or ambiguous genitalia. These disorders are discussed in detail below.

CLINICAL PHENOTYPES

XY Gonadal Dysgenesis (Swyer's Syndrome)

The cause of this phenotype may be absence or mutation of SRY (possibly 20% of cases) or another gene involved in testis differentiation as discussed above. As the testes do not develop, neither androgens nor anti-Mullerian hormone are produced resulting in normal, or slightly infantile, female external and internal genitalia. The gonads are dysgenetic and appear as streaks as two X chromosomes are necessary for normal ovarian development.

The typical patient with XY pure gonadal dysgenesis has a female or some-what eunuchoid habitus and presents with primary amenorrhoea. Secondary sex characteristics, especially breast development are poor (in the case of Simpson *et al.* (1982), the patient did show spontaneous menstruation and breast develop-ment and the authors hypothesised that the hormone production was from the gonadoblastoma that was present). The mean height usually exceeds that of nor-mal females though there have been some patients with short stature which raises the possibility of undetected 45X mosaicism. Similarly, a minority of patients show some stigmata of Turner's syndrome.

The streak gonads do not differ from that seen in Turner's syndrome though the hilar cells may be more abundant and in some cases they resemble Leydig cells. Of the XY gonadal dysgenesis patients described in the literature, at least 30% have developed a dysgerminoma or gonadoblastoma (Verp and Simpson, 1987). These neoplasia often arise in the first or second decade – therefore the gonads should be removed soon after the diagnosis has been made. The uterus and fallopian tubes should be left in situ, even though it is technically easier to remove all of these organs than to extirpate only the streaks. Retention of the uterus allows the possibility of a pregnancy through a donor egg and *in-vitro* fer-tilisation procedure.

The patients are psychologically female and of normal intelligence. The diagnosis is usually made at puberty and patients should be given a full expla-nation – most patients should be given as much information about the condi-tion as they can readily assimilate. After explanation, treatment with cyclical hormones should begin. The result is often good though in some patients breast development tends to remain poor and augmentation mammoplasty may be considered. The details of the clinical management are given elsewhere (see p. 136). These patients may have a poor self-image given their infertility and poorly developed secondary sex characteristics. It is important in coun-selling to use language that reinforces their view of themselves as girls and women.

There have been a number of reports of patients with XY gonadal dysgenesis who have developed chronic renal failure. The term Frasier syndrome has been coined for this association (Moorthy *et al.*, 1987) after the author of the first report (see Table 12.1). The nephropathy of Frasier syndrome is similar to that seen in Denys–Drash syndrome but is usually of later onset (for a review of these syndromes, see Mueller (1994)).

Genetic counselling in XY gonadal dysgenesis depends on the cause. Most cases due to mutations in SRY will be spontaneous but the report of Vilain *et al.* (1992) indicates the importance of checking for the mutation in the father of the affected child before giving a low recurrence risk. Indeed two fathers of XY girls have been reported who were mosaic for mutations in SRY (Schmitt–Ney *et al.*, 1995). In isolated cases with SRY present and no mutation detectable in the gene, counselling is difficult. The majority of cases may be sporadic but as X-linked and autosomal recessive cases occur, one would need to discuss these possibilities with the families.

Abnormal testes

Absence of Leydig cells

Several XY patients have been shown to have complete absence of Leydig cells. Affected siblings have been recognised and consanguinity observed consistent with autosomal recessive inheritance (Saldanha *et al.*, 1987). The phenotype in its extreme form consists of female external genitalia, absent uterus and bilateral testes which are devoid of Leydig cells. The epididymes and vasa deferentia are present. In milder forms of the condition, males may present with hypergonadotrophic hypogonadism and micropenis. Levels of LH are elevated. Recently, Kremer *et al.* (1995) identified a homozygous mutation in the LH receptor gene in one family with this condition.

Undifferentiated Leydig cells require luteinising hormone (LH) for proliferation and differentiation. It may be that the initiation of androgen synthesis in early fetal life is independent of LH and hence the epididymis and vas deferens form. Presumably at a later stage in fetal development, the absence of a functional LH receptor interferes with Leydig cell proliferation and maturation and hence masculinization of the external genitalia is impaired. No abnormal female sex characteristics have been noted in 46XX sisters of these patients, consistent with experimental results that indicate absence of a functional ovarian LH receptor until after birth.

Rudimentary testes

There have been reports of patients with rudimentary testes (Bergada *et al.*, 1962). These patients are phenotypic males with well-formed but very small testes and small penises and affected sibships from consanguineous parents have been described suggesting that at least one form is genetic.

Anorchia

Anorchia describes patients with an XY karyotype who are phenotypic males with normal Wolffian derivatives but absent testes. Many cases probably result from torsion of the testicular arterial supply.

There are however familial cases of anorchia and the pathogenesis is probably that of testicular regression whereby the fetal testes began functioning (and hence produced anti-Mullerian hormone) but then regressed. The phenotype in these patients varies from normal male external genitalia with absent testes (anorchia) to absent gonads, absent or rudimentary Mullerian or Wolffian derivatives and external genitalia usually consisting of a phallus about the size of a clitoris with nearly complete fusion of the labio-scrotal folds (agonadia). Some of these patients have also had craniofacial and vertebral anomalies and mental retardation. Testicular regression syndrome might be the most appropriate name for this condition with the phenotype dependent on the timing of the regression. Autosomal recessive or X-linked recessive inheritance seems likely.

Defective Androgen Biosynthesis

In this group of disorders, the testes differentiate and produce anti-Mullerian hormone but do not produce androgens. The external genitalia are female or ambiguous but internally Mullerian structures are absent. An enzyme deficiency should be suspected if the levels of testosterone or its metabolites are decreased. This may be difficult to determine in infancy because the baseline testosterone levels are normally low and an HCG stimulation test is usually recommended to facilitate diagnosis. The biochemical pathway is illustrated in Fig. 12.1. Deficiencies of 3-beta hydroxysteroid dehydrogenase (HSD), 17-beta HSD, 17-alpha hydroxylase/17,20 lyase or in the system involved in the conversion of cholesterol to pregnenolone (congenital adrenal lipoid hyperplasia) can result in incomplete masculinisation.

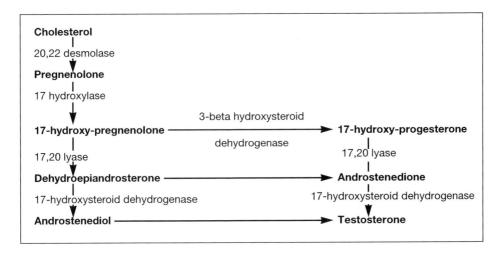

Fig. 12.1 Testosterone biosynthesis.

In congenital adrenal lipoid hyperplasia, it has been thought that this disorder is due to a defect in the cholesterol side-chain cleavage enzyme system responsible for the conversion of cholesterol to pregnenolone, i.e. 20-alpha hydroxylase, 20,22 desmolase or 22-alpha hydroxylase. Recently however, mutations have been identified in the gene encoding the StAR protein (steroidogenic acute regulatory protein), which appears to be involved in the transport of cholesterol from the outer to the inner mitochondrial membrane (Tee *et al.*, 1995). Mutations in the StAR gene appear to be the main cause of this disorder.

These patients have female or ambiguous genitalia and severe salt-wasting. Inheritance is autosomal recessive. Just over 30 cases have been described though most have died in adrenal crises in infancy. One patient that I was involved with recently was diagnosed because a previous sibling had died in the newborn period and the autopsy had demonstrated adrenal lipoid hyperplasia (foamy appearing cells filled with cholesterol in the adrenal glands). She was monitored carefully after birth and when salt-wasting was detected, effective treatment with corticosteroids was instituted. Unfortunately her chromosomes were not checked at that stage and her genetic sex was not discovered until she presented with pubertal failure and was found to have an XY karyotype. In teenage years this sudden discovery created considerable psychological problems.

3-beta HSD deficiency is another autosomal recessive disorder and can result in hypospadias or ambiguous genitalia in genetic males. There is a salt-wasting and a non-salt-wasting form. The genes for the type I and type II isoenzymes have been cloned and mutations in several patients have been identified in the type II 3-beta-HSD gene (Tajima *et al.*, 1995).

P450C17 is a single enzyme that mediates both 17-alpha hydroxylase and 17,20 lyase activity. The subject is reviewed by Yanase *et al.* (1991). Enzyme deficiency in males usually presents with ambiguous genitalia but severe cases can present with female external genitalia. At puberty, gynaecomastia can be a prominent feature. The males usually display normal blood pressure, though this can be elevated due to excess production of corticosterone. Inheritance is autosomal recessive and the gene has been cloned. There are no reports of pre-natal diagnosis.

17-beta HSD deficiency is the most common defect in testosterone biosynthesis and can be recognised on the basis of elevated androstenedione levels (or increased androstenedione: testosterone ratio). Inheritance is autosomal recessive. The enzyme catalyses the conversion of androstenedione to testosterone in the testes, although this reaction is reversible and the testosterone to androstenedione reaction occurs in extragonadal tissues. It is the isoenzyme 17-beta HSD3 which catalyses the process in the testis and the gene encoding this isoenzyme maps to 9q22. Mutations in this gene have been identified in XY females (Geissler *et al.*, 1994). The external genitalia are usually female at birth but mild to moderate ambiguity can be present. If the genitalia are phenotypically female at birth, the diagnosis may be suspected if the gonads are palpable. Internally Wolffian structures develop and no Mullerian structures are present. More often the diagnosis is not made until puberty when the patients fail to menstruate and they masculinize, developing a male body habitus and male secondary sex characteristics, although some have gynaecomastia. Some patients have switched to becoming male after puberty having been raised as females. Surgical repair of the external genitalia can produce good cosmetic and functional results though infertility is inevitable.

It is not understood why, in the absence of testosterone, Wolffian ducts develop in utero in these patients. One possibility is that androstenedione itself can virilise the Wolffian ducts or possibly the androstenedione is converted to testosterone in the placenta where the isoenzyme 17-beta HSD2 is expressed at high levels. It is also not clear why virilisation occurs at puberty. One hypothesis is that there may be peripheral conversion of the high circulating levels of androstenedione to testosterone by isoenzymes 17-beta HSD1 or 17-beta HSD2 or another, as yet unidentified isoenzyme. Whatever the reason, if the diagnosis is made before puberty, the testes can be removed to prevent virilisation.

Androgen Resistance Syndromes

These disorders probably account for the majority of cases of male pseudohermaphroditism. The subject is well reviewed by Griffin (1992).

Complete androgen insensitivity syndrome

This is also known as testicular feminisation syndrome. These individuals have female external genitalia (though occasionally with slight enlargement of the clitoris), bilateral testes (often palpable in the inguinal regions), blind-ending vaginas and absent uterus and fallopian tubes. At puberty, these patients develop normal feminisation with breast development. Most patients are similar in appearance to other girls in the general population though the phenotype has sometimes been described as voluptuously feminine because of their height and excellent breast development. There been one case described who was a famous photographic model. Increased testicular secretion of oestradiol together with peripheral aromatization of testosterone probably account for the breast development at puberty. The breasts contain normal ductal and glandular tissue but the areolae are often pale and underdeveloped. Pubic and axillary hair are sparse or absent but scalp hair is normal. The labia and clitoris are normal or slightly underdeveloped. The vagina ends blindly and may be shorter than usual, though it is rare for it to be very short. The testes are normal in size and histology shows spermatogenesis to be incomplete or absent, although Leydig cells are abundant. The testes may be present in the abdomen, the inguinal canal or the labia. If present in the inguinal canal they can produce inguinal herniae. Dewhurst (1971) reviewed 82 cases collected in the United Kingdom and reported that 32 were diagnosed before the age of 15–20 years with an inguinal hernia that contained a testis, 8 because of a positive family history, 3 had testes palpable in the groins and in 1 case the child had a urethral prolapse and the characteristic features were then recognised. The remaining cases presented in later childhood/early adult life, usually with primary amenorrhoea.

Height is slightly increased over normal women (mean 171.5 cm in one series) with bone age corresponding to chronological age and hands and feet may be relatively large. Plasma testosterone concentrations are within the age-appropriate male range or in some cases may be slightly elevated. Intelligence is normal and psychological development is unmistakably female with regard to behaviour, outlook and maternal instincts.

The frequency of gonadal neoplasia is increased – although one survey tabulated this risk at 22% (Morris and Mahesh, 1963), Verp and Simpson (1987) estimate that this risk is really no higher than 5%. Most agree that the risk is low before 25–30 years of age (unlike patients with gonadal dysgenesis) but increases thereafter. Benign tubular adenomas are especially common in post-pubertal patients and orchidectomy is therefore necessary. It has been the practice to leave testes in situ until after puberty, rather than have to give hormone replacement. There is now a tendency to proceed to gonadectomy earlier, rather than wait for puberty. In general pre-pubertal children tend to be less sexually preoccupied and so there may be some psychological benefit in pre-pubertal surgery. On the other hand the adolescent may have a better cognitive grasp of the issues around the decision to operate, could give informed consent and would not require HRT to induce breast development. All of these issues should be discussed with the family before a decision is made about the timing of surgery.

Estimates of the incidence of this syndrome have varied from 1 in 20 000 to 1 in 65 000 males, this latter figure being mainly based on the frequency of inguinal herniae in females (Jagiello and Atwell, 1962) and the estimate that 1–2% of girls with inguinal herniae have the disorder. New and more accurate figures for prevalence may soon be forthcoming as androgen insensitivity is currently one of the subjects of study undertaken through the auspices of the British Paediatric Surveillance Unit. The evidence that androgen insensitivity occurs because of an abnormality of the androgen receptor was first obtained from assays of androgen binding activity in genital skin fibroblasts. Binding is generally classified as negative, deficient or positive. The majority of patients with CAIS have negative or deficient binding. (Androgen receptor binding assays are only available in specialised centres). The evidence to date suggests that most, if not all cases of CAIS are due to mutations in the androgen receptor gene which maps to the X chromosome at Xq11–12. The gene was cloned in 1988 and contains 8 exons encoding 3 clearly identifiable functional domains. The C terminal domain is encoded by 5 exons (D-H) and is responsible for receptor binding to androgen. The central domain is encoded by 2 exons (B and C) and is involved in binding the receptor to chromosomal DNA and the N terminal domain is encoded by one large exon (A) and is involved in the receptor's role in gene regulation. A number of mutations have now been identified in the gene and the vast majority are point mutations. From the viewpoint of genetic counselling, this is an X-linked condition with zero reproductive fitness and it is assumed that 1 in 3 cases arise as new mutations. Finding the mutation may be very helpful in carrier detection. Carrier females do not usually have symptoms or signs although Sai *et al.* (1990) point out that a minority of female carriers have had delayed menarche – a finding they observed in 4 out of 26 families that they studied. Gayral (quoted in McKusick, 1992) described a case of an obligate carrier female who had breast asymmetry and no pubic hair to the right of the midline. These patchy changes represent the effect of lyonisation.

Partial androgen insensitivity syndrome (PAIS)

This is also known as incomplete androgen receptor deficiency or Reifenstein syndrome. Typically this disorder presents at birth with genital ambiguity but the clinical phenotype is highly variable. At the mildest end of the spectrum, there may be hypospadias or even infertility in otherwise normal males. At the other end of the spectrum, the child might have predominantly female external genitalia with clitoromegaly and labial fusion. Even within the same family, there is considerable phenotypic variation with almost opposite extremes occurring. The reason for this variation is unknown but Batch *et al.* (1993) suggest that it may reflect variable androgen production at critical stages of uterogenital development.

Pelvic ultrasound scanning generally shows absence of female internal genitalia and the main differential diagnosis is then between a testosterone biosynthetic defect or 5-alpha reductase deficiency. The investigations which need to be performed to clarify the diagnosis are itemised below.

Subsequent management depends on the sex of rearing – most patients have been reared as males but if a female sex of rearing is chosen, appropriate genital surgery and gonadectomy should be performed early with oestrogen replacement at the time of puberty.

PAIS is usually associated with positive androgen binding to receptors in genital skin fibroblasts though qualitative defects in binding are found in 10% of cases. In some cases, mutations in the androgen receptor gene have been identified (Bevan *et al.*, 1996) but not in others. It is possible that PAIS may be due to mutations in other genes in some cases, particularly where no androgen binding abnormality is present. Genetic counselling is therefore unreliable in this condition unless there is an X-linked pedigree or a mutation is found in the androgen receptor gene. Such a mutation would allow accurate carrier detection and prenatal diagnosis if requested. It is more likely that pre-natal diagnosis would be requested in PAIS than CAIS because of the significant risk of genital ambiguity. Prenatal diagnosis by assay of androgen receptors in amniocytes is unreliable. The disorder has been detected in utero by documenting the absence of male genitalia in a 46XY fetus (Stephens, 1984).

5-alpha reductase deficiency

Failure to convert testosterone to dihydrotestosterone results in genital ambiguity at birth. The external genitalia are nevertheless predominantly female i.e. a phallus that more resembles a clitoris than a penis and a blind ending perineal orifice that resembles a vagina with a separate perineal urethral orifice. The condition has been termed pseudovaginal perineoscrotal hypospadias. At puberty, these patients virilise as pubertal virilisation can be achieved by testosterone alone. This is a serious problem for those affected individuals who are raised as girls as the degree of pubertal virilisation can be dramatic. For these girls, the management should be as for PAIS with removal of the testes, oestrogen/progestogen treatment at puberty and vaginoplasty where appropriate. There are some patients who have been raised as girls and then reversed their roles and functioned as men after puberty.

The disorder is inherited as an autosomal recessive trait. It is rare as evidenced by the high frequency of consanguinity in reported cases. There are two functional 5-alpha reductase genes in man and a deletion has been reported in one of these genes in two related individuals with pseudohermaphroditism (Andersson *et al.*, 1991).

SUMMARY OF THE INVESTIGATIONS IN AN XY FEMALE

The above discussion indicates the possible diagnoses to be considered and their main features. A summary is given in Table 12.2. A general approach to the problem is as follows:

(a) *Clinical history/family history/physical examination.* This may diagnose a multiple anomaly syndrome or at least indicate a pattern of inheritance. Clues to a diagnosis may be forthcoming e.g. Turner's features may suggest cryptic 45X mosaicism, palpable testes would rule out gonadal dysgenesis etc.

Table 12.2   Summary of differential diagnosis

	External	*Internal*	*Testosterone*	*Luteinising hormone (LH)*
XY gonadal dysgenesis	Female	Streak gonads Uterus and tubes present No Wolffian structures	Low	High
Leydig cell agenesis	Female	Testes Absent uterus No Wolffian structures	Low	High
Testicular regression	Abnormal	Absent gonads Rudimentary structures	Low	High
Androgen biosynthesis	Abnormal/ female	Testes	Low	High
CAIS	Female	Testes Absent uterus No Wolffian structures	Normal/high	High*
PAIS	Abnormal	Testes Absent uterus Wolffian structures usually present	Normal/high	High*
5-alpha reductase deficiency	Female (may virilise at puberty)	Testes Absent Mullerian Wolffian present	Normal	Normal or just raised

* LH levels high due to diminished feedback at the pituitary, because of androgen resistance at the hypothalamic–pituitary level.

(b) *Detailed karyotype*. This should be done to exclude sex chromosome mosaicism or abnormal Y or X or an autosomal anomaly if there are multiple abnormalities.

(c) *Pelvic ultrasound/genitogram/laparotomy*. If the internal genitalia are female, this would suggest gonadal dysgenesis. The gonads would need to be removed and the histology and chromosomes of the gonads checked. A mutation in the SRY gene could be sought.

If female internal genitalia are absent, androgen resistance or biosynthetic defect is suggested. Measurement of testosterone levels and an HCG stimulation test will help distinguish these.

The HCG stimulation test may be performed as follows (Hughes, 1986). Baseline blood samples for plasma testosterone, androstenedione and dihydrotestosterone levels are taken as well as a 24-hour urine sample for measurement of steroid precursor metabolites. HCG is then given (2000 units i.m. daily) for three days and on day 4, repeat blood and 24-hour urine samples are taken (i.e. 24 hours after the last injection).

Plasma testosterone should increase at least 2-3-fold after HCG stimulation. The response is actually more marked in the first 6 months of life and in early to mid-puberty. Normal testosterone production is a prerequisite for the diagnosis of PAIS. A biosynthetic defect will result in increased precursor steroid secretion.

Measurement of testosterone and dihydrotestosterone in plasma together with their 5-alpha and 5-beta reduced metabolites in the urine will diagnose 5-alpha reductase deficiency. Odame *et al.* (1992) demonstrate that measurement of plasma dihydrotestosterone and testosterone : dihydrotestosterone ratios alone can be unreliable (even after HCG stimulation) in the early neonatal period. They comment on the value of a trial of dihydrotestosterone cream applied twice daily to the phallus – phallic growth in response to this treatment provides indirect confirmation of the diagnosis of 5-alpha reductase deficiency as well as improving the appearance and aiding reconstructive surgery in those children raised as males.

Androgen receptor and mutation studies in the androgen receptor gene are important in CAIS and PAIS.

MANAGEMENT

The medical management of each disorder or group of disorders is discussed above. For patients and their families there is the additional problem of the psychological management. The issue of gender is a major one in any family – knowledge of the infant's gender shapes parents' and others' attitudes to the child, consciously and unconsciously, in their expectations of behaviour, role modelling and aspirations for the future of the child. It is therefore important to consider the counselling of the parents as well as the child when the diagnosis is made. A full explanation is essential stressing that their child is phenotypically *and* psychologically female. The parents themselves need time to come to terms with several issues common to families with genetic disorders:

- acknowledging that there is a problem with their child and mourning for the loss of the idea of a 'perfect' child.
- confronting the guilt which many families feel if the disorder has been genetically transmitted by the parents.
- mourning the loss of the continuing family line as the child will not produce grandchildren. In addition the parents may have to confront the issue of what is female/maleness.

It has been explained above that these patients are psychologically female. Children develop awareness of male/femaleness in infancy and certainly by age 2–3 years and this has generally been felt to be irreversible, although some have claimed successful reassignment in adolescence (Diamond, 1965). It is important therefore that these patients are regarded and referred to as girls and treated with the utmost sensitivity. A recent 'personal view' written in the *British Medical Journal* (1994) by a patient with CAIS emphasises some of the distress which can be caused by inappropriate comments from doctors and nurses. Terms like 'pseudohermaphrodite' should be avoided.

Most parents are at a loss as to how to explain the nature of their medical condition to their daughter without implying that she 'really is a boy'. Where this has occurred, Dewhurst and Grant (1984) suggest telling the child that the ovaries or testes had to be removed because they were 'unhealthy or producing the wrong balance of hormones' and that hormone treatment will be needed to bring along the correct changes of puberty and that fertility is not possible. In androgen insensitivity it is necessary to add that they were born without a uterus and so menstruation will not occur. These explanations may suffice early on but a full explanation is necessary at the time of adolescence. The 'personal view' referred to above (1994) claims, 'there was a reluctance to explain clearly and unambiguously to me the nature of the condition and its manifestations. Allied to this was the ignorance of the nursing staff and their ill-advised comments . . . . . the patient must be told the nature of the condition. The genetic explanation is vital for understanding but it must be explained that although the patient is chromosomally male and that the genotype is male, the phenotype is female'.

For those patients diagnosed in early childhood, Goodall (1991) feels that it is advisable to unfold the truth stage by stage, matching simple statements to the child's conceptual growth until the personal implications are finally realised as part of a maturing process. This is likely to be kinder to the child than the sudden delivery of information during the vulnerable teenage years. She describes this process in the counselling of one of her patients who presented at birth with ambiguous genitalia. In pre-school and early school years the parents were advised to tell their child that she needed an operation when she was a baby and to indicate its site but not to attempt any further explanation. By the age of 8–9 years the girl's sister had noticed differences between their genitalia but both girls were satisfied with the explanation about the earlier operation. At this stage the parents were advised to take opportunities to casually mention that not all people can have children of their own. She was shown a diagram to explain the names and functions of parts of the body, including the external genitalia. At 11 years of age she was commenced on hormone replacement which enabled her to develop pubertal changes before her younger sister. The introduction of therapy was explained on the basis that 'some people need such treatment to help change shape'. At 12 years of age, the girl was mature enough to have a fuller discussion which in this case involved watching a film about a patient with CAIS with her mother and paediatrician.

All children are different and mature at different rates but this case history provides a useful framework for families to follow in this difficult situation. It is important to reinforce the positive features of the condition – normal sex life/ possibility of having children by donor egg in those cases where a uterus is present – as well as explaining the problems. Involvement of the whole family is to be encouraged as isolation is a danger as emphasised by the patient who wrote her personal view – 'mine was a dark secret kept from all outside the medical profession (family included) but this is not an option as it increases the feelings of freakishness and the sense of isolation. It also neglects the counselling of siblings'.

It helps to have a diagnosis in order to give as full an explanation as possible as to why the disorder has occurred. Such explanations take time and it is helpful to have a nurse/counsellor who can arrange follow-up visits to reinforce the information given. It is my policy to offer to write to patients and put the information down in a letter which she can then refer to. Patient support groups can also provide helpful literature and back-up. Support needs to be long-term as the psychological problems can be long-lasting – 'I spent a large part of my early twenties feeling repugnance towards myself and I have had to work hard to push it to the back of my mind' (Personal View, 1994).

ACKNOWLEDGEMENTS

I would like to thank Dr Tina Routh, Department of Child Psychiatry, Alder Hey Childrens Hospital for useful comments on the psychological management of these patients.

SUPPORT GROUPS IN THE UNITED KINGDOM

- Androgen Insensitivity Syndrome (AIS) Support Network, c/o Mrs Jackie Burrows, 2 Shirburn Avenue, Mansfield, Nottinghamshire NG18 2BY.
- Vaginoplasty Support Network (North), c/o Sheila Naish, Royd Well Counselling, 35 Royd Terrace, Hebden Bridge, West Yorkshire HX7 7BT.

- Vaginoplasty Support Network (South), c/o Hilary Everett, Gynaecology Social Worker, Social Services Department, St Bartholomews Hospital, London EC1A 7BE.

REFERENCES

Andersson S, Berman BM, Jenkins EP, Russell DW, 1991: Deletion of steroid 5-alpha reductase 2 gene in male pseudohermaphroditism. *Nature* **354**, 159–161.

Baird PN, Santos A, Groves N *et al.* 1992: Constitutional mutations in the WT1 gene in patients with the Denys–Drash syndrome. *Human Molecular Genetics* **1**, 301–306.

Bardoni B, Zanaria E, Guioli S *et al.* 1994: A dosage sensitive locus at chromosome Xp21 is involved in male to female sex reversal. *Nature Genetics* **7**, 497–501.

Batch JA, Davies HR, Evans BAJ, Hughes IA, Patterson MN, 1993: Phenotypic variation and detection of carrier status in the partial androgen insensitivity syndrome. *Archives of Diseases in Childhood* **68**, 453–457.

Bergada C, Cleveland WW, Jones HW Jr, Wilkins L, 1962: Variants of embryonic testicular dysgenesis: bilateral anorchia and the syndrome of rudimentary testes. *Acta Endocrinologica* **40**, 521–536.

Bernstein R, Koo GC, Wachtel SS, 1980: Abnormality of the X chromosome in human 46XY female siblings with dysgenetic ovaries. *Science* **207**, 768–769.

Berta P, Hawkins JR, Sinclair AH *et al.* 1990: Genetic evidence equating SRY and the testis-determining factor. *Nature* **348**, 448–450.

Bevan CL, Brown BB, Davies HR, Evans BAJ, Hughes IA, Patterson MN, 1996: Functional analysis of six androgen receptor mutations identified in patients with partial androgen insensitivity syndrome. *Human Molecular Genetics* **5**, 265–273.

Brondum-Neilson K, Langkjaier F, 1982: Inherited partial X chromosome duplication in a mentally retarded male. *Journal of Medical Genetics* **19**, 222–236.

Brosnan PG, 1980: A new familial syndrome of 46 XY gonadal dysgenesis with anomalies of ectodermal and mesodermal structures. *Journal of Pediatrics* **97**, 586–590.

Capel B, Rasberry C, Dyson J *et al.* 1993: Deletion of Y chromosome sequences located outside the testis determining region can cause XY female sex reversal. *Nature Genetics* **5**, 301–307.

Chang HJ, Clark RD, Bachman H, 1990: The phenotype of 45X\46 XY mosaicism: an analysis of 92 prenatally diagnosed cases. *American Journal of Human Genetics* **46**, 156–167.

Coles K, MacKenzie M, Crolla J *et al.* 1992: A complex rearrangement associated with sex reversal and the Wolff-Hirschorn syndrome: a cytogenetic and molecular study. *Journal of Medical Genetics* **29**, 400–406.

Dewhurst CJ, 1971: The XY female. *American Journal of Obstetrics and Gynaecology* **109**, 675–688.

Dewhurst J, Grant DB, 1984: Intersex problems. *Archives of Disease in Childhood* **59**, 1191–1194.

Diamond M, 1965: A critical evaluation of the ontogeny of human sexual behaviour. *Quarterly Review of Biology* **40**, 147–175.

Drash A, Sherman F, Hartmann WH, Blizzard RM, 1970: A syndrome of pseudohermaphroditism, Wilms tumour, hypertension and degenerative renal disease. *Journal of Pediatrics* **76**, 585–593.

Eicher EM, Washburn LL, 1986: Genetic control of primary sex determination in mice. *Annual Reviews of Genetics* **20**, 327–360.

Ferguson-Smith MA, 1992: Abnormalities of human sex determination. *Journal of Inherited Metabolic Disorders* **15**, 518–525.

Foster JW, Dominguez MA, Guioli S *et al.* 1994: Campomelic dysplasia and autosomal sex reversal caused by mutations in an SRY-related gene. *Nature* **372**, 525–530.

Frasier SD, Bashore RA, Mosier HD, 1964: Gonadoblastoma associated with pure gonadal dysgenesis in monozygotic twins. *Journal of Pediatrics* **64**, 740–745.

Friedman AL, Finlay JL, 1987: The Drash syndrome revisited; diagnosis and follow-up. *American Journal of Medical Genetics* **Suppl. 3**, 293–296.

Geissler WM, Davis DL, Wu L *et al.* 1994: Male pseudohermaphroditism caused by muta-tions of testicular 17beta hydroxysteroid dehydrogenase 3. *Nature Genetics* **7**, 34–39.

German J, Simpson JL, Chaganti RSK, Summitt RL, Reid LB, Merkatz IR, 1978: Genetically determined sex-reversal in 46, XY humans. *Science* **202**, 53–56.

Goodall J, 1991: Helping a child to understand her own testicular feminisation. *Lancet* **337**, 33–35.

Greenberg F, Gresik MV, Carpenter RJ, Law SW, Hoffman LP, Ledbetter DH, 1987: The Gardner–Silengo–Wachtel or genito-palato-cardiac syndrome; male pseudohermaphro-ditism with micrognathia, cleft palate and conotruncal cardiac defect. *American Journal of Medical Genetics* **26**, 59–64.

Griffin JE, 1992: Androgen resistance – the clinical and molecular spectrum. *New England Journal of Medicine* **326**, 611–618.

Haning HV, Chesney RW, Moorthy AV, Gilbert EF, 1985: A syndrome of chronic renal fail-ure and XY gonadal dysgenesis in young phenotypic females without genital ambiguity. *American Journal of Kidney Diseases* **6**, 40–48.

Hastie ND, 1992: Dominant negative mutations in the Wilms tumour (WT1) gene causes Denys–Drash syndrome – proof that a tumour suppressor gene plays a crucial role in nor-mal genitourinary development. *Human Molecular Genetics* **1**, 293–296.

Hodgkin J, 1990: Sex determination compared in Drosophila and Caenorhabiditis. *Nature* **344**, 721–728.

Hoo JJ, Salafsky IS, Lin CC, Pinsky L, 1989: Possible location of a recessive testis forming gene on 9p24. *American Journal of Medical Genetics* **45**, A78.

Houston CS, Opitz JM, Spranger JW *et al.*, 1983: The campomelic syndrome: review, report of 17 cases, and follow-up on the currently 17-year old boy first reported by Maroteaux *et al.* in 1971. *American Journal of Medical Genetics* **15**, 3–28.

Hu L-J, Laporte J, Kress W *et al.* 1996: Deletions in Xq28 in two boys with myotubular myopathy and abnormal genital development define a new contiguous gene syndrome in a 430 kb region. *Human Molecular Genetics* **5**, 139–143.

Hughes IA, 1986: *Handbook of endocrine tests in children*. Wright, Bristol.

Hunter CP, Wood WB, 1992: Evidence from mosaic analysis of the masculinizing gene her-1 for cell interactions in *C. Elegens* sex determination. *Nature* **355**, 551–555.

Irons M, Elias ER, Salen G, Tint GS, Batta AK, 1993: Defective cholesterol biosynthesis in Smith–Lemli–Opitz syndrome. *Lancet* **341**, 1414.

Jager RJ, Anvret M, Hall K, Scherer G, 1990: A human XY female with a frameshift muta-tion in the candidate testis-determining gene SRY. *Nature* **348**, 452–453.

Jagiello G, Atwell JD, 1962: Prevalence of testicular feminisation. *Lancet* **i**, 329.

Kremer H, Kraaij R, Toledo SPA *et al.* 1995: Male pseudohermaphroditism due to a homozygous missense mutation of the luteinizing hormone receptor gene. *Nature Genetics* **9**, 160–164.

Maaswinkel-Mooij PD, Stokvis-Brantsma WH, 1992: Phenotypically normal girl with male pseudohermaphroditism, hypoplastic left ventricle, lung aplasia, horseshoe kidney and diaphragmatic hernia. *American Journal of Medical Genetics* **42**, 647–648.

Mann JR, Corkery JJ, Fisher HJW *et al.* 1983: The X-linked recessive form of XY gonadal dysgenesis with a high incidence of gonadal germ cell tumours: clinical and genetic studies. *Journal of Medical Genetics* **20**, 264–270.

McElreavy K, Vilain E, Abbas N *et al.* 1992: XY sex reversal associated with a deletion 5′ to the SRY 'HMG box' in the testis-determining region. *Proceedings of the National Academy of Sciences, USA* **89**, 11016–11020.

McElreavy K, Vilain E, Abbas N, Herskowitz I, Fellous MA, 1993: A regulatory cascade hypothesis for mammalian sex determination: SRY represses a negative regulator of male development. *PNAS* **90**, 3368–3372.

McKusick VA, 1992: *Mendelian inheritance in man*, 10th edn. Baltimore: Johns Hopkins University Press.

Moorthy AV, Chesney RW, Lubinsky M, 1987: Chronic renal failure and XY gonadal dysgenesis: 'Frasier' syndrome – a commentary on reported cases. *American Journal of Medical Genetics* **Suppl.3**, 297–302.

Morris JM, Mahesh VB, 1963: Further observations on the syndrome 'testicular feminisation'. *American Journal of Obstetrics and Gynaecology* **87**, 731–748.

Mueller RF, 1994. The Denys–Drash syndrome. *Journal of Medical Genetics* **31**, 471–477.

Narahara K, Kodama Y, Kimura S *et al.* 1979: Probable inverted tandem duplication of Xp in a 46, Xp+ Y boy. *Japanese Journal of Human Genetics* **24**, 105–110.

Ninomiya S, Isomura M, Narahara K, Seino Y, Nakamura Y, 1996: Isolation of a testis-specific cDNA on chromosome 17q from a region adjacent to the breakpoint of t(12;17) observed in a patient with acampomelic campomelic dysplasia and sex reversal. *Human Molecular Genetics* **51**, 69–72.

Nivelon A, Nivelon J-L, Mabille J-P *et al.* 1992: New autosomal recessive chondrodysplasia-pseudohermaphroditism syndrome. *Clinical Dysmorphology* **1**, 221–227.

Odame I, Donaldson MDC, Wallace AM, Cochran W, Smith PJ, 1992: Early diagnosis and management of 5-alpha reductase deficiency. *Archives of Disease in Childhood* **67**, 720–723.

Ogata T, Hawkins JR, Taylor A, Matsuo N, Hata J, Goodfellow PN, 1992: Sex reversal in a child with a 46 X,Yp+ karyotype: support for the existence of a gene(s), located in Xp21, involved in testis formation. *Journal of Medical Genetics* **29**, 226–230.

Ogata T, Matsou O, 1994: Testis determining gene(s) on the X chromosome short arm: chromosomal localisation and possible role in testis determination. *Journal of Medical Genetics* **31**, 349–350.

Ogawa O, Eccles MR, Yun K *et al.* 1993: A novel insertional mutation at the third zinc finger coding region of the WT1 gene in Denys–Drash syndrome. *Human Molecular Genetics* **2**, 259–264.

Page DC, Mosher R, Simpson EM *et al.* 1987: The sex-determining region of the human Y chromosome encodes a finger protein. *Cell* **51**, 1091–1104.

Personal View, 1994: Once a dark secret. *British Medical Journal* **308**, 542.

Sai T, Seino S, Chang C *et al.* 1990: An exonic point mutation of the androgen receptor gene in a family with complete androgen insensitivity. *American Journal of Human Genetics* **46**, 1095–1100.

Saldanha PH, Arnold IJP, Mendonca BB, Bloise W, Toledo SPA, 1987: A clinico-genetic investigation of Leydig cell hypoplasia. *American Journal of Medical Genetics* **26**, 337–344.

Scherer G, Schempp W, Baccicchetti C *et al.* 1989: Duplication of an Xp segment that includes the ZFX locus causes sex inversion in man. *Human Genetics* **81**, 291–294.

Schipper JA, Delemarre-v d Waal HA, Jansen M, Sprangers MAJ, 1991: Case report: testicular dysgenesis and mental retardation in two incompletely masculinized XY-siblings. *Acta Paediatrica Scandinavia* **80**, 125–128.

Schmitt-Ney M, Thiele H, Kaltwasser P, Bardoni B, Cisternino M, Scherer G, 1995: Two novel SRY missense mutations reducing DNA binding in XY females and their mosaic fathers. *American Journal of Human Genetics* **56**, 862–869.

Simpson JL, 1990: Disorders of the gonads and internal reproductive tracts. In Emery AEH, Rimoin DL, (eds), *Principles and practice of medical genetics,* 2nd edn, Edinburgh: Churchill Livingstone. 1593–1617.

Simpson JL, Blagowidow N, Martin AO, 1981: XY gonadal dysgenesis: genetic heterogeneity based upon clinical observations, H-Y antigen status and segregation analysis. *Human Genetics* **58**, 91–97.

Simpson JL, Chaganti RSK, Mourdian J, German J, 1982: Chronic renal disease, myotonic dystrophy and gonadoblastoma in XY gonadal dysgenesis. *Journal of Medical Genetics* **19**, 73–76.

Sinclair AH, 1995: New genes for boys. *American Journal of Human Genetics* **57**, 998–1001.

Sinclair AH, Berta P, Palmer MS *et al.* 1990: A gene from the human sex-determining region encodes a protein with homology to a conserved DNA-binding motif. *Nature* **346**, 240–244.

Stephens JD, 1984: Prenatal diagnosis of testicular feminisation. *Lancet* **ii**, 1038.

Stern HJ, Garrity AM, Saal HM, Wangsa D, Disteche CM, 1990: Duplication Xp21 and sex reversal: insight into the mechanism of sex determination. *American Journal of Human Genetics* **47** (suppl), 1.81 (0153).

Sternberg WH, Barclay DL, Kloepfer HW, 1968: Familial XY gonadal dysgenesis. *New England Journal of Medicine* **278**, 695–700.

Swain A, Zanaria E, Hacker A, Lovell-Badge R, Camerino G, 1996: Mouse DAXI expression is consistent with a role in sex determination as well as in adrenal and hypothalamus function. *Nature Genetics* **12**, 404–409.

Tajima T, Fujieda K, Nakae J *et al.* 1995: Molecular analysis of type 11 3beta-hydroxy-steroid dehydrogenase gene in Japanese patients with classical 3beta-hydroxysteroid dehydrogenase deficiency. *Human Molecular Genetics* **4**, 969–971.

Tee M-K, Lin D, Sugawara T *et al.* 1995: T-A transversion 11bp from a splice acceptor site in the human gene for steroidogenic acute regulatory protein causes congenital lipoid adrenal hyperplasia. *Human Molecular Genetics* **4**, 2299–2305.

Tint GS, Lyons M, Elias ER *et al.* 1994: Defective cholesterol biosynthesis associated with the Smith–Lemli–Opitz syndrome. *New England Journal of Medicine* **330**, 107–113.

Toriello HV, Higgins JV, 1992: Report of another child with sex reversal and cardiac, pulmonary and diaphragm defects (letter). *American Journal of Medical Genetics* **44**, 252.

Verloes A, Gillerot Y, Delfortrie J *et al.* 1990: Male pseudohermaphroditism with persistent Mullerian structures, mental retardation and Borjesson–Forssman–Lehmann–like features. A new syndrome? *Genetic Counselling* **1**, 219–225.

Verp MS, Simpson JL, 1987: Abnormal sexual differentiation and neoplasia. *Cancer Genetics Cytogenetics* **25**, 191–218.

Vilain E, Le Fiblec B, Morichon-Delvallez N *et al.* 1994: SRY-negative XX fetus with complete male phenotype. *Lancet* **343**, 240–241.

Vilain E, McElreavy K, Jaubert F, Raymond JP, Richaud F, Fellous M, 1992: Familial case of with sequence variant in the testis-determining region associated with two sex phenotypes. *American Journal of Human Genetics* **50**, 1008–1011.

Wagner T, Wirth J, Meyer J *et al.* 1994: Autosomal sex reversal and campomelic dysplasia are caused by mutations in and around the SRY-related gene SOX9. *Cell* **79**, 1111–1120.

Wilkie AOM, Campbell FM, Daubeney P *et al.* 1993: Complete and partial XY sex reversal associated with terminal deletion of 10q: Report of 2 cases and literature review. *American Journal of Medical Genetics* **46**, 597–600.

Yanase T, Simpson ER, Waterman MR, 1991: 17-alpha-hydroxylase/17,20-lyase deficiency: from clinical investigation to molecular definition. *Endocrinology Reviews* **12**, 91–108.

PART IV

GYNAECOLOGICAL PROBLEMS THROUGHOUT CHILDHOOD AND ADOLESCENCE

CHAPTER 13

Abdominal pain

DAVID A. LLOYD AND PAUL D. LOSTY ───────────────

Abdominal pain in the adolescent female is a common problem and a frequent cause of hospital admission and parental anxiety (O'Donnell, 1985). The differential diagnosis faced by clinicians is more diverse than in males, and must take into account an understanding of the female internal genital anatomy, as well as the physiological hormonal changes that herald the beginning of reproductive life. This Chapter provides a practical approach to the diagnosis and management of abdominal pain in the adolescent female. Relevant pathological disorders are discussed.

ACUTE ABDOMINAL PAIN

Acute abdominal pain demands prompt diagnosis and management. The pain requires adequate, effective analgesia and the possibility that a potentially life-threatening disorder may exist must always be borne in mind. Diagnosis in most situations is arrived at by a thorough clinical history and physical examination, together with the appropriate use of ancillary laboratory and radiological studies. The differential diagnosis is extensive and the commonly encountered conditions are listed in Table 13.1.

History and Physical Examination

An adequate clinical history should record the chronological sequence of events leading up to presentation: the location of the pain and its radiation; any associated gastrointestinal upset; urinary tract infection and/or other systemic disorders should all be noted. A menstrual, sexual and contraceptive history is mandatory in the adolescent. Physical examination should be conducted methodically in an unhurried manner, and time spent gaining the patient's confidence is often worthwhile. The presence of a nurse (chaperone) or the mother at the initial examination is important. A general examination should be done initially, then specific attention should focus on the abdomen in order to localise the site of the pain and elicit signs of peritoneal irritation, tenderness, guarding and/or signs of

Table 13.1   Differential diagnosis of acute abdominal pain in adolescent females

Gynaecological pathology	Pelvic inflammatory disease
	Rupture of physiological–functional ovarian cyst
	Tubo-ovarian torsion
	Ectopic pregnancy
	Tumour
	Endometriosis
	Congenital vaginal anomalies
	Mittelschmertz
Gastrointestinal pathology	Appendicitis
	Acute non-specific abdominal pain
	Meckel's diverticulitis
	Mesenteric adenitis
	Intestinal obstruction
	Gastroenteritis
Urinary tract disorders	Urinary tract infection
	Urinary calculus disease
	Obstructive uropathies

intestinal obstruction. Pelvic and rectal examination are not required as a routine in the adolescent girl, but occasionally are necessary. In an apprehensive girl the examination may be done under general anaesthesia.

Diagnostic Studies

Laboratory studies should include a full blood count with differential profile, C-reactive protein (CRP) measurement, urinalysis including microscopy and urine culture, bacteriological cultures of any vaginal discharge and a pregnancy test when appropriate (Ashcraft and Holder, 1993; Stovroff *et al.*, 1994).

Leucocytosis and a raised CRP suggest an infective or inflammatory process, and torsion of an adnexal appendage must also be considered. A negative pregnancy test does not exclude the possibility of an intrauterine or ectopic pregnancy (Goldstein, 1989). Ultrasound examination will help confirm the presence or absence of an intra-abdominal or pelvic mass, in addition to providing information about the morphology of the ovaries and uterus, including intrauterine or ectopic pregnancy, and the presence of calcification or intra-peritoneal air or fluid (Goldstein, 1989; Moss *et al.*, 1993). Abdominal X-ray may be helpful if there is a faecolith (Fig. 13.1) or intestinal obstruction. Computerised tomography (CT) and magnetic resonance imaging (MRI) are playing an increasingly important role in diagnosis, particularly when neoplasia is suspected. Serum in such patients should be reserved for analysis of the tumour markers β-human chorionic gonadotrophin (β-HCG) and alpha-fetoprotein (AFP), which are also useful for follow up surveillance. Finally, the availability of laparoscopy has

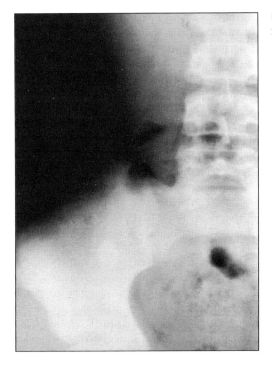

Fig. 13.1 Plain abdominal X-ray showing the presence of a faecolith.

seen further advances in diagnosis and definitive patient care (Gans and Austin, 1988; Shaler *et al.*, 1991; Héloury *et al.*, 1992).

Management – General Principles

Definitive management depends on the clinical findings and diagnostic studies as well as sound clinical judgement. The following diagnostic scenarios may arise:

- *Surgical emergencies that necessitate prompt laparotomy.* Diagnosis in these situations includes acute appendicitis or perforated appendicitis with peritonitis, tubo-ovarian pathology such as a torsion or abscess, and acute haemoperitoneum as a result of a ruptured ectopic pregnancy. Other less common gastrointestinal emergencies should also be borne in mind.
- *Acute abdominal conditions* not *requiring urgent operation.* Examples include infective gastroenteritis, inflammatory bowel disease, and pelvic inflammatory disease (PID).
- *Conditions mimicking the 'acute abdomen'.* Included in this category are urinary tract infection, lobar pneumonia and spinal disorders.
- *Events related to ovulation and menstruation.* These include rupture of an ovarian follicular or corpus luteal cyst and disorders related to menstruation, such as dysmenorrhoea.
- *Acute abdominal pain of undetermined origin.* It is within this group that most confusion and difficulty can arise. The clinician is often faced by the

questions 'Is this appendicitis?' 'Could this be a twisted ovary?', 'Does this patient have an ectopic pregnancy?'. In such patients laparoscopy has a valuable role to play. Laparoscopy permits an immediate diagnosis that can direct further management. Furthermore, with the advances in laparoscopic instrumentation, it is now technically feasible to perform definitive procedures such as appendicectomy, cyst puncture, biopsy of suspicious intraperitoneal lesions and laparoscopic 'fixation' of ovarian and adnexal tissues following torsion (Gans and Austin, 1988; Shaler *et al.*, 1991; Héloury *et al.*, 1992; Ashcraft and Holder, 1993). It is important to recognise that included within this category are adolescents with the characteristic features of acute non-specific abdominal pain (*vide infra*).

SPECIFIC DISORDERS CAUSING ACUTE ABDOMINAL PAIN (Refer to Table 13.1)

Gynaecological Pathology

Pelvic inflammatory disease (PID)

PID results from infection of the uterus, fallopian tubes, ovaries, and the pelvic peritoneum, vascular structures and connective tissues (Khoiny, 1989). Excluding infection following teenage pregnancy, involvement of the uterus is unusual. The adnexa are common sites for primary infection, the usual mode of transmission being ascending infection through the cervix. Sexually transmitted diseases (STD) have been identified as key elements in PID (Khoiny, 1989; Shafer and Sweet, 1989). Congenital anomalies of the urogenital tract (septate uterus, rudimentary uterine horns or cloacal anorectal disorders) may also predispose to infection. Adolescent females between the ages of 15 and 19 years, are a high risk group for PID; impaired immune host defences are frequently cited as risk factors for this age group. Organisms usually implicated are *Neisseria gonorrhoea* and *Chlamydia trachomatis*. Once infection reaches the fallopian tubes and ovaries, tubo-ovarian abscess formation may occur. The Fitz-Hugh–Curtis syndrome (infectious perihepatitis), may affect up to 30% of infected females and arises when purulent peritoneal exudate tracks along the parietal peritoneal surfaces to the liver capsule and undersurface of the diaphragm, producing extensive intra-abdominal adhesions (Khoiny, 1989). Several factors link the onset of PID to the menstrual cycle; breakdown of the protective cervical mucus barrier and the culture medium provided by the menstrual flow are cited as aetiological factors (Washington *et al.*, 1985).

Clinical features

PID disease can present as acute or chronic abdominal pain (Khoiny, 1989; Shafer and Sweet, 1989). Acute PID is characterised by a short clinical history, usually of less than 3 weeks duration. Chronic presentation is less well defined.

The clinical features are variable. The adolescent girl with acute PID usually presents with lower abdominal pain, malaise, fever, dysuria and vaginal discharge. In patients with the Fitz-Hugh–Curtis syndrome there may be right upper quadrant abdominal tenderness. Other patients have unilateral or bilateral iliac fossa tenderness and guarding. In the presence of purulent peritonitis, guarding and rebound tenderness are common. Patients who develop a tubo-ovarian abscess may have a palpable abdominal mass (Khoiny, 1989; Shafer and Sweet, 1989) which, on the right side, must be distinguished from an appendix abscess.

Diagnosis

The diagnosis is based on the history, physical examination and clinical suspicion. Laboratory studies include full blood count with differential profile, erythrocyte sedimentation rate (ESR) or CRP, culture of the vaginal discharge and endocervical swab and pregnancy test. Ultrasound has a key role to play in the diagnosis of tubo-ovarian abscess formation (Fig. 13.2) and in excluding ectopic pregnancy or retained intrauterine products (Khoiny, 1989; Shafer and Sweet, 1989).

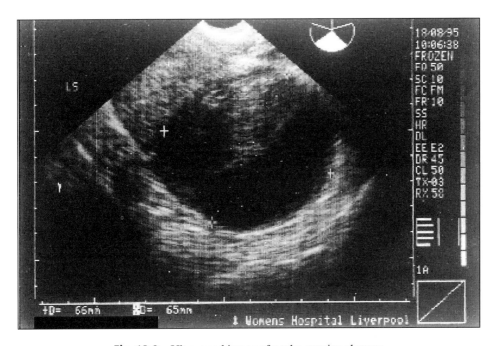

Fig. 13.2   Ultrasound image of a tubo-ovarian abscess.

Treatment

Antibiotic therapy should be commenced promptly after diagnosis. Recommended agents are a combination of tetracycline with a cephalosporin or a combination of clindamycin and gentamicin. Antibiotics are continued until symptoms and signs subside, usually in 5–7 days. Management should be further guided by the results of culture studies. Non-responders may require laparotomy or a laparoscopic assisted drainage procedure. Long-term sequelae include adhesions, tubal stenosis, ectopic pregnancy and infertility (Khoiny, 1989; Shafer and Sweet, 1989).

Rupture of a physiologic (functional) ovarian cyst

With the onset of puberty, physiological hormonal changes lead to maturation of the female internal reproductive organs. In the ovaries, follicles develop and it is not surprising that cystic ovaries are frequently seen in this age group. Rupture of a follicular or corpus luteal cyst may occur during midcycle or may herald the onset of menstruation. Ultrasound is invaluable in assessing such situations. Management is expectant and full resolution of symptoms can be anticipated. Increasing severity of symptoms suggests other pathology such as haemorrhage, torsion or ruptured ectopic pregnancy (*vide infra*).

Tubo-ovarian torsion

Torsion of the ovary or the fallopian tube may present with acute or subacute lower abdominal pain (Mordehai *et al.*, 1991; Kurzbart *et al.*, 1994). Predisposing factors include enlargement of the ovary due to cystic disease or a neoplasm, excess mobility of the adnexa due to an abnormally long mesosalpinx or mesovarium, adnexal venous congestion and tubal disease, such as hydrosalpinx (James *et al.*, 1970; Evans, 1978; Mordehai *et al.*, 1991).

Urgent recognition of torsion is essential if the ovary is to be salvaged (Fig. 13.3) but accurate pre-operative diagnosis can be difficult. Symptoms and signs depend on the degree of torsion and can vary from intermittent lower abdominal pain or cramps to an acute abdominal crisis. Anorexia, nausea, vomiting, fever and leucocytosis may be present, particularly if infection and necrosis occur with abdominal tenderness and guarding on the side of the torsion. A mass may be palpated. Right-sided torsion can mimic early acute appendicitis or acute non-specific abdominal pain (ANSAP); as a result the diagnosis frequently is delayed.

Urgent ultrasound scanning is essential when tubo-ovarian torsion is suspected and may reveal diffuse ovarian enlargement, a complex pelvic mass, and occasionally free fluid in the pouch of Douglas (Mordehai *et al.*, 1991) (Fig. 13.4). Laparoscopy provides an immediate diagnosis in the difficult case.

Definitive treatment is emergency surgery if the ovary is to be salvaged. At laparotomy, the torted adnexa are untwisted (Mordehai *et al.*, 1991; Kurzbart *et al.*, 1994). Infarcted, necrotic tissue should be excised. It is important to fix the contralateral ovary (Mordehai *et al.*, 1991). It is now technically feasible to perform some of these procedures by laparoscopy (Shaler *et al.*, 1991).

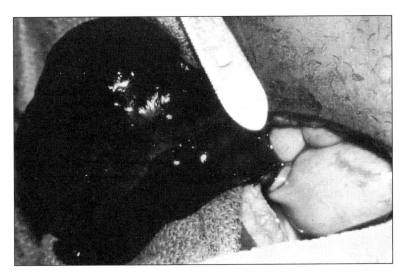

Fig. 13.3   Infarcted, necrotic ovary and tube as a result of torsion.

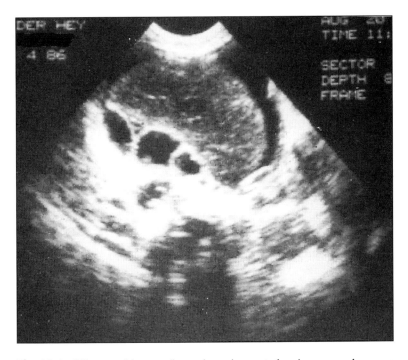

Fig. 13.4   Ultrasound image of torted ovarian cyst showing a complex mass surrounded by free fluid.

Ectopic pregnancy

Ectopic (tubal) pregnancy is an ever increasing problem encountered in sexually active adolescents (Ammerman *et al.*, 1990). In the United States of America, the incidence has increased five-fold in the last 20 years, from 18 000 cases in the 1970s to 88 000 cases in the late 1980s (Ammerman *et al.*, 1990). Ectopic pregnancy is now the leading cause of death in the first trimester of pregnancy (Ammerman *et al.*, 1990). Predisposing factors include tubal abnormalities, notably salpingitis, congenital anomalies, adhesions, prior tubal surgery and endometriosis (Marchbanks *et al.*, 1988; Taylor, 1988). Mortality is highest in adolescence, primarily due to delay in recognition by the patient that she may be pregnant, and failure of attending medical personnel to suspect pregnancy in the young adolescent (Ammerman *et al.*, 1990).

Clinical features

The cardinal symptoms of ectopic pregnancy include abdominal pain, amenorrhoea and vaginal bleeding. The abdominal pain varies in intensity and may be localised to the side of the pregnancy. Pain becomes more diffuse and severe when tubal rupture occurs. Syncope, shoulder tip pain and shock may follow as a result of haemoperitoneum. A history of amenorrhoea and vaginal bleeding or 'spotting' is reported by 75% of patients. Vital signs usually are well maintained until late into the course of the illness. A pelvic mass is identifiable in 50% of patients (Ammerman *et al.*, 1990).

Diagnosis and treatment

The urinary pregnancy test, which provides a result within minutes, is important in the emergency situation. Reliability is increased when urinary specific gravity is greater than 1.015. Ideally, serum should also be drawn for quantitative estimation of β-HCG to confirm that the patient is pregnant and if so, whether it is a normal intrauterine pregnancy. β-HCG, produced by the placenta, is first detected in maternal serum 10 days following conception and has a doubling time in serum of 1.9–2.0 days within the first 30 days of a normal gestation (Ammerman *et al.*, 1990). Ectopic tissue is known to produce HCG at lower rates. This, therefore, can be used to predict the likelihood of the pregnancy being intrauterine or ectopic.

Ultrasound, in combination with a positive pregnancy test, is diagnostic (Fig. 13.5). At 6.5 weeks, the yolk sac can be identified, and at 7 weeks following the last menstrual period, the embryo can be visualised clearly (Nyberg *et al.*, 1985). Laparoscopy may also be used for diagnosis (Ammerman *et al.*, 1990). Increasing emphasis is now placed on tubal preservation, when possible, to maximise future fertility potential (Hallat, 1986). Following resuscitation and stabilisation, surgical management by laparoscopic or open technique includes salpingotomy, evacuation of the ectopic pregnancy and tubal repair. Failing this, salpingectomy is performed.

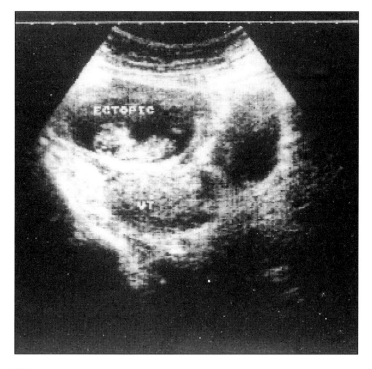

Fig. 13.5 Ultrasound image of an ectopic pregnancy in the left adnexa. The fetus, which was viable, was clearly seen. It is unusual to see a viable fetus in an ectopic pregnancy, more usually the diagnosis is made by the finding of a positive pregnancy test in the absence of an intra-uterine pregnancy. UT= uterus.

Neoplasms

In adolescent girls, neoplasms of the ovary are rare and most lesions encountered in paediatric surgical practice are benign (Schwobel and Stauffer, 1991; Brown *et al.*, 1993; Skinner *et al.*, 1993; Van Winter *et al.*, 1994). Abdominal pain may be a presenting feature and can on occasions simulate appendicitis. The pain usually is chronic and often is accompanied by abdominal distension. In the pre-adolescent female with an oestrogen-secreting tumour, precocious puberty may occur. Weight loss, anaemia and ill health are ominous findings suggesting malignancy. A neoplasm may also present acutely as a result of complications, notably torsion or haemorrhage. Ovarian neoplasms are discussed in Chapter 15.

Diagnosis and treatment

Measurement of β-HCG and AFP levels will identify tumours of germ cell origin (Schwobel and Stauffer, 1991; Brown *et al.*, 1993; Skinner *et al.*, 1993; Van Winter *et al.*, 1994). Inhibin and Mullerian-inhibiting substance (MIS) are elevated in some patients with granulosa cell tumours (Gustafson *et al.*, 1992, 1993; Lappohn *et al.*, 1993). All of these serum protein markers play an important role in tumour follow up.

A plain abdominal radiograph may reveal calcification in a soft tissue mass consistent with a tumour (Moss *et al.*, 1993). Ultrasound can further differentiate the lesion as solid, cystic or of mixed composition (Thind *et al.*, 1989). CT scanning and MRI studies may provide further information. A chest radiograph is essential for identifying possible metastases (Schwobel and Stauffer, 1991; Brown *et al.*, 1993; Skinner *et al.*, 1993; Van Winter *et al.*, 1994). Benign lesions should be managed by conservative surgical methods, namely ultrasound guided cyst puncture, cystectomy or partial oophorectomy where possible, in order to preserve future reproductive and endocrine potential. A benign cyst less than 5 cm in diameter should be managed non-operatively with serial clinical and radiographic follow up.

Malignant disease requires surgery, chemotherapy and/or radiotherapy depending on the type of tumour and stage at presentation (Schwobel and Stauffer, 1991; Brown *et al.*, 1993; Skinner *et al.*, 1993) (see Chapter 14).

Endometriosis (see p. 149)

Endometriosis, a condition characterised by the presence of ectopic endometrial tissue, may present with acute or chronic abdominal pain. The most frequent sites for ectopic endometrial implantation are the uterosacral ligaments, the pouch of Douglas and the ovaries, where the lesions may lead to internal haemorrhage and cyst formation. Clinical presentation in the adolescent girl is often associated with lower abdominal pain and heavy menstruation. In sexually active girls, coitus can provoke pelvic pain (Cuschieri and Bouchier, 1989).

Ultrasonography, CT scanning and MRI play a minor role in diagnosis (Togashi *et al.*, 1991). However, laparoscopy permits direct visualisation of the affected organs (Vercellini *et al.*, 1989).

Definitive treatment is by surgery. In milder cases, pharmacological hormonal manipulation can be carried out using oestrogen–progestogen preparations or the anti-gonadotrophin agent, danazol.

Congenital vaginal anomalies (see p. 137)

Rarely, congenital abnormalities of the vagina may present in adolescence with acute or chronic abdominal pain. An imperforate hymen may not be detected until medical attention is sought because of amenorrhoea and abdominal pain. Physical examination in such circumstances may reveal a lower abdominal mass (the distended uterus) and a bulging hymenal membrane. Ultrasound examination demonstrates vaginal and uterine distension. Under anaesthesia, the visible bulging hymenal membrane is incised in a cruciate manner, draining the retained menstrual and vaginal secretions.

Uterine duplication and vaginal septation may be seen as isolated abnormalities or as part of a more complex cloacal anorectal anomaly. In the latter, the abnormality is readily identified at birth. In isolated cases, presentation may be delayed until adolescence, when symptoms develop after the onset of menstruation. Pain arises if there is obstruction of the hemi-vagina which becomes distended by the menstrual flow. Examination under anaesthesia reveals a patent vagina, a visible cervix and a paravaginal mass. Ultrasound or CT reveals a dilated hemi-vagina with its own uterus and fallopian tube. Division of the septated vagina creates a single vagina with a double cervix and uterus.

Gastrointestinal Pathology

Appendicitis

Acute appendicitis is the most common condition which requires emergency surgery in paediatric surgical practice. The incidence is 1.9 per 1000 females compared to 1.5 per 1000 males and predominantly is seen in the 20–30-year-old age group (Cuschieri and Bouchier, 1989). Specific problems may arise in adolescent females, as a result of incorrect assumptions that a gynaecological disorder exists, resulting in delay in diagnosis and definitive treatment and a subsequent increase in morbidity.

Clinical features

Acute appendicitis follows a sequential clinical pattern, the predominant early symptoms being vomiting and abdominal pain. The initial pain is typically periumbilical, following which it localises to the right iliac fossa. Nausea, vomiting, anorexia and thirst invariably accompany the pain. Fever and tachycardia become prominent as the disease process further evolves. Variations in symptomatology may be accounted for by the anatomical location of the appendix. For example, urinary symptoms of dysuria and frequency may arise if a retrocaecal appendix is resting alongside the ureter. Similarly, symptoms of an inflamed pelvic appendix, provoking diarrhoea through rectal irritation, may mimic gastroenteritis.

Physical findings

The cardinal physical finding in acute appendicitis is localised point tenderness, usually at McBurneys's point. Generalised tenderness implies advanced disease with generalised peritonitis as a result of perforation. Involuntary guarding indicates peritoneal inflammation; gentle shaking or percussion of the abdomen can also be used to demonstrate this. Asking the patient to 'sit up', 'hop out of bed', or 'jump up and down' are useful manoeuvres in the apprehensive child, when the diagnosis may be in doubt (O'Donnell, 1985). A number of the so-called 'classic signs' of appendicitis, such as Rovsing's sign (pain in the right iliac fossa when pressure is applied to the left iliac fossa), or the presence of hyper-aesthesia in Sherren's triangle, are of historical rather than practical significance. An appendiceal mass may be palpated in the advanced stage of appendicitis. Rectal examination rarely is required in the child to make a diagnosis of appendicitis and is not recommended as a routine.

Investigations

Appendicitis is essentially a clinical diagnosis. In doubtful circumstances the white cell count can be useful but a normal leucocyte count does not exclude appendicitis (Cuschieri and Bouchier, 1989). Elevation of the CRP level indicates an inflammatory process is present (Stovroff *et al.*, 1994). Urinalysis may reveal a pyuria as a result of ureteric or bladder irritation.

Imaging is unnecessary in most patients. In the adolescent female, however, ultrasound has a major role to play in excluding tubo-ovarian pathology. Typical ultrasound findings in appendicitis include thickening or distension of the appendix, which may be surrounded by dilated, non-contracting loops of intestine; an appendix abscess may also be identified (Fig. 13.6) (Wong *et al.*, 1994). On plain X-ray the presence of a calcified faecolith, found in 20% of cases, may be helpful when the diagnosis is uncertain.

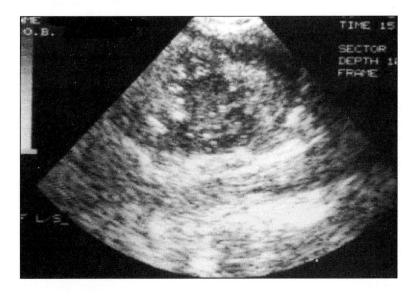

Fig. 13.6 Ultrasound image of complex appendix mass.

Differential diagnosis

The following differential diagnosis need to be considered: acute gynaecological disorders (notably torsion of ovarian cyst, salpingitis, ruptured follicular cyst, tumour and ectopic pregnancy), urinary tract infection and Meckel's diverticulitis.

Treatment

Early appendicectomy, under prophylactic antibiotic cover, is the definitive treatment. Adequate pre-operative preparation of the patient is mandatory. There is little to gain from rushing a dehydrated, pyrexial patient to the operating theatre (O'Donnell, 1988). Adequate volumes of crystalloid or colloid should be administered intravenously, together with broad spectrum antibiotics when perforation is suspected. Analgesia and antipyretics should not be withheld. In complicated cases, a nasogastric tube may be required for gastrointestinal decompression and a urinary catheter for monitoring urinary output. At operation, the appendix should be removed. In the presence of perforation with general contamination, saline lavage is carried out. This helps to rinse out infected debris within the peritoneal cavity. We close all wounds primarily using subcuticular sutures and have found, like others, a low incidence of wound infection (Surana and Puri, 1994). Drains are used only to drain an abscess cavity.

Appendiceal mass

If, on initial examination, a fixed appendiceal mass is palpated, appendicectomy is postponed (O'Donnell, 1988). A 5–7 day course of antibiotics is given, and provided the mass and systemic features resolve, the patient may be discharged. Interval appendicectomy may be performed electively 4–6 weeks later (O'Donnell, 1988).

   If an appendix mass is palpated when the patient is already under anaesthesia, we proceed with the operation to drain the abscess, using an extraperitoneal approach. The appendix is removed if this can be done easily, otherwise it is left *in situ*. If a faecolith is present it should be removed if possible. Pus is removed by suctionand a penrose drain is left in the abscess cavity. Some surgeons, on palpating a fixed mass under anaesthesia, may defer the operation, treat with antibiotics and perform a delayed appendicectomy (O'Donnell, 1988).

Antibiotic therapy

In cases of uncomplicated acute appendicitis, our policy is to administer prophylactic antibiotics (currently we use a broad spectrum cephalosporin and metronidazole) on induction of anaesthesia and then 8-hourly for a total of 3 doses only. With perforated appendicitis, the antibiotic therapy is commenced immediately in the pre-operative resuscitation period. Peritoneal swab cultures and the clinical post-operative course of the patient will determine the need for additional or alternative antibiotics such as an aminoglycoside. We continue antibiotic therapy for a minimum of 48 hours post-operatively in cases of gangrenous appendicitis and 5 days if perforation with generalised peritoneal contamination has occurred.

Complications

The most significant complication following appendicectomy is infection, which includes local wound infection and pelvic or abdominal sepsis, with or without abscess formation. This usually develops within 4 days after operation. Infection may be suspected from the presence of a painful red wound, pyrexia, or paralytic ileus. With abscess formation, a swinging temperature develops accompanied by elevation of the white blood cell count. Ultrasound scanning may demonstrate the abscess cavity. A small abscess may resolve with antibiotic therapy. Abscess collections which persist should be drained, either percutaneously under ultrasound guidance, or locally if pointing occurs at the wound site or in the rectum. Intestinal obstruction may develop early as a manifestation of sepsis, or as adhesive obstruction months or years following appendicectomy. Stump 'blowout' is a rare occurrence (Ashcraft and Holder, 1993). Scarring and obstruction of the fallopian tubes has been reported as a potential complication in females with pelvic sepsis (Mastroianni, 1978). Infertility has been reported in some series, although others have found evidence to the contrary, refuting such claims, provided there is sufficient evidence to exclude prior tubal inflammatory disease in such patients (Powley, 1965; Thompson and Lynn, 1971; Mastroianni, 1978; Wiig *et al.*, 1979; Puri *et al.*, 1984).

Acute non-specific abdominal pain

This condition represents the commonest cause of acute abdominal pain in paediatric surgical practice, and accounts for well over 50% of hospital admissions in certain series (O'Donnell, 1985). The aetiology is not known, but is attributed to viral infection, although cause and effect remain to be proven. Typical symptoms and signs include central non-radiating abdominal pain, which is more of a constant ache and has a gradual onset. There are few, if any, positive abdominal findings apart from mild peri-umbilical or hypogastric tenderness. Guarding rarely is present. A policy of 'active observation' involving periodic clinical examination coupled with an adequate explanation to the parents and patient of the benign self-limiting course of this disorder, helps to allay anxiety. In most patients complete resolution of symptoms occurs in 24–36 hours. Fewer than 1% of patients go on to develop acute appendicitis (O'Donnell, 1985).

Mesenteric adenitis

Mesenteric adenitis refers to a condition in which there is pathological enlargement of the mesenteric lymph nodes in association with central colicky abdominal pain. Characteristic of this condition is the presence of a high pyrexia (39°C or more), which tends to be out of proportion to the findings on abdominal examination. A history of recent upper respiratory tract infection or sore throat may be obtained. The presence of a red throat, pustular or erythematous tonsils and cervical adenopathy is diagnostic in typical cases. In the thin teenage female, enlarged nodes may be palpable on abdominal examination. In such circumstances operation can be avoided. A benign self-limiting course (24–48 hours) is predictable and appropriate use of a mild antipyretic analgesic (for example, paracetamol) usually suffices, with antibiotics only rarely indicated. Patients whose clinical features are not typical or in whom doubt exists, require a laparoscopy or laparotomy to confirm the diagnosis. The presence of a normal appendix and fleshy enlarged mesenteric nodes is characteristic (O'Donnell, 1985). The appendix should be removed and submitted for histological examination.

Meckel's diverticulitis

This remnant of the embryonic vitello-intestinal duct is found in approximately 2% of the population, and in most it remains asymptomatic. The complications which may occur are bleeding due to peptic ulceration, intestinal obstruction by bands, or abdominal pain due to diverticulitis. The latter simulates acute appendicitis; indeed, the symptoms and signs are indistinguishable and the diagnosis usually is made at laparotomy. Perforation may complicate diverticulitis or can develop as a result of peptic ulceration. On occasions, intussusception can occur. Volvulus of a narrow-based Meckel's or the entire midgut as a result of a congenital Meckel's band obstruction is also possible.

Diagnosis and treatment

Abdominal pain secondary to Meckel's diverticulitis invariably is attributed to appendicitis until the true cause is revealed at laparotomy. Scintiscanning may be useful for gastrointestinal bleeding associated with Meckel's diverticulum. Radiolabelled technetium-99 is taken up preferentially by the ectopic gastric mucosa (Fig. 13.7) (Harden *et al.*, 1967; Jewett *et al.*, 1970); the sensitivity and specificity range between 50 and 92% (Fries *et al.*, 1984; Ashcraft and Holder, 1993). In the symptomatic patient with diverticulitis or haemorrhage, definitive treatment is diverticulectomy including a margin of normal ileum. When intussusception has occurred, operative reduction and resection of the diverticulum are required.

Intestinal obstruction

Intestinal obstruction from a variety of causes can precipitate acute abdominal pain in any age group. Likely causes include congenital band obstruction, intussusception secondary to a Meckel's diverticulum, small or large bowel tumours, or an intramural haematoma complicating Henoch Schonlein purpura. Strangulated internal hernia through a mesenteric defect or an external groin hernia are other possibilities. Malrotation with volvulus rarely presents in this age group. The characteristic features of obstruction are bilious vomiting, intestinal colic, abdominal distension and constipation. Plain abdominal X-ray will demonstrate features of obstruction: additional imaging by ultrasound scan or contrast studies may be needed to establish the cause of the obstruction. Definitive management is determined by the underlying pathology. Most patients will require laparotomy.

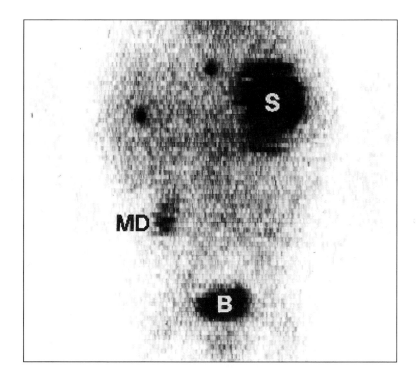

Fig. 13.7   Technetium (^{99}Tc) scintiscan in a patient with a bleeding Meckel's diverticulum (MD). Note increased isotope uptake in the ectopic gastric mucosa of the diverticulum located in the right iliac fossa. Normal uptake and isotope excretion is demonstrated in the stomach (S) and bladder (B).

Gastroenteritis

A clear history of abdominal pain, nausea, vomiting and diarrhoea suggests infective gastroenteritis. Food of suspect quality may have been eaten recently, and the diagnosis is further strengthened by associated illness in other family members or associates.

Urinary Tract Disorders

Urinary tract infection

Urinary tract infection is an uncommon cause of acute abdominal pain in females. In the absence of definitive urinary tract symptoms, such as dysuria or frequency, the clinician should be cautious in labelling the patient with this diagnosis (O'Donnell, 1985). Urinary infection should be documented by microscopic and culture studies. The presence of bacteriuria, pyuria (greater than five white blood cells per high power field) and cultures yielding more than 10^5 organisms confirms the diagnosis. In girls, an underlying cause should be sought, particularly vesico-ureteric reflux, if more than one infection has occurred in the past.

Urinary calculus disease

Urinary tract calculi in the adolescent female often are infective in origin. Calculi therefore usually present with features of infection, or as renal or ureteric obstruction. A history of colicky loin pain radiating to the groin is characteristic of ureteric obstruction, and there may be associated haematuria and urinary infection. The plain abdominal X-ray may demonstrate a radio-opaque calculus (Fig. 13.8). Ultrasound scan will show the calculus and dilatation of the renal pelvis and ureter proximal to the calculus. Calculi less than 5 mm in size often pass spontaneously. Larger calculi currently are managed using a combination of extracorporeal shock wave lithotripsy, percutaneous extraction techniques, Dormia basket extraction or open operation (Losty *et al.*, 1993).

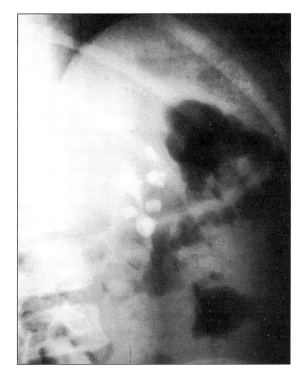

Fig. 13.8 Plain abdominal X-ray showing renal calculus.

Obstructive Uropathies

Chronic obstruction of the urinary tract rarely presents as an acute abdomen unless complicated by infection or bleeding. Loin pain and/or the presence of haematuria following trivial trauma suggests an obstructive hydronephrosis.

Ultrasound scan and isotope renal excretion studies assist the diagnosis. Definitive treatment will depend on the cause.

DISORDERS CAUSING CHRONIC ABDOMINAL PAIN

Chronic abdominal pain in adolescent females is equally frustrating and difficult for the patient, family and clinician alike (Apley, 1975; O'Donnell, 1985; Goldstein, 1989). The differential diagnosis is extensive and includes several organ systems (Table 13.2). It must be remembered that underlying functional, emotional and psychological disorders are prevalent in this age group. By definition, the diagnosis of chronic abdominal pain is made when at least three distinct episodes of abdominal pain have occurred within a three month period (Apley and Naish, 1958; Apley, 1975; O'Donnell, 1985; Goldstein, 1989). Symptoms may be characterised by ill defined, poorly localised, abdominal pain. Pelvic pain and gastrointestinal and menstrual disturbances may be prominent. Absenteeism from school, frequent use of proprietary analgesics and frequent general practitioner consultations are not uncommon. An organised, sympathetic and systematic approach is required, in order to gain patient confidence and parental support (O'Donnell, 1985).

Table 13.2   Differential diagnosis of chronic abdominal pain in female adolescents*

Psychogenic	Recurrent abdominal pain in childhood
Gynaecologic disorders	Pelvic inflammatory disease Endometriosis Ovarian cyst Mittelschmertz Dysmenorrhoea Congenital anomalies
Gastrointestinal tract disorders	Chronic constipation Irritable bowel syndrome Inflammatory bowel disease Chronic appendicitis Postoperative adhesions
Urinary tract disorders	Urinary infection Calculus disease Obstructive uropathies
Spinal disorders	Discitis Herniation of intervertebral disc Congenital spinal disorders

* Some of these conditions may present with acute abdominal pain and have been discussed in that section of the chapter.

History and Physical Examination

The clinical history should review the nature of the problem, including a full description and location of the pain, exacerbating and relieving factors, and menstrual, gastrointestinal, urinary and musculoskeletal symptoms. Past medical and surgical history, results of previous investigations (laboratory or radiological) and treatment should be reviewed. A detailed family and social history should be sought, in order to uncover any family stress, for example medical problems in other family members, or psychosocial problems including alcoholism or depression.

Physical examination is carried out to exclude a general disorder, and specifically to ascertain the presence of abdominal tenderness, organomegaly or an abdominal mass. Musculoskeletal examination is important, to avoid overlooking potential causes of referred abdominal pain, notably discitis (Leahy *et al.*, 1984). If gynaecological pathology is suspected, pelvic and vaginal examination by a gynaecologist may be appropriate (Goldstein, 1989).

Diagnostic Studies

Laboratory investigations or radiological studies are used only where necessary to exclude organic disease. Special emphasis should be directed at attempting to uncover potential psychogenic causes. A full blood count, with differential profile, and ESR and CRP may be obtained. Urine microscopy and culture studies are performed when infection is suspected. Stool analysis for ova and parasites and faecal occult blood studies may prove useful. Abdominal ultrasonography is used for initial screening for intra-abdominal or retroperitoneal abnormalities. However, the benefits derived from performing this examination in children with recurrent abdominal pain remains to be proven (*vide infra*). It has been reported that, rather than allaying parental anxiety, such studies can have the opposite effect (Shanon *et al.*, 1990). Special studies, such as gastrointestinal endoscopy, contrast studies and skeletal radiographs are indicated when there is a possibility of, for example, inflammatory bowel disease or spinal pathology. Laparoscopy can play an important role in evaluating the adolescent with chronic abdominal pain in whom organic symptomatology seems genuine, or even, on occasion, if not (Gans and Austin, 1988; Vercellini *et al.*, 1989).

Recurrent Abdominal Pain in Childhood

Recurrent abdominal pain (RAP) in childhood is a common problem affecting 10% of schoolchildren in Western societies (Apley and Naish, 1958; Apley, 1975; O'Donnell, 1985; Bury, 1987). Organic disease is found in fewer than 10% of these children and it is apparent that functional, emotional and psychological disorders are prevalent (Apley, 1975). The adolescent female with chronic abdominal pain falls within this category. The clinical picture may resemble the irritable bowel syndrome (*vide infra*) (Hyams *et al.*, 1995).

Diagnosis is arrived at after detailed interview of the patient and parents. Absence of a parental figure at the initial interview may serve as a clue to diagnosis (O'Donnell, 1985). The use of a specific clinical questionnaire helps gain patient and parental confidence and sets the scene for the interview and clinical examination (O'Donnell, 1985). The patient and parents thus quickly realise that RAP is a common problem, and this has a positive effect on the consultation. Little is gained by a hasty approach to the situation. Usually, identified problems in adolescents include eating disorders, ambitious personality types, difficulties at school, and domestic psychosocial problems, such as alcoholism, anxiety and depression, chronic family illness and recent family bereavements.

Management involves a sympathetic explanation to the patient and parents of the benign self-limiting nature of RAP, which may require reinforcement on more than one consultation. Specific laboratory or radiologic investigations are not required. In refractory cases psychotherapy may be appropriate.

Chronic Constipation

Constipation of long duration is a potential cause of chronic abdominal pain in children. In some constipated individuals pain may not be significant initially but the excessive unsupervised use of laxatives may precipitate attacks of severe abdominal colic. A massive faecaloma may be palpated as an abdominal mass or seen on abdominal X-ray.

Management involves appropriate dietary adjustment to increase the fibre content, and a supervised laxative programme to ensure adequate bowel emptying. Lactulose and docusate are effective stool softeners if used in adequate doses, while the sennosides, picosulphate and bisacodyl are useful stimulant laxatives. Persistent severe constipation may warrant evaluation by contrast enema, endoscopy and rectal biopsy to exclude an underlying abnormality such as Hirschsprung's disease.

Irritable Bowel Syndrome (IBS)

IBS is a term used to describe symptoms of abdominal pain and altered bowel habit in the absence of any anatomical or physiological abnormalities.

Clinical features

Although IBS may be regarded as a diagnosis of exclusion, such a negative approach may be counterproductive. A positive diagnosis is important for successful management and can be reached based on symptom patterns rather than exhaustive exclusion of other disorders. The diagnostic criteria for IBS have been defined by an international panel (Table 13.3). The symptoms typically have a gradual onset during late adolescence. Abdominal pain is usually

Table 13.3   Symptom criteria for irritable bowel syndrome

At least 3 months, continuous or recurrent symptoms of abdominal pain or discomfort which is

- relieved by defaecation
- and/or associated with a change in frequency of stool
- and/or associated with a change in consistency of stool

plus

Two or three more of the following, on at least a quarter of occasions or days

- altered stool frequency*
- altered stool form (lumpy/hard or loose/watery)
- altered stool passage (straining, urgency or feeling of incomplete evacuation)
- passage of mucus
- bloating or feeling of abdominal distension

---

* For research purposes 'altered' can be defined as >3 bowel movements/day or <3 bowel movements/week (from Thompson *et al.*, 1989).

intermittent but can be continuous with superimposed crampy symptoms and may be worse approximately one hour after meals. Disturbances in the passage of stools include alterations in stool frequency, consistency (hard or loose) or passage (straining, urgency, feeling of incomplete evacuation). With constipation-predominant IBS, the stools are typically narrow and hard, while with diarrhoea-predominant IBS, the stools are loose and frequent but small in volume. On physical examination, there may be no significant abnormality, but there may be signs of anxiety and the sigmoid colon or a tender bowel loop may be palpated (Weber and McCallum, 1992). IBS is often associated with gynaecological symptoms (Longstreth, 1994).

Investigations should be limited to excluding infections by means of stool culture, and anatomical disorders of the gastrointestinal tract by means of contrast X-rays and endoscopy.

Management

IBS is a frustrating disorder to treat. An explanation of IBS and reassurance about its functional and benign nature are important to allay the anxiety that usually is present. Medications are prescribed to relieve gastrointestinal symptoms that persist in spite of counselling and dietary manipulations. Patients with constipation-predominant IBS may benefit from increased dietary fibre and, if necessary, osmotic laxatives or stool softeners. Stimulant laxatives are not advised. Cisapride may be helpful for patients with colonic inertia. For diarrhoea-predominant IBS, factors such as lactulose intolerance and food sensitivity should be excluded. Useful medications include loperamide and cholestyramine. The abdominal pain may be relieved by agents including anti-cholinergic drugs or mebeverine. Anti-depressants may also be helpful. For many patients, a confident diagnosis combined with education, reassurance, dietary modifications and a compassionate physician, prove effective (Weber and McCallum, 1992; Thompson, 1993).

Inflammatory Bowel Disease

Crohn's disease and ulcerative colitis may present with chronic abdominal pain, often associated with the passage of blood and mucus per rectum. There may be features of partial intestinal obstruction. Growth may be impaired, and puberty delayed. Extra-intestinal manifestations of the disease may be apparent, including uveitis, arthralgia, erythema nodosum and oral and peri-anal aphthous ulceration. The diagnosis is made by contrast radiography and endoscopy. Management requires a multidisciplinary team approach employing medical and surgical therapies (Fonkalsrud, 1995; Telander, 1995).

Chronic Appendicitis

The entity of chronic appendicitis is controversial (O'Donnell, 1985; Cuschieri and Bouchier, 1989). There are instances in which chronic right iliac fossa pain has been relieved following appendicectomy in girls and microscopic examination may demonstrate chronic inflammatory changes. Many would argue, however, that such symptoms frequently have a psychological basis. Thorough evaluation is important, including gynaecological investigation, before making this diagnosis. Evidence of a faecolith on abdominal X-ray supports the diagnosis. In selected patients, diagnostic laparoscopy can help resolve the issue (Gans and Austin, 1988). When no other cause is found for the pain, and appendiceal pathology cannot be excluded, laparoscopic or open appendicectomy may be justified.

Post-operative Adhesions

The peritoneal reaction that follows laparotomy can give rise to post-operative adhesion formation and intermittent bouts of sub-acute intestinal obstruction. Abdominal pain in such patients may be of long duration. Diagnosis is suspected by noting the presence of a previous abdominal incision and plain film radiological evidence of incomplete intestinal obstruction. Management is non-operative in the first instance, with nasogastric decompression and appropriate intravenous fluid support. In persistent cases, laparotomy or laparoscopy, and adhesiolysis is required.

Spinal Disorders

Discitis, an inflammatory lesion affecting the intervertebral disc, is an uncommon cause of abdominal pain in children (Leahy *et al.*, 1984). In typical cases fever, difficulty in walking and back pain are characteristic. Occasionally, abdominal pain can be the sole presenting symptom. Symptoms are presumed to arise as a result of referred nerve root pain and retro-peritoneal inflammation. Narrowing of the disc space, a raised ESR and a 'hot spot' on a radiolabelled technetium isotope bone scan is diagnostic. Blood cultures may reveal the infective organism. Treatment includes bed rest and appropriate antibiotics. Disc prolapse and congenital spinal disorders may similarly provoke abdominal pain as a result of nerve root entrapment and/or referred pain. Management will depend on the underlying pathology, for example, corrective spinal surgery for severe scoliosis (Goldstein, 1989).

REFERENCES

Ammerman S, Shafer MA, Synder D, 1990: Ectopic pregnancy in adolescents: A clinical review for pediatricians. *Journal of Pediatrics* **117**, 677–686.

Apley J, 1975: *The child with abdominal pains*. London: Blackwell Scientific Publications.

Apley J, Naish N, 1958: Recurrent abdominal pains: a field survey of 1000 school-children. *Archives of Disease in Childhood* **33**, 165–170.

Ashcraft KW, Holder TM, 1993: *Pediatric surgery*. Philadelphia: WB Saunders Company.

Brown MF, Hebra A, McGeehin K, Ross III AJ, 1993: Ovarian masses in children: a review of 91 cases of malignant and benign masses. *Journal of Pediatric Surgery* **28**, 930–932.

Bury RG, 1987: A study of 111 children with recurrent abdominal pain. *Australian Paediatric Journal* **23**, 117–119.

Cuschieri A, Bouchier IAD, 1989: The small intestine and vermiform appendix. In Cuschieri A, Giles GR, Moossa AR, (eds), *Essential surgical practice*. Bristol: Wright, PSG 933–953.

Evans JP, 1978: Torsion of normal uterine adnexa in premenarchial girls. *Journal of Pediatric Surgery* **13**, 195–196.

Fonkalsrud EW, 1995: Surgery for pediatric ulcerative colitis. *Current Opinion in Pediatrics* **7**, 323–327.

Fries M, Mortensson W, Robertson B, 1984: Technetium pertechnetate scintigraphy to detect ectopic gastric mucosa in Meckel's diverticulum. *Acta Radiologica Diagnostica* **25**, 417–422.

Gans SL, Austin E, 1988: Laparoscopy in infants and children. In Spitz L, Nixon HH, (eds), *Rob & Smith's operative surgery – paediatric surgery*. London: Butterworths, 260–267.

Goldstein DP, 1989: Acute and chronic pelvic pain. In *Adolescent gynecology*. Philadelphia: WB Saunders Company.

Gustafson ML, Lee MM, Asmundson L, MacLaughlin DT, Donahoe PK, 1993: Mullerian inhibiting substance in the diagnosis and management of intersex and gonadal abnormalities. *Journal of Pediatric Surgery* **28**, 439–444.

Gustafson ML, Lcc MM, Scully RE, Moncure MD, Hirakawa TH, Goodman A, Muntz HG, Donahoe PK, MacLaughlin DT, Fuller AF, 1992: Mullerian inhibiting substance as a marker for ovarian sex-cord tumour. *New England Journal of Medicine* **326**, 466–471.

Hallat JG, 1986: Tubal conservation in ectopic pregnancy: a study of 200 cases. *American Journal of Obstetrics and Gynecology* **70**, 1216–1221.

Harden RM, Alexander WD, Kennedy I, 1967: Isotope uptake and scanning of stomach in man with 99m Tc-pertechnetate. *Lancet* **1**, 1305–1307.

Héloury Y, Guiberteau V, Sagot P, Plattner V, Baron M, Rogez JM, 1992: Laparoscopy in adnexal pathology in the child: a study of 28 cases. *European Journal of Pediatric Surgery* **3**, 75–78.

Hyams JS, Treem WR, Justinich CJ, David P, Shoup M, Burke G, 1995: Characterisation of symptoms in children with recurrent abdominal pain: resemblance to irritable bowel syndrome. *Journal of Paediatric Gastroentrology and Nutrition* **20**, 209–214.

James DF, Barber HRK, Graber EA, 1970: Torsion of normal uterine adnexa in children. *Obstetrics and Gynecology*, **35**, 226–230.

Jewett TCJ, Duszynski DO, Allen JE, 1970: The visualization of Meckel's diverticulum with 99m Tc-pertechnetate. *Surgery* **68**, 567–570.

Khoiny FE, 1989: Pelvic inflammatory disease in the adolescent. *Journal of Pediatric Health Care* **3**(5), 230–236.

Kurzbart E, Mares AJ, Cohen Z, Mordehai J, Finaly R, 1994. Isolated torsion of the fallopian tube in premenarchal girls. *Journal of Pediatric Surgery* **29**, 1384–1385.

Lappohn RE, Burger HG, Bouma J, Bangah M, Krans M, 1992: Inhibin as a marker for granulosa cell tumor. *Acta Obstetrics Gynecology Supplement* **155**, 61–65.

Leahy AL, Fogarty EE, Fitzgerald RJ, Regan BF, 1984: Discitis as a cause of abdominal pain in children. *Surgery* **95**, 412–414.

Longstreth GF, 1994: Irritable bowel syndrome and chronic pelvic pain. *Obstetric and Gynecological Survey* **49**, 505–507.

Losty P, Surana R, O'Donnell B, 1993: Limitations of extracorporeal shock wave lithotripsy for urinary tract calculi in young children. *Journal of Pediatric Surgery* **28**, 1037–1039.

Marchbanks PA, Annegers JF, Coulam CB, *et al.* 1988: Risk factors for ectopic pregnancy: a population-based study. *JAMA* **259**, 1823–1828.

Mastroianni L, 1978: Tubal occlusion. In Keller PJ, (ed.) *Female infertility*. Basel: Karger, 114–131.

Mordehai J, Mares AJ, Barki Y, Finaly R, Meizner I, 1991: Torsion of uterine adnexa in neonates and children: a report of 20 cases. *Journal of Pediatric Surgery* **26**, 1195–1199.

Moss EH, Carty H, Sprigg A, 1993: A retrospective study of large ovarian masses in paediatric practice. *European Journal of Radiology* **17**, 159–165.

Nyberg DA, Filly RA, Mahony BS, *et al.* 1985: Early gestation: correlation of HCG levels and sonographic identification. *American Journal of Roentgenology* **144**, 951–954.

O'Donnell B, 1985: *Abdominal pain in children* (First Edition). Oxford: Blackwell Scientific Publications.

O'Donnell B, 1988: Appendicectomy. In Spitz L, Nixon HH, (eds), *Rob & Smith's operative surgery: paediatric surgery*, London: Butterworths 392–335.

Powley PH, 1965: Infertility due to pelvic abscess and pelvic peritonitis in appendicitis. *Lancet* 27–29.

Puri P, Guiney EJ, O'Donnell B, McGuinness EPJ, 1984: Effects of perforated appendicitis in girls on subsequent fertility. *British Medical Journal* **288**, 25–26.

Schwobel MG, Stauffer UG, 1991: Surgical treatment of ovarian tumors in childhood. *Progress in Pediatric Surgery* **26**, 113–123.

Shafer MA, Sweet RL, 1989: Pelvic inflammatory disease in adolescent females. In Strasburger VC, (ed.), *Adolescent gynecology:* Philadelphia: WB Saunders, 513–533.

Shalev E, Mann S, Romano S, Rahav D, 1991: Laparoscopic detorsion of adnexa in childhood: a case report. *Journal of Pediatric Surgery* **26**, 1193–1194.

Shanon A, Martin DJ, Feldmann W, 1990: Ultrasonographic studies in the management of recurrent abdominal pain. *Pediatrics* **86**, 35–38.

Skinner MA, Schlatter MG, Heifetz SA, Grosfeld JL, 1993: Ovarian neoplasms in children. *Archives in Surgery* **128**, 849–854.

Stovroff M, Ricketts RR, Heiss KF, 1994: *C-reactive protein: a role in the diagnosis of suspected appendicitis.* Twenty-Fifth Annual Meeting of the American Pediatric Surgical Association, Tuscon, Arizona.

Surana R, Puri P, 1994: Primary wound closure after perforated appendicitis in children. *British Journal of Surgery* **81**, 440.

Taylor RN, 1988: Ectopic pregnancy and reproductive technology. *JAMA* **259**, 1862–1864.

Telander RL, 1995: Surgical management of Crohn's disease in children. *Current Opinion in Pediatrics* **7**, 328–334.

Thind CR, Carty HML, Pilling DW, 1989: The role of ultrasound in the management of ovarian masses in children. *Clinical Radiology* **40**, 180–182.

Thompson WG, 1993: Irritable bowel syndrome: pathogenesis and management. *Lancet* **341**, 1569–1572.

Thompson WG, Dotevall G, Drossman DA, Heaton KW, Kruis W, 1989: Irritable bowel syndrome; guidelines for the diagnosis. *Gastroenterology International* **2**, 92–95.

Thompson WM, Lynn HB, 1971: The possible relationship of appendicitis with perforation in childhood to infertility in women. *Journal of Pediatric Surgery* **6**, 458–461.

Togashi K, Nishimura K, Kimura I, Tsuda Y, *et al.* 1991: Endometrial cysts: diagnosis with MR imaging. *Radiology* **180**, 73–78.

Van Winter JT, Simmons PS, Podratz KC, 1994: Surgically treated adnexal masses in infancy, childhood and adolesence. *American Journal of Obstetrics and Gynecology* **170**, 1780–1789.

Vercellini P, Fedele L, Arcaini L, Bianchi S, Rognoni MT, Candiani GB, 1989: Laparoscopy in the diagnosis of chronic pelvic pain in adolescent women. *Journal of Reproductive Medicine* **34**, 827–830.

Washington AE, Sweet RL, Shafer MB, 1985: Pelvic inflammatory disease and its sequelae in adolescents. *Journal of Pediatric Health Care* **6**, 298–310.

Weber FH, McCallum RW, 1992: Clinical approaches to irritable bowel syndrome. *Lancet* **341**, 1447–1452.

Wiig JN, Janssen CW, Fuglesang P, 1979: Infertility as a complication of perforated appendicitis. *Acta Chirurgica Scandinavica* **145**, 409–410.

Wong ML, Casey SO, Leonidas JC, Elkowitz SS, Becker J, 1994: Sonographic diagnosis of acute appendicitis in children. *Journal of Pediatric Surgery* **29**, 1356–1360.

CHAPTER 14

Gynaecological tumours

ANNE S GARDEN

INTRODUCTION

Gynaecological tumours are rare in childhood and adolescent years. Malignant genital tract tumours are particularly rare. Their rarity, however, compounds the problem as often the diagnosis is not considered until the disease is well advanced. The commonest presenting symptom of malignant tumours of the lower genital tract in childhood and adolescence is vaginal bleeding, underlying the necessity for careful examination under anaesthesia for all girls presenting with this symptom. Tumours of the ovary present with an abdominal mass or less commonly, abdominal pain. Ovarian tumours are the commonest gynaecological neoplasms in this age group.

Two things should be borne in mind when considering childhood gynaecological tumours: those which present in the neonatal period or in early infancy may be embryological in derivation and, unlike malignant tumours in adults which are usually carcinomas, malignant tumours in childhood are much more likely to be sarcomas. Both of these factors will influence the behaviour of tumours which present in childhood compared to those presenting in adult life.

A further general point worth making is that all girls and adolescents who require radiotherapy as either a total or an adjunctive treatment for pelvic malignancies will be at high risk of ovarian failure depending on the dose received. If this occurs, they will require hormone replacement therapy (HRT) and, where necessary, hormonal induction of puberty (see p. 136). None of the malignant genital tract tumours of childhood are oestrogen-dependent and so there is no risk of causing tumour progression. Those looking after girls who have had pelvic radiotherapy should be aware of this possibility so that early diagnosis may be made and treatment started to prevent additional problems for this unfortunate group of girls. Girls having pelvic surgery prior to radiotherapy should have their ovaries transposed out of the pelvis to try to prevent their being damaged by the field of radiation.

Included in this Chapter will be those lesions which, while not truly tumours, present with a lump or swelling and therefore have the initial appearance of a tumour.

TUMOURS OF THE VULVA

True tumours

While tumours of the genital tract in childhood are uncommon, tumours of the vulva are particularly uncommon. The commonest are haemangiomas. Other tumours such as squamous cell carcinoma, malignant melanoma, and sarcoma boitryoides of the vulva are so rare in childhood and adolescent years that they will not be considered.

Haemangiomas

Haemangiomas may occur on any part of the body and are found not infrequently on the vulva. They may be capillary or cavernous in nature although there is overlap in the histological features of the two types.

Mixed haemangiomas (strawberry naevus) usually appear within the first few weeks of life (Fig. 14.1). Growth is rapid over the first six months of life but then slows. Most lesions begin to decrease in size after one year of age with complete

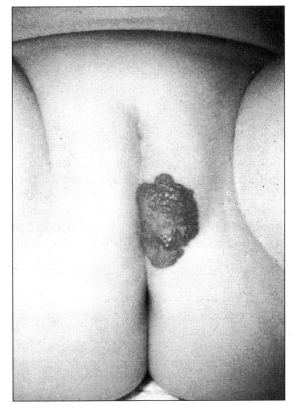

Fig. 14.1   Strawberry naevus involving the vulva.

regression in 80% of cases by the age of five (MacColum and Martin, 1956). Regression of the tumour is due to thrombosis of the vessels and is associated with the appearance of a grey area in the centre of the lesion. The majority of haemangiomas in the body have disappeared by puberty although this is perhaps less likely for those situated on the vulva.

Mixed haemangiomas are typically lobulated, well-demarcated and usually bright red in appearance. Histology shows proliferation of immature capillaries. Although haemangiomas are generally asymptomatic, those on the vulva may become ulcerated, particularly in the first six months of life during the period of active growth. Ulceration may lead to infection and local scarring and in-patient treatment will be required. Reassurance that the lesions are likely to disappear, is usually the only treatment required, although intralesional steroids have been used in the treatment of these tumours where spontaneous resolution has not taken place. Excision of the residual lesion may be necessary.

Cavernous haemangiomas, in contrast, are normally present at birth and grow proportionately with the girl's body growth. They occur in the deeper structures of the vulva and so appear as elevated, soft tumours with blue discoloration of the overlying skin. Cut section of the tumour shows a spongelike appearance and histology shows large vascular channels. Some cavernous haemangiomas will undergo spontaneous regression but this is less likely than with mixed types.

Excision of these tumours may be possible, although difficult. Pretreatment by embolisation under angiographic control may be required prior to surgery.

Vulvar lesions presenting as tumours

Hymenal tags

Hymenal tags are common, vary in size and are usually asymptomatic. If they do cause symptoms they usually present with irritation from rubbing on nappies or underwear. Adolescent girls who are sexually active may present with discomfort on intercourse. The diagnosis is made by close inspection which shows that the tags are attached to the hymen. If they are asymptomatic, explanation and reassurance may be all that is necessary. If, however, they are symptomatic or reassurance is not sufficient, they may be excised; usually this is possible under local anaesthetic.

Hymenal cysts

Hymenal cysts are thin-walled cystic swellings of the hymen. They are usually found on routine examination after birth and are asymptomatic (Fig. 14.2). Their main importance is that, if they are of significant size, they may be mistaken for hydrocolpos. the ability to pass a fine probe through the hymen will confirm the diagnosis. Hymenal cysts often regress spontaneously, but if removal is required, incision and drainage should be performed.

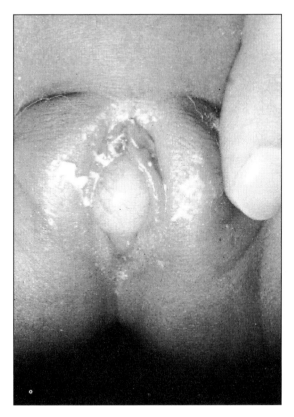

Fig. 14.2 Hymenal cyst in a new-born child (courtesy of Dr P Dunn).

Paraurethral cysts

Paraurethral cysts are unusual but when present are situated dorsal to the lower third of the urethra in the vaginal wall and are lined with squamous or transitional epithelium. Their position differentiates them from the more common mesonephric (Gartner's duct) cysts which are located in the lateral walls of the vagina, and from paramesonephric cysts which are situated near the cervix. The aetiology of paraurethral cysts is unknown but they have been variously attributed to Wolffian duct remnants or invagination of the vaginal mucosa.

Paraurethral cysts are usually small and asymptomatic but, rarely, may be of sufficient size to displace or compress the urethra or to block the vaginal opening. They are usually found by chance or on routine examination after birth.

Treatment is by marsupialisation. If they are asymptomatic and not interfering with micturition, treatment can be delayed until menarche when the structures are larger and more easily identified. It is usually recommended that they are dealt with at puberty even if asymptomatic as they may rupture during intercourse, which although not serious, can be very frightening. If the cyst recurs after marsupialisation, excision of the cyst may be considered but must be performed with care due to the risk of damage to the urethra.

Ectopic ureterocoeles not infrequently present with the appearance of para-urethral cysts. It is, therefore, advisable to perform a complete urological examination, including imaging, prior to surgery (Blaivas *et al.*, 1976).

Urethral prolapse

A urethral prolapse usually presents as a painless pink or red mass in the vulva which is often mistaken for a tumour. The cause of the prolapse is not known but is usually attributed to redundancy of the urethral mucosa. Increased intra-abdominal pressure may be a factor in a minority of cases. It is usually found in pre-pubertal girls.

The presence of urethral prolapse may be accompanied by bleeding – in fact the mass may first be noted because of a bloodstained discharge or spotting. Examination of the vulva shows a doughnut-like circumferential eversion of the mucosa which is soft and extremely tender on palpation. The prolapse is treated by excision of the redundant mucosa at the level of the external meatus and suture of the cut edge of the urethra to the mucosa of the vestibule. It is important that undue traction is not used prior to excising the redundant mucosa, otherwise the cut edge will retreat making suturing impossible. Prior insertion of a Foley catheter into the bladder is useful to control the retraction.

Hydrocolpos (see also p. 51)

Hydrocolpos is caused by the accumulation of secretions in the vagina behind an imperforate hymen. This causes the appearance of a bulging tumour at the vaginal orifice (Fig. 14.3).

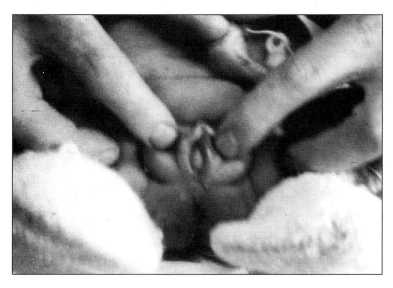

Fig. 14.3   Hydrocolpos presenting as a cystic mass at the vulva (courtesy of Dr P Dunn).

A hydrocolpos is generally asymptomatic and noticed at routine neonatal examination when examination of the external genitalia reveals a tense mass at the introitus which is grey/white in colour. Treatment is by excision of the hymen with drainage of the fluid.

If the diagnosis is not made in the newborn period, the hydrocolpos resolves due to resorption of the fluid. In these circumstances, the girl will probably not present again until puberty when the onset of menstruation causes a haematocolpos. If the mother is unwilling for surgery in the newborn period, she should be advised to bring her daughter back at the first sign of puberty when examination under anaesthetic and, if necessary, incision of the hymen can be performed.

Occasionally, a very large hydrocolpos may present as an abdominal mass (Fig. 14.4). Vaginal examination, therefore, is an essential part of the assessment of all newborn girls with an abdominal mass. An incorrect diagnosis leads to unnecessary imaging studies and possibly to laparotomy which has been associated with a perioperative mortality as high as 35% (Gravier, 1969). Occasionally, hydrocolpos has been reported as part of an autosomal recessive syndrome – the McKusick–Kaufman syndrome. These girls, in addition to the hydrocolpos, present with uterovaginal duplication, anorectal anomalies, post-axial polydactyly and congenital heart disease (Robinow and Shaw, 1979).

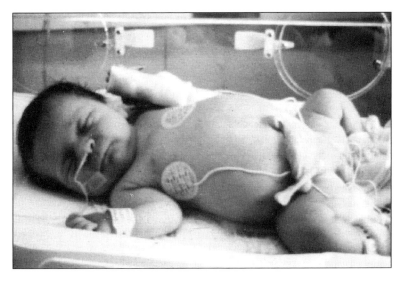

Fig. 14.4   Hydrocolpos presenting as a large abdominal mass (courtesy of Dr P Dunn).

Haematocolpos

This condition, where menstrual blood collects behind a vaginal septum, is much less likely to present as a mass because the cyclical abdominal pain and primary amenorrhoea usually lead to early presentation (see p. 138). Examination of the vulva, however, will reveal a bulging bluish mass at the introitus. Treatment is by excision of the hymen with release of the altered blood.

Congenital hydrocoele and hernia

Hydrocoeles, or cysts of the Canal of Nuck, arise in a patent processus vaginalis. The processus vaginalis is an outpouching of the peritoneum which extends along the round ligament into the labium majus. It usually disappears except for a thin strand of tissue in the third trimester of pregnancy, but it occasionally remains patent and fills with peritoneal fluid forming a cystic swelling. As the left processus vaginalis closes before the right, most abnormalities are right-sided.

A hydrocoele of the processus vaginalis, therefore, presents as a smooth, round, fluctuant swelling, usually of the right labium majus. It can be differentiated from a Bartholin's cyst by its more anterior situation. In addition, Bartholin's cysts are extremely rare in childhood, usually not being seen until adolescence. Very occasionally, an ovary may prolapse into the processus vaginalis being found as a hernia, which is usually not reducible, in the labium majus. Palpation of this hernia will reveal a firm mass allowing it to be differentiated from a hydrocele. A loop of bowel may also herniate into the processus vaginalis.

Treatment of a hydrocoele is surgical with exposure, ligation and excision of the sac. A hernia should be treated without delay because of the risk of strangulation.

Bartholin's cyst

Bartholin's gland cysts or abscesses are extremely rare in childhood but occasionally occur in adolescent life after the glands have developed their secretory function with the onset of puberty. They occur due to blockage of the duct opening onto the vulva with subsequent accumulation of secretions. Infection of the cyst will lead to abscess formation.

Diagnosis of a Bartholin's cyst is made by the position of the cyst on the lower inner aspect of the labium majus pointing in towards the vestibule. Treatment is by marsupialisation of the cyst taking care to leave a sufficiently wide opening to the gland to allow drainage of the secretions and prevent recurrence.

TUMOURS OF THE VAGINA

Lesions which present as tumours of the vagina in childhood and adolescence fall into two main types – those that result from embryological structures, which are usually cystic, and those that are the result of maternal hormone ingestion. They need to be differentiated from condylomata which are due to viral infection but which usually present as a vulvar mass. If there is any doubt as to the nature of this lesion, biopsy may be performed but the macroscopic appearance is usually diagnostic. Condylomata are discussed more fully on p. 173.

True tumours of the vagina

Hormone related tumours

It was in 1970 that the first association between *in utero* exposure to diethylstil-boestrol (DES) and vaginal adenosis or clear cell adenocarcinoma of the vagina in young women was first described (Herbst and Scully, 1970; Herbst *et al.*, 1971). DES usage had been advocated in the late 1940s for the prevention of mis-carriages, preterm labour, pregnancy induced hypertension and stillbirth (Smith, 1948). It was banned by the United States Food and Drug Administration in 1971 after publication of Herbst's report, but not until an estimated two to three million women had received it in pregnancy (Stillman, 1982). Its use in the United Kingdom was never so widespread as in the United States of America – one study suggested only 7500 women had received the drug (Kinlen *et al.*, 1974) – and its use was discontinued by the Committee on Safety of Medicines in 1973. The fact that it has not been used in either country for over 20 years means that it is unlikely that new cases of DES exposed vaginal adenosis or clear cell adenocar-cinoma will be seen in childhood and adolescent years in the late 1990s. However, two thirds of the patients with clear cell adenocarcinoma of the vagina registered in an international registry had been exposed to DES (Horwitz *et al.*, 1988) and it has been estimated that the risk of DES exposed girls developing the cancer is between 0.14 and 1.4 per 1000 (Herbst, 1979).

In addition to the risk of developing clear cell adenocarcinoma of the vagina, DES exposure *in utero* causes a variety of structural abnormalities of the genital tract including uterine hypoplasia, cervical hoods, cockscomb deformity of the cervix and pseudopolyps. The most common abnormality associated with DES, however, is vaginal adenosis.

Vaginal adenosis

Vaginal adenosis is the occurrence of glandular tissue in or under the vaginal epithelium. The glandular tissue produces heaped up areas on the vagina which is initially red in colour. Squamous metaplasia usually occurs causing the vagina to return to its normal pale pink appearance but maintaining the heaped up con-figuration. Occasionally, dysplastic changes may occur within the area of squa-mous metaplasia.

Vaginal adenosis is usually asymptomatic and found during routine examina-tion or on follow-up of DES exposed girls. Those girls with symptoms usually complain of a clear mucus discharge. Sexually active adolescent girls may present with dyspareunia or more commonly, post-coital bleeding. Treatment is usually expectant. Surgery, with excision of the affected epithelium, may be necessary if there is profuse discharge or bleeding.

Vaginal adenosis has been reported in up to 90% of girls exposed to DES (Stafl *et al.*, 1974) and is found in 13% of adolescents and young adults not exposed to DES (Kurman and Silly, 1974). The risk of developing clear cell adenocarcinoma calculated from birth to the age of 34 is estimated to be about 1 : 1000 women exposed *in utero* (Melnick *et al.*, 1987). The risk is dependent on the gestational age at the time of exposure to DES. Girls exposed to DES before 12 weeks gestation have a relative risk of developing malignancy which is three times higher than those exposed after 13 weeks (Herbst *et al.*, 1986). It is, however, recommended that all girls exposed *in utero* to DES are screened at yearly intervals from the menarche. These girls are advised to use tampons for three to six months prior to examination to facilitate colposcopic examination. Careful digital examination of the vagina should first be performed to exclude any nodular areas that may be suggestive of clear cell adenocarcinoma. An appropriate sized speculum should be then be used to visualise the vaginal walls. Samples for cytology should be taken from the cervix, endocervical canal and all four vaginal walls. Colposcopy should then be performed. Careful recording of the findings should be made, including photography, but biopsies are rarely necessary (Emens, 1994).

Clear cell adenocarcinoma

Clear cell adenocarcinoma presents with abnormal vaginal discharge or bleeding although in early stages it may be asymptomatic. Examination shows a firm, polypoid lesion usually in the upper third of the anterior vaginal wall which may be ulcerated. The cervix may also be involved. The tumour spread is local and to the lymph nodes which may be involved at an unexpectedly early stage of tumour growth. Diagnosis is by biopsy, the histology showing clear and 'hobnail' tumour cells. Treatment is by extended hysterectomy, vaginectomy (with replacement by split skin graft) and lymph node dissection. Radiotherapy may be required if there is lymph node involvement. Advanced disease is treated with radiotherapy. Senekjian *et al.* (1987) however, concluded from their study of 219 patients that a combination of wide local excision with retroperitoneal pelvic lymphadenopathy, followed by local irradiation is an effective treatment for vaginal clear cell adenocarcinoma where the initial lesion is less than 2 cm in diameter.

Survival is related to the stage at diagnosis, with a five year survival of 90% for those who had Stage I disease but with poor survival for those with Stage IV disease.

Non-hormone related tumours

The other malignant tumour of the vagina found in childhood and adolescence is the mixed mesodermal tumour or sarcoma botryoides. This tumour will be considered in the section on cervical tumours (p. 253).

An extremely rare vaginal tumour in infancy is the endodermal sinus tumour, more commonly, although still rarely, found in the ovary. Less than 50 reports of the vaginal tumour have been documented in the world literature (Collins *et al.*, 1989). Presentation is with vaginal bleeding and discharge. A polypoid mass may be found at the introitus not dissimilar in appearance to sarcoma botryoides. Diagnosis is by biopsy, which typically shows a reticular, solid or tubular pattern and which will differentiate it from the more common sarcoma botryoides. The tumour will also test positive for alpha-fetoprotein and serum alpha-fetoprotein levels may be used to monitor response to therapy. Because of the rarity of the tumour, experience of treatment is limited. Earlier management was by radical surgery, but more recent work suggests that chemotherapy may be used in place of surgery, or at least prior to surgery, allowing a less radical procedure to be performed (Anderson *et al.*, 1985; Collins *et al.*, 1989).

VAGINAL LESIONS PRESENTING AS TUMOURS

Cysts arising from embryological structures

Gartner's duct cyst

Gartner's duct cysts, the commonest cause of a vaginal mass, arise from the remnants of the mesonephric duct. In embryonic life, the mesonephric duct runs lateral to the paramesonephric or Mullerian duct. With the fusion of the paramesonephric duct to form the uterus and vagina, the mesonephric duct regresses. Failure of regression of the duct may cause the appearance of a cyst along the line of the duct. Gartner's duct cysts cause signs and symptoms dependent on the situation and size of the cyst.

In childhood a Gartner's duct cyst may present as a dome-shaped swelling at the introitus. It may be difficult to differentiate from an imperforate hymen with hydrocolpos but the ability to pass a fine probe alongside the swelling will confirm the patency of the vagina and suggest the diagnosis.

If not diagnosed in early childhood by the appearance mentioned above, Gartner's duct cysts will probably not become apparent until the girl becomes sexually active. At this time, they may cause dyspareunia but are more likely be noticed, as a chance finding, at the first cervical smear or pelvic examination. The cyst is then seen on either lateral aspect of the vagina, at any point from the cervix to the introitus, as a fluctuant swelling. The cyst is usually unilocular and contains mucoid material. It is lined with cuboidal or columnar epithelium and commonly has an overlying thin muscular layer.

If the cyst is asymptomatic, no treatment other than reassurance as to the benign nature of the lesion is required. If surgery is required, either as a result of the symptoms or due to anxiety on the part of the girl or her parents, marsupialisation of the cyst is adequate.

Paramesonephric cysts

Paramesonephric cysts are much less common than mesonephric cysts and, while present from birth, usually do not normally cause symptoms until puberty. They occur as a result of failure of fusion of the paramesonephric or Mullerian duct. Failure of fusion of the Mullerian ducts normally causes duplication of the uterus or vagina, but in some cases, one of the paramesonephric ducts fails to differentiate into uterus, cervix and vagina and remains as a cystic structure lined with columnar epithelium. If the paramesonephric duct, in addition to the columnar epithelium, also contains endometrial elements, then the onset of menstruation will cause the cyst to be filled with menstrual blood.

The girl, therefore, presents with pain and dysmenorrhoea. On examination a cystic swelling is seen bulging into the vagina. Ultrasound scan will show a cystic swelling extending from the lower vagina up into the pelvis. Excision of a paramesonephric cyst is difficult and initial treatment should probably be by excision of the cyst wall allowing drainage into the vagina. A sufficiently large opening is required to allow continued drainage. Excision of the paramesonephric cyst may be carried out when the girl is older.

TUMOURS OF THE CERVIX

Both benign and malignant tumours of the cervix are extremely rare in childhood and adolescence.

Cervical papillomas

A few cases of benign cervical papillomas have been reported in children. They present with the usual non-specific symptoms of vaginal bleeding and discharge and are found at the time of examination under anaesthesia. Treatment is by surgical removal, although this can be difficult due to limited access. The use of a paediatric cystoscope to remove the polyp may be helpful. In the one patient seen by the author, the trauma resulting from the difficult removal of the polyp resulted in a secondary infection associated with vaginal bleeding which was heavier than at the initial presentation. Prophylaxis with antibiotics at the time of surgery may be helpful in preventing this.

Carcinoma of the cervix

Carcinoma of the cervix – either squamous or adenocarcinoma – is extremely rare in childhood and adolescence, although probably less rare than benign papillomas of the cervix. The pathogenesis of and screening for squamous carcinoma of the cervix is considered in Chapter 9. Squamous carcinoma of the cervix is related to sexual activity and such cases that have been reported in this age group are in adolescents. The youngest case reported was in a girl of 16 (Lisa and Cornwall, 1926).

There is no screening programme for adenocarcinoma and the pathogenesis (other than those related to DES exposure) is not known. Although rare, it affects all age groups. Symptoms of cervical carcinoma, irrespective of histological type, are vaginal bleeding and offensive vaginal discharge. Diagnosis is by visual inspection, under anaesthetic in young girls and those not sexually active. Anaesthesia allows a biopsy to be taken for histological diagnosis and staging of the tumour to be carried out.

Carcinoma of the cervix appears as either an ulcerative, necrotic lesion or as a fungating lesion. Adenocarcinoma of the cervix in the earlier stages may be confined to the endocervical canal in which case no lesion will be visible but palpation of the cervix will reveal it to be hard, indurated and, classically, barrel-shaped. Tumour spread is local to the pelvic side wall, vagina and draining lymph nodes. In later stages, bladder and bowel may be involved. Treatment is by radical hysterectomy with conservation of the ovaries. Adjuvant radiotherapy may be necessary in advanced lesions which may result in ovarian failure. The ovaries should therefore be transfixed out of the pelvis at the time of initial surgery to prevent ovarian failure occurring. Squamous cell carcinoma of the cervix is relatively radio-responsive, adenocarcinoma of the cervix does not respond well to radiotherapy.

Sarcoma botryoides

The most common tumour of the vagina and cervix in childhood and early adolescence is sarcoma botryoides, a highly malignant rhabdomyosarcoma of the mixed mesodermal type (Copeland *et al.*, 1985). The tumour occurs most commonly in girls below the age of two, with 90% of the tumours occurring in girls below five years of age (Blaustein and Sedlis, 1982). Cases have even been reported at birth. The tumour is found more commonly in the vagina in younger girls and on the cervix in adolescents and young women, although frequently at time of presentation it is not possible to ascertain the origin of the tumour.

The presenting symptoms are the common presentation of most genital tract tumours of childhood and adolescence – vaginal bleeding and discharge. The amount of bleeding is not a guide to the seriousness or otherwise of the lesion.

Occasionally, in older girls, the presenting symptom may be an abdominal mass. Young girls may be first seen with a friable mass at the introitus. Rarely, the initial presentation may be when a piece of the tumour is passed vaginally.

Sarcoma botryoides originates in the subepithelial layer of the cervical or vaginal epithelium and spreads widely within this layer producing a characteristic polypoid appearance before invading the vaginal wall itself. The subepithelial nature of the tumour with normal mucosa overlying it and the loose oedematous appearance of the stroma, which does not appear strikingly malignant, may result in the diagnosis being initially missed both clinically and histologically.

Examination of the mass, usually under anaesthesia, shows classically a friable polypoid tumour said to resemble a bunch of grapes. The colour varies from pale pink to a dark haemorrhagic red. It may vary in size from a small simple polyp to that of a large bulky mass filling the whole vagina. The tumour usually appears on the anterior vaginal wall and spreads rapidly to the posterior wall of the bladder and urethra and to other structures in the pelvis. Later spread is by blood and lymphatics to lung, liver and bone. In terminal stages of the disease, tumour may spread to the vulva and perineum.

Biopsy is essential for diagnosis as the clinical appearance of the tumour is similar to that of the rarer endodermal sinus tumour (see p. 268). Biopsy is best performed under anaesthesia, even for those tumours which are visible at the introitus as this allows full evaluation of the tumour and its spread. Anaesthesia also allows a good representative biopsy to be taken of the tumour which is essential given the often misleading clinical and histological appearance. Several cases have been reported where the diagnosis has been missed and treatment delayed because initial microscopic examination of the tumour was reported as benign. Further evaluation of tumour spread includes cystoscopy, bimanual vaginal examination and rectal examination. Investigations should include chest X-ray, bone scan, intravenous urogram, pelvic CT scan and, more debatably nowadays, lymphangiogram.

The histological appearance of the tumour is varied. The main features are of oedematous stroma containing poorly differentiated spindle cells. In addition, there are large, vacuolated, eosinophilic, multinucleated cells known as rhabdomyoblasts. The WHO classification requires that these rhabdomyoblasts are present for the diagnosis of sarcoma botryoides to be made. Some cells show the striations of smooth muscle which are characteristic of mixed mesodermal tumours, although these may be difficult to find. Other features of mixed mesodermal tumours in adults, such as cartilage and bone, are rare in mixed mesodermal tumours of the vagina and cervix in children. The tumour shows marked pleomorphism with the components of oedematous stroma, sarcomatous stroma and rhabdomyoblasts being present in varying proportions – one feature may predominate to the exclusion of others.

The treatment of sarcoma botryoides has undergone a marked change over the last 20 years. Formerly, the only hope of cure was with early and extensive surgery often incorporating anterior and posterior exenteration or palliative surgery and radiation. More recently, however, after a report in 1976 (Kumar *et al.*, 1976), combined treatment with chemotherapy, radiotherapy and more limited, although still extensive, surgery has become normal practice (Bell *et al.*, 1986).

Treatment is with triple chemotherapy – vincristine, actinomycin D and cyclophosphamide (VAC) given intravenously at two or three week intervals for a six month period, at doses appropriate for the girl's weight and height. Response to therapy is monitored clinically and by CT scan. If the response to chemotherapy is not maximal, radiotherapy may be added after three months but may impair growth of the pelvis. Cases have been reported of complete tumour remission after chemotherapy but in most girls, surgery is also recommended by the Intergroup Rhabdomyosarcoma Study (Mayrer *et al.*, 1977) to prevent local recurrence. Surgery is extended hysterectomy with vaginectomy and lymph node dissection. Following surgery, further courses of VAC are given for six to 24 months, depending on response. The prognosis for girls with sarcoma botryoides on this regime is extremely good and justifies the intensive treatment. The Intergroup Rhabdomyosarcoma Study reported two deaths in a group of 24 girls using this multimodality approach over a surveillance period of up to 10 years

(Hays *et al.*, 1985). Prior to the use of this combined therapy, the 10 year survival rate was 18% (Hilgers *et al.*, 1970).

Cases have been reported of conservative treatment of girls with vaginal or vulvar sarcoma botryoides which has allowed them subsequently to become pregnant (Flamamnt *et al.*, 1990). While preservation of reproductive function is obviously important, it is even more important that girls with this condition receive curative therapy and the decision for conservative therapy should only be made by a practitioner with experience in managing these tumours. Recurrences can be treated with further doses of combination chemotherapy, but, in general, the prognosis is poor. Sarcoma botryoides should, if at all possible, be treated in a centre with experience of the condition in order to maximise the outcome.

UTERINE TUMOURS

Tumours of the uterine corpus, whether benign or malignant are the most rare of the already rare tumours of the genital tract in childhood. Because of that the greatest difficulty is actually making the diagnosis.

Uterine fibroids

Fibroids or leiomyomas of the uterus are the most common benign tumour in adult women, but are extremely uncommon in girls. Individual cases have been reported (Wiscot *et al.*, 1969). Presentation is the same as in adults with heavy periods or with an abdominal mass. Treatment is surgical by myomectomy with every attempt made to preserve reproductive function.

Carcinoma of the endometrium

Carcinoma of the endometrium is extremely rare in young girls. It presents with irregular vaginal bleeding and discharge. Treatment is by hysterectomy. The main problems with this tumour are its extreme rarity and that it is not visible at examination under anaesthesia. Diagnosis in adults is normally by hysteroscopy and dilatation and currettage. This is not appropriate in young girls because of the risk of uterine perforation and damage to the cervix with the risk of cervical incompetence in later life. Ultrasound examination of the uterus and measurement of the endometrial thickness is probably the first investigation to consider in such girls with instrumentation of the uterus reserved for those in whom a thickened endometrium is found on ultrasound.

Uterine sarcoma

The most common of this rare group of tumours are the uterine sarcomas, particularly the mixed mesodermal tumours. Sarcoma of the uterus presents as a rapidly growing abdominal mass with irregular uterine bleeding. The girl may also complain of abdominal pain. Gentle curettage will provide tissue for diagnosis allowing pre-operative chemotherapy to be given. More usually, the diagnosis is made at laparotomy for an abdominal mass. Histology shows oedematous tissue with sarcomatous elements. Heterotopic tissue is usually present including cartilage and bone. Further evaluation is with pelvic ultrasound and CT scan. Treatment is with chemotherapy and radical surgery.

OVARIAN TUMOURS

Ovarian tumours are the most common genital tract tumours in girls and adolescents although they constitute no more than 1% of all tumours of girls under 16 years of age. Of the ovarian cysts, the most common are teratomas which account for about a quarter to a third of the total number.

Although ovarian tumours are the commonest genital tract tumour, not all of them are neoplastic and, more importantly, not all of them require removal. Breen and Maxson (1977) in a review of 1309 ovarian masses in girls found 36% to be non-neoplastic. Of the neoplasms, 35% were malignant.

While the most important aspect of the management of ovarian tumours is that the correct treatment be given to ensure a good outcome, just as important is that non-neoplastic functional cysts of less than 5 cm are not removed 'just because they have been found' on ultrasound as part of the investigation of a girl with lower abdominal pain. It is also important that surgeons operating on a girl with suspected appendicitis do not remove simple cysts noted at the time of surgery 'just because they are there'. Simple unilocular cysts of less than 5 cm do not cause pain unless they have undergone torsion or haemorrhage.

It is essential that radiographers and radiologists give the dimensions of ovarian cysts noted on ultrasound scan and not use misleading phrases such as 'ovarian cyst occupying the whole ovary' which on laparotomy is found to be a simple follicular cyst of 3 cm maximum dimension. It is preferable, if the size of the unit permits, to have one radiologist performing all of the paediatric gynaecology ultrasound examinations.

Fetal and neonatal ovarian cysts (see also p. 75)

With the continuing improvement in definition of images obtained with ultrasound and with the increasing use of antenatal ultrasound screening for congenital abnormalities, the diagnosis of fetal ovarian cysts is being made more frequently. In a review of eight cases of fetal ovarian cyst, the histology reported was either of a follicular or a theca–lutein cyst (Landrum *et al.*, 1986) while a similar review of neonatal ovarian cysts showed the histology to be that of a follicular cyst (Widdowson *et al.*, 1988). These cysts probably develop in response to the high levels of circulating maternal human chorionic gonadotrophin (HCG).

Treatment in the fetal and neonatal period should be expectant, with monitoring of the size of the cyst with ultrasound. Intra-uterine aspiration of the cyst may be required in the rare event of the size of a fetal ovarian cyst compromising fetal lung development with subsequent risk of pulmonary hypoplasia (Fig. 14.5). Intra-uterine aspiration, however, is not without its risks (Purkiss *et al.*, 1988) and should be restricted to those in whom the risk of pulmonary hypoplasia is a significant one.

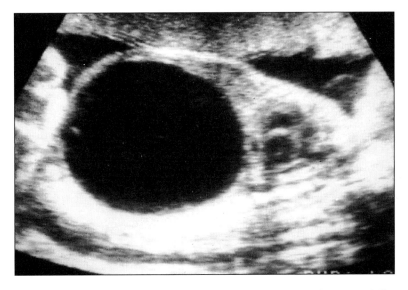

Fig. 14.5 Ultrasound image of a large fetal ovarian mass causing upward displacement of the diaphragm and potential restriction in growth of the fetal lungs.

In the neonatal period, management is also expectant. Widdowson *et al.* (1988) found that complications such as torsion, or rupture, only occurred in cysts of more than 5 cm. They recommended simple aspiration with ultrasound follow-up of cysts larger than 5 cm in diameter and ultrasound monitoring alone for those less than this size. They recommended that surgery should be reserved for cysts which were recurrent or had complications such as torsion.

Other than in the fetal and neonatal period, when ovarian masses are likely to be a chance finding, ovarian masses, irrespective of their pathology, usually present with abdominal pain or an abdominal mass. As the ovaries are an abdominal organ in early childhood, ovarian masses in this age group tend to cause pain in the peri-umbilical area, while in older girls and teenagers, the pain is more likely to be in either iliac fossa or in the supra-pubic area. In the absence of complications such as torsion or haemorrhage, pain is more likely to be a feature of fast growing tumours, particularly malignant tumours, whereas the finding of an abdominal mass is more likely in slow-growing benign tumours. Ovarian tumours in childhood are likely to be germ cell in derivation, while the pattern in adolesence is similar to that in adult life.

Further non-specific symptoms associated with ovarian tumours are nausea, vomiting and less often, diarrhoea. In the rarer group of hormone-secreting tumours, symptoms and signs secondary to hormone production will be present.

Ovarian cysts in childhood seem to be more prone to complications than those in adolescence and adult life. Common complications are torsion, rupture or haemorrhage. These complications will present with acute abdominal pain and signs of peritonism.

The main investigation of a suspected ovarian cyst is an ultrasound scan. Particular attention should be paid to the size of the tumour, whether it is unilocular and whether there are any solid elements present. If there is a suspicion of malignancy on ultrasound, an intravenous urogram or renal ultrasound may be helpful to exclude ureteric compression. Hormone assays will be required in tumours which are hormone-secreting and tumour markers will be helpful, not so much for diagnosis as for follow-up, in malignant neoplasms. If there is difficulty in ascertaining the nature of an ovarian cyst on ultrasound, direct visualisation with laparoscopy may be of value.

FUNCTIONAL CYSTS

Follicular Cysts

The presentation of follicular cysts in the fetal and neonatal period has already been considered. Follicular cysts, however, may occur at any time in a woman's life. Ultrasound examination shows a unilocular cyst with no solid components. They are usually small, normally less than 5 cm but can be as large as 10 cm in diameter. They are lined with granulosa cells which often have a flattened appearance (Fig. 14.6). Treatment is as already described – expectant with ultrasound monitoring for cysts of less than 5 cm, aspiration of cysts greater than 5 cm (with cyst fluid sent for cytological examination to exclude malignancy) and surgery reserved for those which are recurrent or complicated.

If surgery is required, it should be as conservative as possible, with enucleation of the cyst and preservation of the ovarian tissue. The ovary should be reconstructed with 2–0 catgut to achieve haemostasis within the substance of the ovary and with fine (6–0, if possible) nylon to the capsule.

Corpus Luteum Cyst

The corpus luteum is formed following ovulation and secretes progesterone. Normally, the corpus luteum does not exceed 3 cm in diameter and structures larger than this are referred to as corpus luteum cysts, although they, too, are small and rarely exceed 5 cm. Persistent cysts will continue to secrete

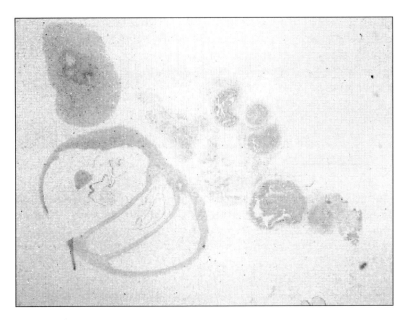

Fig. 14.6 Low power magnification of a follicular ovarian cyst showing the small size of the cyst and the flattened appearance of the epithelium.

progesterone and therefore are associated with delayed menstruation. Ultrasound scan will show a simple, fluid-filled unilocular cyst. As these cysts are associated with ovulation, they are only found in post-pubertal girls. Treatment is expectant as these tumours almost always resolve spontaneously.

Corpus luteum cysts are, however, prone to rupture and haemorrhage and may present as an acute abdomen. The combination of delayed menstruation and acute abdominal pain results in the main differential diagnosis being an ectopic pregnancy but this can be excluded by a pregnancy test. Surgery should be conservative. Laparoscopy will show whether the cyst is continuing to bleed actively. If there is no active bleeding, aspiration of the haemoperitoneum via the laparoscope is all that is required. Continued bleeding requires laparotomy to allow either cautery or oversewing of the bleeding vessel.

Theca Lutein Cysts

Theca lutein cysts are the least common of the functional ovarian cysts and are found in association with raised levels of HCG. They develop from unruptured ovarian follicles. In practical terms, this means that they are found in fetal life, as already described, or in the presence of a hydatidiform mole or choriocarcinoma which makes them an extremely unusual finding in childhood or adolescence. Ultrasound examination will show a unilocular, or more likely a multilocular, fluid-filled cyst which can be quite large – diameters up to 25 cm are not unusual. Histology shows the wall to be lined with an inner layer of luteinized theca interna and granulosa cells, and an outer layer of theca externa cells. These cysts require only symptomatic treatment, however, as a fall in HCG levels will bring about resolution of the tumour.

BENIGN TUMOURS AND NEOPLASMS

Teratoma

The commonest benign ovarian tumour in girls and young women is a teratoma. These are usually small – rarely more than 10 cm in diameter – and appear as partly solid, partly cystic structures on ultrasound examination (Fig. 14.7). They are usually unilateral but are bilateral in 10–15% of patients – either at the time of initial presentation or later in reproductive life.

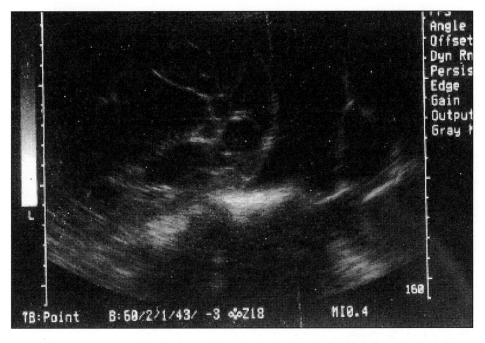

Fig. 14.7   Ultrasound image of an ovarian teratoma showing the solid and cystic components.

Teratomas are derived from totipotential primordial germ cells so that on histological examination, derivatives of all three germ cell layers may be identified. There is usually a predominance of tissue of ectodermal origin with the cyst wall lined with squamous epithelium containing sebaceous (Fig. 14.8) and sweat

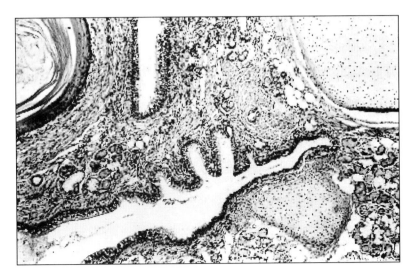

Fig. 14.8 Histological appearance of a mature cystic teratoma showing the different types of tissue involved particularly squamous tissue.

glands. Incision of such a tumour reveals sebaceous material and hair giving rise to the common name of dermoid cyst. The presence of bone, teeth (Fig. 14.9) and cartilage gives the tumour a characteristic appearance on X-ray.

A not uncommon component of teratoma is thyroid tissue, which if present in sufficient amounts, may cause symptoms of thyrotoxicosis. A teratoma almost completely composed of thyroid tissue is known as 'struma ovarii', although the

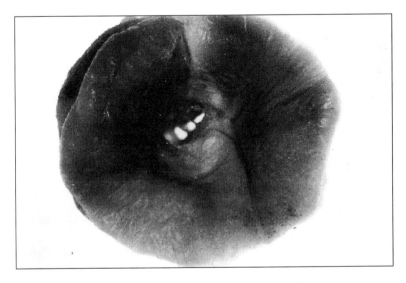

Fig. 14.9 Dermoid cyst containing teeth.

term is increasingly used for tumours which are only predominantly, as opposed to completely, thyroid tissue.

It is unusual for teratomas to be malignant in childhood, but as there is a small risk of malignancy, the teratoma must be removed. If the teratoma is less than 5 cm in size, this can probably be performed by enucleation with preservation of the remaining ovarian tissue. This is particularly important because of the chance of the tumour being bilateral. It is important in enucleating the tumour, that care is taken to remove all the teratomatous tissue otherwise it will recur. It is unlikely that tumours larger than 5 cm can be enucleated as the residual ovarian tissue is so attenuated that it is difficult to identify but this is well worth attempting. It is essential that the other ovary is inspected to exclude a bilateral tumour.

Endometrioma

An endometrioma is a cystic neoplasm in the ovary with walls lined by endometrial cells and containing altered blood with a chocolate appearance. Endometriosis is considered on p. 149 and is rare in adolescents. Endometriosis sufficient to cause an endometrioma is even rarer. Treatment is by a combination of medical regimes as outlined in the above Chapter followed by surgery.

Mucinous cystadenoma

This is the most common benign ovarian neoplasm found in adults and as such may be found in older adolescents. They can grow to extremely large sizes (Fig. 14.10), in older women filling the whole abdominal cavity, although it is unusual to find that size in adolescents. Ultrasound examination shows a multiloculated cyst. These cysts contain mucinous material which varies in colour from clear to dark brown. Histology shows the loculi to be lined with columnar cells. These tumours are benign but if they rupture, either spontaneously or during removal, the patient is at risk of developing myxoma peritonei – a recurring collection of mucinous producing cells in the abdominal cavity which may eventually, despite repeated surgery, prove fatal.

Serous cystadenoma

Serous cystadenoma are occasionally found in adolescents. They do not grow as big as mucinous cystadenoma usually being no larger than 15 cm. On ultrasound, they will appear as unilocular or occasionally, multilocular, fluid-containing cysts. Histological examination shows them to be lined with tall, ciliated, columnar epithelial cells. The cyst is not infrequently lined with papillary excrescences which may also appear on the outer surface of the cyst. This, however, does not imply malignancy.

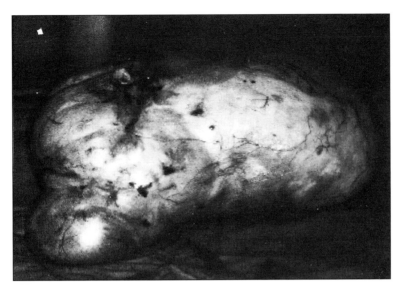

Fig. 14.10 A huge mucinous cystadenoma removed from an 18-year-old girl. The mass had been up to her xyphisternum.

Both serous cystadenoma and mucinous cystadenoma may undergo malignant change in the adult but this has not been reported in adolescents.

SEX-CORD TUMOURS

Gonadoblastoma

This is a relatively rare tumour found in adolescent or young adult women and arises from a dysgenetic gonad usually in a patient with a Y chromosome or fragment in her karyotype (Fig. 14.11). The tumour is usually benign but frequently contains islands of germ cells which may form a malignant germ cell tumour, particularly dysgerminomas. For this reason, it is important that girls whose karyotype includes a Y chromosome or a Y fragment have their gonads removed. The risk of malignancy in these women has been estimated to be around 5% (Verp and Simpson, 1987).

Gonadoblastomas are solid, smooth tumours which are unilateral in 70% of cases. They are usually small, often microscopic, and only rarely reach sizes of 10 cm. Histological examination shows them to consist of islands of large germ cells, with granulosa and Sertoli cells mixed with smaller sex-cord cells. Foci of calcification are a feature of this tumour. Treatment is by surgical excision of both gonads.

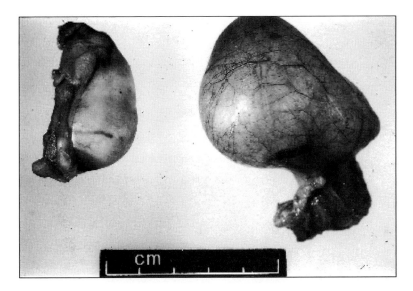

Fig. 14.11   Gonads removed from a girl who was 46XY showing a normal testis and a gonadoblastoma.

Fibroma

Although fibromas are rare, they are probably the most common sex-cord tumour in young girls. They are small solid tumours which histologically are composed of bundles of spindle cells. They are normally benign but large fibromas may present with ascites and pleural effusion – Meig's syndrome. Treatment is by surgical excision.

Granulosa/Theca Cell Tumour

Granulosa cell tumours are uncommon prior to puberty with only 1% of them presenting before 10 years of age (Evans *et al.*, 1986). They are usually unilateral. Ultrasound examination shows a solid tumour with numerous cystic areas which on direct vision are found to contain serosanguinous fluid and blood. Histologically, the cells may appear in a diffuse pattern, in the so-called 'moire silk' pattern, or in a solid pattern with small round spaces (Call–Exner bodies), or in a microfollicular pattern (Figs. 14.12 and 14.13). They are of low malignancy.

Thecomas are also rare before puberty but are usually bilateral. They are firm and rubbery in consistency and are frequently small, only being visible when the ovary is bisected. The histological appearance is of large oval cells admixed with spindle cells. There is abundant lipid in the cells and thus staining for cell fat is necessary to make the diagnosis.

Although thecomas are rare prior to puberty, they are of significance in this age group as they are oestrogen-producing. Precocious puberty is the presenting

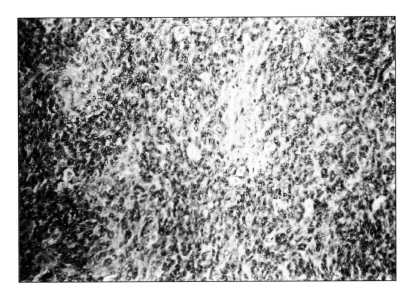

Fig. 14.12   Low power histological view of a granulosa cell tumour showing the moire silk appearance.

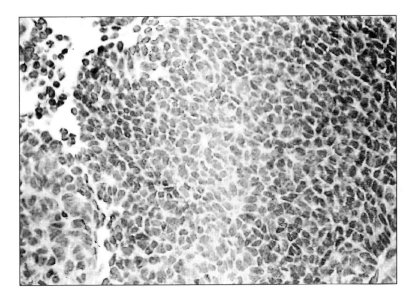

Fig. 14.13   High power histological view of a granulosa cell tumour.

symptom in 70% of girls with these tumours (Young *et al.*, 1984). Treatment is by unilateral oophorectomy with combination chemotherapy for those with metastatic tumour. Oestrogen levels may be useful as a marker to monitor the progress of the tumour.

Sertoli–Leydig Tumours

Sertoli–Leydig tumours (arrhenoblastoma) are rare but important as they produce androgens and so cause virilisation. They are of low malignant potential. The tumours are semi-solid, semi-cystic and can be extremely large. Presentation is with symptoms of virilisation – male pattern baldness, hirsutism, clitormegaly and in post-pubertal girls, breast atrophy. Histological examination shows Sertoli cell tubules with intervening Leydig cells, the ease of recognising this pattern depending on the degree of differentiation. Treatment is by unilateral oophorectomy.

Gynandroblastoma

This extremely rare tumour consists of granulosa–theca cells and Sertoli–Leydig cells. They produce either androgens causing virilisation or oestrogens or a mixture of the two. They are benign.

MALIGNANT OVARIAN TUMOURS

As with benign ovarian tumours, malignant ovarian tumours in childhood and adolescence are more likely to be of germ cell origin, rather than the epithelial tumours found in adults. The commonest malignant tumours found in this group are dysgerminoma, endodermal sinus tumour, malignant teratoma, embryonal carcinoma, primary ovarian choriocarcinoma and mixed germ cell tumour, in order of frequency.

The correct management of malignant ovarian disease in young girls and adolescents is critical to achieve both the highest cure rate and maintain fertility.

The use of tumour markers in the management of these tumours is extremely helpful. Markers such as alpha-fetoprotein (AFP) and HCG are produced by some germ cell tumours and monitoring their serum levels is an extremely helpful means of assessing response to therapy.

Laparotomy for potentially malignant ovarian tumours should be carried out with a midline abdominal incision to allow sufficient exposure and to ensure that an adequate staging laparotomy can be carried out. At laparotomy, the tumour is inspected to ascertain if it is benign or malignant. A tumour with an intact smooth capsule which is predominantly cystic is likely to be benign. A frozen section may be helpful although the interpretation of the histology of ovarian tumours is notoriously difficult. If in doubt as to whether a tumour is benign or malignant in a young girl, it is better to err on the side of caution and remove only the affected ovary. If subsequent histology shows the tumour to be malignant, consideration can be given as to whether further surgery is required but it is not possible to re-implant a removed ovary!

If there is any doubt as to the nature of the tumour, a staging laparotomy must be performed with aspiration of peritoneal fluid or washings; exploration of the liver and diaphragm, with consideration to the use of diaphragmatic smears; inspection and biopsy of the omentum; and palpation and sampling of para-aortic nodes. Staging of ovarian malignancy is shown in Table 14.1.

Table 14.1 Staging for carcinoma of the ovary

Stage 1 Growth limited to the ovaries

a	Growth limited to one ovary; no malignant cells in ascites or washings; capsule intact.
b	Growth limited to both ovaries; no malignant cells in ascites or washings; capsule intact.
c	Tumour as in 1a or 1b but tumour present on surface/capsule ruptured; malignant cells in ascites or washings.

Stage 2 Growth involving one or both ovaries, with pelvic extension.

a	Involving uterus/tubes.
b	Involving other pelvic tissues.
c	As 2a or 2b with tumour present on surface/capsule ruptured; malignant cells in washings or ascites.

Stage 3 Tumour involving one or both ovaries with spread outside pelvis/node involvement.

Stage 4 Distant metastases.

Dysgerminoma

Dysgerminoma is the commonest malignant ovarian tumour in childhood and also occurs most frequently in young women – 60% of these tumours being found in young women under 20. It is usually unilateral and grows rapidly to a considerable size – 15–20 cm is not unusual. Ultrasound examination shows a solid tumour. Macroscopic examination of a dysgerminoma reveals a yellow–white, encapsulated, nodular but smooth tumour. Frequently, there are areas of cystic degeneration, haemorrhage or necrosis on section. The degree of malignancy varies and, although most girls presenting with a dysgerminoma have a good prognosis, ascites with spread to the contralateral ovary and elsewhere on the peritoneum may be present and is a bad prognostic sign. Histologically, a dysgerminoma consists of clusters of large neoplastic cells with irregular nuclei and abundant, pale cytoplasm. The cells are arranged in either cords or nests with strands of connective tissue running between them. This connective tissue is infiltrated with lymphocytes and occasionally eosinophils. A granulomatous reaction may be present with Langhan's giant cells similar to that found in seminoma. Areas of choriocarcinoma, immature teratoma or endodermal sinus tumour may be present. A pure dysgerminoma does not produce any tumour markers.

Initial treatment is operative. Surgery should be conservative in stage 1a of the disease, with removal of only the affected ovary, provided that the girl does not have a Y chromosome or part of a Y chromosome in her karyotype. However, as the tumour in the contralateral ovary may be very small, it is prudent to inspect and biopsy the remaining ovary to exclude bilateral disease. Take care not to jeopardise the blood supply. Biopsy may be performed using a Trucut biopsy needle which will allow histological examination of the ovarian stroma while causing minimal damage to the ovarian tissue and minimum adhesion formation. The tumour is extremely chemo- and radio-sensitive. Combination chemotherapy with bleomycin, etopside and the platinum group of agents may be very successful and has the advantage over radiotherapy of not damaging fertility. If it has not been possible to remove all the tumour at initial surgery, a second laparotomy following chemotherapy may allow any residual tumour to be removed.

The prognosis for girls with dysgerminoma is good. Overall five-year survival rates of 85% have been reported (Thomas *et al.*, 1987) and a five-year survival of 96% for early disease treated with unilateral oophorectomy (Kurman and Norris, 1977). If, however, other tumour elements are present such as choriocarcinoma, then the prognosis is dependent on the most malignant element of the tumour.

Endodermal Sinus Tumour

This tumour, also called a yolk sac tumour, is the second most common ovarian tumour in this age group. They are extremely aggressive and malignant tumours, the patients presenting with abdominal pain and mass, often accompanied by low grade fever. The tumour is one almost exclusively of girls and teenagers with a median age of presentation of 19 years (Gerherson *et al.*, 1983). The tumours are large, usually over 10 cm and ultrasound appearances are of a solid tumour, often with cystic areas due to necrosis. Alpha-fetoprotein (AFP) levels may be raised. Macroscopically, the tumour is grey–white in appearance with areas of haemorrhage and necrosis. On microscopic examination, the tumour is seen to consist of a background of microcysts and the classic Schiller–Duval bodies – a central capillary in a mesenchymal core surrounded by cuboidal tumour cells and projecting into a space communicating with the microcysts. Eosinophilic hyaline globules which immunostain for AFP are also present.

Treatment is by surgical removal of the tumour followed by aggressive chemotherapy using VAC. Bleomycin and the platinum group of chemotherapy agents have also been used with some success (Athaniker *et al.*, 1989). If elevated AFP levels allow its use as a tumour marker, chemotherapy should be continued for two courses after normal levels have been reached. Radiotherapy is used in the treatment of recurrent disease.

Malignant Teratoma

Most ovarian teratomas in girls are benign but two forms of malignancy exist. The more common is the immature teratoma which occurs most frequently in the first two decades of life. Approximately 8% of all ovarian tumours in children under 15 years are immature teratomas (Neven *et al.*, 1993). The median age of presentation is 21 (Kouios *et al.*, 1989) Embryonic forms of all three germ cell layers may be present with the most common being neuro-ectodermal tissue. Presentation and ultrasound appearance is similar to that found in benign teratoma. Tumour markers are usually negative unless choriocarcinoma is present where HCG levels will be raised. Treatment is surgical, with removal of the tumour and sampling of peritoneal implants which may be of a different histological grade (either higher or lower) than the original tumour. Combination chemotherapy with VAC is used post-operatively. The prognosis depends on the size of the tumour and the amount of immature tissue present.

The other form of malignancy is malignant change in one of the tissue elements of tumour, particularly in squamous cells. This form of malignancy, although more common than the immature form in adults, is rarely found in children.

Embryonal Carcinoma

This is a rare tumour but is probably the most aggressive of the malignant ovarian tumours in childhood. It affects a younger age group than the other tumours, the mean age being 14 (Kurman *et al.*, 1976). They are large solid tumours although scan appearance may show cystic areas due to tumour necrosis. Elevated levels of AFP and HCG may be present. Histologically the tumour consists of pleomorphic epithelial like cells with eosinophilic cytoplasm. As with all the malignant germ cell tumours, treatment is by surgery and a combination chemotherapy of VAC. Good results have also been reported using cisplatin.

Choriocarcinoma

Primary ovarian choriocarcinoma is extremely rare and has a poor prognosis. HCG levels are raised. Treatment is by tumour debulking followed by combination chemotherapy which includes methotrexate.

Mixed Germ Cell Tumour

Mixed germ cell tumours may contain elements of all the germ cell tumours, the most common being dysgerminoma. Treatment is with surgery and chemotherapy.

In summary, true tumours of the genital tract are rare in childhood and adolescence. They must always be considered, however, as most are associated with a good prognosis if diagnosed early.

REFERENCES

Anderson WA, Sabio H, Durso N, Mills SE, Levien M, Underwood PB, 1985: Endodermal sinus tumor of the vagina – the role of primary chemotherapy. *Cancer* **56**, 1025–1027.

Athaniker N, Saika TK, Rankrishnan G, Nair CN, Nadkarni KS, Advani SH, 1989: Aggressive chemotherapy in endodermal sinus tumor. *Journal of Surgical Oncology* **40**, 17–20.

Bell J, Averette H, Davis J, Toledano S, 1986: Genital rhabdomyosarcoma: Current management and review of the literature. *Obstetrical and Gynecological Survey* **41**, 257–263.

Blaivas JG, Pais VM, Retik AB, 1976: Paraurethral cysts in female neonate. *Urology* **7**, 504–507.

Blaustein A, Sedlis A, 1982: Diseases of the vagina. In Blaustein A (ed.), *Pathology of the female genital tract.* 2nd edn. New York: Springer Verlag, 59–98.

Breen JL, Maxson WS, 1977: Ovarian tumours in children and adolescents. *Clinical Obstetrics and Gynaecology* **20**, 607–623.

Collins HS, Burke TW, Heller PB, Olson TA, Woodward JE, Park RC, 1989: Endodermal sinus tumour of the infant vagina treated exclusively by chemotherapy. *Obstetrics and Gynecology* **73**, 507–509.

Copeland LJ, Gershenson DM, Saul PB, Sneige N, Stringer CA, Edwards CL, 1985: Sarcoma botryoides of the female genital tract. *Obstetrics and Gynecology* **66**, 262–266.

Emens JM, 1994: Continuing problems with diethylstilboestrol. *British Journal of Obstetrics and Gynaecology* **101**, 748–750.

Evans AT, Gaffey TA, Malkasian GD, Annegers JF, 1986: Clinicopathologic review of 118 granulosa and 82 theca cell tumours. *Obstetrics and Gynecology* 231–237.

Flamamnt F, Gerbaulet C, Nihoul-Fekete C, *et al.*, 1990: Long-term sequelae of conservative treatment by surgery, brachytherapy and chemotherapy for vulvar and vaginal rhabdomyosarcoma in children. *Journal of Clinical Oncology* **8**, 1847–1853.

Gerherson DM, del Junco G, Herson J, Rutledge FN, 1983: Endodermal sinus tumour of the ovary: the MD Anderson experience. *Obstetrics and Gynecology* **61**, 194–202.

Gravier L, 1969: Hydrocolpos. *Journal of Pediatric Surgery* **4**, 563–568.

Hays DM, Shimada H, Raney RB Jnr, *et al.*, 1985: Sarcomas of the vagina and uterus. The Intergroup Rhabdomyosarcoma Study. *Journal of Pediatric Surgery* **20**, 718–724.

Herbst AL, 1979: Current status of the DES problem. *Obstetrical and Gynecological Survey* **34**, 844–850.

Herbst AL, Anderson D, Hubby MM, Haenszel WM, Kaufman RH, Noller KL, 1986: Risk factors for the development of diethylstilboestrol-associated clear cell adenocarcinoma: a case control study. *American Journal of Obstetrics and Gynecology* **154**, 814–822.

Herbst AL, Scully RE, 1970: Adenocarcinoma of the vagina in adolescence: a report of seven cases including six clear cell carcinomas (so called mesonephromas). *Cancer* **25**, 745–757.

Herbst AL, Ulfelder H, Poskanzer DC, 1971: Adenocarcinoma of the vagina. Association of maternal stilboestrol therapy with tumour appearance in young women. *New England Journal of Medicine* **284**, 878–881.

Hilgers RD, Malkasian GD, Soule EH, 1970: Embryonal rhabdomyosarcoma (botryoid type) of the vagina. A clinicopathological review. *American Journal of Obstetrics and Gynecology* **107**, 484–501.

Horwitz RI, Viscoli CM, Merino M, Brennan TA, Flannery JT, Robboy SJ, 1988: Clear cell adenocarcinoma of the vagina and cervix: incidence, undetected disease, and diethylstilbestrol. *Journal of Clinical Epidemiology* **41**, 593–597.

Kinlen LJ, Badaracco MA, Moffett J, Vessey MP, 1974: A survey of the use of oestrogens during pregnancy in the United Kingdom and of the genito-urinary cancer mortality and incidence rates in young people in England and Wales. *Journal of Obstetrics and Gynaecology of the British Commonwealth* **81**, 849–855.

Kouios JP, Hoffman JF, Steinhoff MM, 1989: Immature teratoma of the ovary. *Gynecological Oncology* **34**, 46–49.

Kumar APM, Wrenn EL, Fleming ID, Hustu HO, Pratt CB, 1976: Combined therapy to prevent complete pelvic exenteration for rhabdomyosarcoma of the vagina or uterus. *Cancer* **37**, 118–122.

Kurman R, Scully R, 1974: The incidence and histogenesis of vaginal adenosis. An autopsy study. *Human Pathology* **5**, 265–276.

Kurman RJ, Norris HJ, 1977: Malignant germ cell tumours of the ovary. *Human Pathology* **8**, 551–564.

Kurman, RJ, Norris HJ, 1976: Endodermal sinus tumour of the ovary. A clinical and pathological analysis of 71 cases. *Cancer* **38**, 2404–2419.

Landrum B, Ogburn PL, Feinberg S *et al.*, 1986: Intrauterine aspiration of a large fetal ovarian cyst. *Obstetrics and Gynecology* **68**(Suppl 3), 11S–14S.

Lisa J, Cornwall LH, 1926: Carcinoma of the uterus in early life. *Proceedings of the New York Pathological Society* **26**, 46–55.

MacColum DW, Martin JW, 1956: Hemangioma in infancy and childhood. A report based on 6479 cases. *Surgical Clinics of North America* **36**, 1647–1663.

Maurer HM, Moon T, Donaldson M, *et al.*, 1977: The Intergroup Rhabdomyosarcoma study: a preliminary report. *Cancer* **40**, 2015–2026.

Melnick S, Cole P, Anderson D, Herbst A, 1987: Rates and risks of diethylstilboestrol related to clear cell adenocarcinoma of the vagina and cervix. *New England Journal of Medicine* **316**, 514–516.

Neven P, Shepherd JH, Lowe DG, 1993: Gynaecological malignancies in childhood. In Studd J and Jardine-Brown C (eds), *The year book of the Royal College of Obstetricians and Gynaecologists*. London: RCOG Press, 157–167.

Purkiss S, Brereton RJ, Wright VM, 1988: Surgical emergencies after prenatal treatment for intra-abdominal abnormality. *Lancet* **i**, 289–209.

Robinow M, Shaw A, 1979: The McKusick–Kaufman syndrome: recessively inherited vaginal atresia, hyrometrocolpos, uterovaginal duplications, anorectal anomalies, post-axial polydactyly and congenital heart disease. *Journal of Pediatrics* **94**, 776–778.

Senekjian EK, Frey FW, Anderson D, Herbst AL, 1987: Local therapy in Stage 1 clear cell adenocarcinoma of the vagina. *Cancer* **60**, 1319–1324.

Smith OW, 1948: Diethylstilboestrol in the prevention and treatment of complications of pregnancy. *American Journal of Obstetrics and Gynecology* **56**, 821–834.

Stafl A, Mattingly RF, Foley DV, Fetherston WC, 1974: Clinical diagnosis of vaginal adenosis. *Obstetrics and Gynecology* **43**, 118–128.

Stillman RJ, 1982: In utero exposure to diethylstilbestrol: adverse effects on the reproductive tract and reproductive performance in male and female offspring. *American Journal of Obstetrics and Gynecology* **142**, 994–1005.

Thomas GM, Dembo AJ, Hacker NF, DePetrillo AD, 1987: Current therapy for dysgerminoma of the ovary. *Obstetrics and Gynecology* **70**, 268–275.

Verp MS, Simpson JL, 1987: Abnormal sexual differentiation and neoplasia. *Cancer Genetics and Cytogenetics* **25**, 1991–2218.

Widdowson DJ, Pilling DW, Cook RCM, 1988: Neonatal ovarian cysts: therapeutic dilemma. *Archives of Disease in Childhood* **63**, 737–742.

Wiscot AL, Neimand KM, Rosenthal AH, 1969: Symptomatic myoma in a 13-year-old girl. *American Journal of Obstetrics and Gynecology* **105**, 639–641.

Young RH, Dickersin GR, Scully RE, 1984: Juvenile granulosa cell tumour of the ovary. A clinico-pathological analysis of 125 cases. *American Journal of Clinical Pathology* **8**, 575–596.

CHAPTER 15

Endocrine disorders

ANNE S GARDEN AND COLIN SMITH ————————————

ENDOCRINE PROBLEMS

While an understanding of basic endocrinology is necessary for all paediatric gynaecological practice, particularly when dealing with disorders of puberty, there are specific problems which demand a greater understanding of endocrinology. The most common of these are ambiguous genitalia at birth, sexual precocity and problems due to excess androgen stimulation, hirsutism and virilism. These are conditions which require to be dealt with by a paediatrician with specialist knowledge. The object of this Chapter is not to provide that specialist knowledge but to provide an overview of the conditions. The background information to this Chapter is contained in Chapter 1.

AMBIGUOUS GENITALIA

This problem is arguably the one which requires the most sensitive handling in the whole of paediatric gynaecology. The first thing any couple asks after delivery is the sex of the child and the inability to answer what is seen as the most simple of questions is incomprehensible to them.

It is understandable that anyone in the situation of not being able to tell the sex of a child wants to give the parents an answer and so there is a great temptation to make a guess at what seems to be the likeliest sex. This temptation must be resisted and the parents told sensitively that it is not possible at this point to determine the sex of the child and that further investigations will be necessary. It is also important at this point that the parents do realise that their child does have a gender and is not some indeterminate third sex or that the child is destined to remain in some sort of gender limbo indefinitely. A fuller discussion of the sort of psychological problems experienced by parents of children whose gender is initially uncertain is found in Chapter 6.

The clinical approach to a child with this problem is a team one with input from a clinical geneticist, paediatric endocrinologist, urologist and gynaecologist as well as the appropriate support and counselling. The parents should be given as full an explanation as possible with the facts available and warned that it may take a week before the complete answer can be given, although the information required to assign the sex of rearing is usually available within 48–72 hours (Meyers–Seifer and Charest, 1992).

The main causes of indeterminate genitalia are seen in Table 15.1. The clinical presentation is not dependent on the cause. The child has a phallus which is larger and wider than a normal clitoris but not so large as a penis. There is a varying degree of fusion of the labio-scrotal folds giving an appearance of rather rugose labia with variable degrees of fusion. The urethral opening is usually on the perineum at the base of the phallus, although it may be anywhere on a line from the ventral surface of the phallus to its normal female position on the perineum. Occasionally, there is a second urethral opening but in most instances when a girl has been masculinised, an overgrowth of the perineum occurs which results in a single opening on the perineum onto which the urethra and vagina open at a higher level. It is not therefore possible to tell on inspection whether these appearances are due to masculinisation of a female or undermasculinisation of a male.

Table 15.1 Causes of indeterminate genitalia

	Chromosomes	*Gonad*	*Cause*
Masculinised female	46XX	Ovary	CAH Iatrogenic Androgen secreting tumour
Undermasculinised male	46XY	Testis	PAIS Mixed gonadal dysgenesis Testicular failure
Hermaphrodite	46XX 46XY Mosaic	Ovotestis	?

The commonest situation is masculinisation of a female fetus. The development of the external genitalia of a fetus is androgen-dependent and the presence of androgens, whether exogenous or endogenous, will cause the genital tubercle to develop into a penis rather than the clitoris and the genital swellings to fuse to form the scrotum rather than the labia. This process is complete by 12 weeks gestation. The most usual reason for masculinisation of the female fetus is congenital adrenal hyperplasia (CAH). The use of androgenic drugs in pregnancy is less common. Drugs which have been reported as causing this are danazol, used for the treatment of maternal endometriosis, and the more androgenic progestogens, such as norethisterone. Nowadays, norethisterone is only given in pregnancy if a woman presents with bleeding in the early stages and this is mistaken by the medical practitioner for dysfunctional uterine bleeding. The masculinisation caused by drug intake in these instances is usually not severe as most drugs are not strongly androgenic and taking the drug is stopped as soon as the woman realises that she is pregnant. Androgen producing ovarian or adrenal tumours in either the mother or the fetus are extremely rare.

Undermasculinisation of a male fetus is less common than the masculinisation of a female fetus. Possibly the commonest cause of an undermasculinised male child is partial androgen insensitivity (PAIS). In this condition, the child has normal testes producing normal levels of testosterone, but the end-organ (in this instance the tissues of the genital area) fails to respond. In the complete form of the disorder, the child is phenotypically female and presents at puberty with primary amenorrhoea. In the partial form, there is a wide diversity of presentation, from the child with grossly abnormal genitalia at birth; through those who appear normal at birth but present with virilism at puberty when the testes begin to produce androgens, to those who are phenotypically normal males but may have poor sperm production. The condition is an X-linked recessive one and is due to mutations on the androgen receptor.

Undermasculisation of the male fetus can also be due to mixed gonadal dysgenesis in which the child has one streak gonad and one dysgenetic testis. In this circumstance, the degree of masculinisation depends on the amount of Leydig cell function present. Testicular failure prior to 12 weeks gestation may also be a cause. Another cause of poor masculinisation of a male child is 5-alpha-reductase deficiency. This enzyme converts testosterone (necessary for the development of the epididymis, vas deferens and seminal vesicles) to dihydrotestosterone (necessary for the development of the external genitalia). Such children have poorly developed external genitalia but are potentially fertile. They develop normally to puberty with the exceptions of the development of facial and body hair and penile development.

True hermaphroditism is exceptionally rare. Ovotestes are usually present although they can have separate gonads. Most have a normal female karyotype but a wide variety of mosaic forms have also been reported (Simpson, 1987).

CONGENITAL ADRENAL HYPERPLASIA

Congenital adrenal hyperplasia (CAH) results from a variety of enzyme defects which result in reduced cortisol and variably reduced aldosterone production. This causes loss of inhibition of adrenocorticotropic hormone (ACTH) production and therefore increased production of steroid precursors from which androgens may be synthesised. ACTH has melanocyte-stimulating properties causing pigmentation of the skin, particularly in the labio-scrotal area and around the areola.

The most frequent enzyme defect is 21-hydroxylase deficiency which is responsible for about 95% of cases and occurs in about 1 : 12 000 births (Miller, 1991). The other enzyme defects causing masculinisation are 11-beta-hydroxy-lase deficiency which has an incidence of around 1 : 100 000 and the much rarer 17-alpha-hydroxylase deficiency, 3-beta-hydroxysteroid dehydrogenase (HSD) deficiency and 20,22 desmolase deficiency. The latter is particularly rare and almost always fatal. The pathways leading to CAH are seen in Fig. 15.1. All the causes of CAH are autosomal recessive and potentially diagnosable pre-natally. The first description of pre-natal diagnosis of CAH occurred when apparently male external genitalia were seen on ultrasound in a fetus who was known by amniocentesis to be female. DNA probes for the 21-hydroxylase gene are now available allowing earlier diagnosis by chorionic villus sampling. Early diag-nosis has the advantage that it allows treatment *in utero* by giving the mother dexamethasone (Forest *et al.*, 1989). This may prevent masculinisation of the fetus and so prevent the need for major surgery both neonatally and possibly later in the girl's life.

Not only is CAH the most common cause of ambiguous genitalia, it has to be the diagnosis first considered as about two-thirds of affected children have the clinically significant salt-losing form which is fatal if not diagnosed and treated. The management of this aspect of the syndrome is beyond the scope of this Chapter.

Absence of 21-hydroxylase prevents conversion of 17-hydroxy-progesterone to 11-desoxycortisol. Low levels of cortisol and desoxy-cortisol are therefore produced and a buildup of 17-hydroxy-progesterone (which is the basis of diag-nosis), androstenedione, oestrone and testosterone results.

11-beta-Hydroxylase deficiency results in decreased conversion of 11-deoxy-cortisol to cortisol, with resultant increased levels of desoxycortisol and testos-terone. The high levels of desoxycortisol and desoxycorticosterone make the child at high risk for developing hypertension. Treatment of CAH is with gluco-corticoid therapy. Mineralocorticoids will also be required in the salt-losing con-dition.

MANAGEMENT OF AMBIGUOUS GENITALIA

The purpose of examination and investigation of a child with ambiguous geni-talia is two-fold to make a diagnosis of the condition and to decide the gender in which the child should be raised.

Examination of the infant must include palpation to try to identify the gonads which may be present in the inguinal region or in the labio-scrotal sac. Palpation of the gonads, however, does not guarantee normal male develop-ment as, very rarely, the gonad palpated may be an ovary (Rowe and Lloyd, 1986) or even if testes, they may be dysgenetic. Ultrasound may be helpful in differentiating between ovary and testes in inguinal masses (Munden *et al.*, 1995).

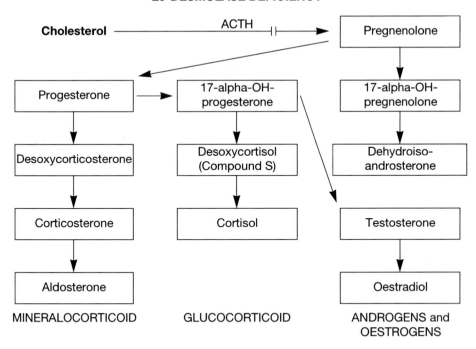

20-DESMOLASE DEFICIENCY

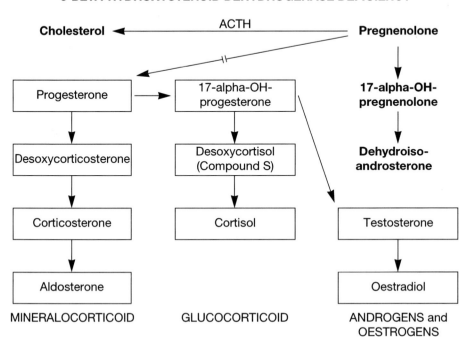

3-BETA-HYDROXYSTEROID DEHYDROGENASE DEFICIENCY

Fig. 15.1 The different enzyme defects which result CAH.

17-ALPHA HYDROXYLASE DEFICIENCY

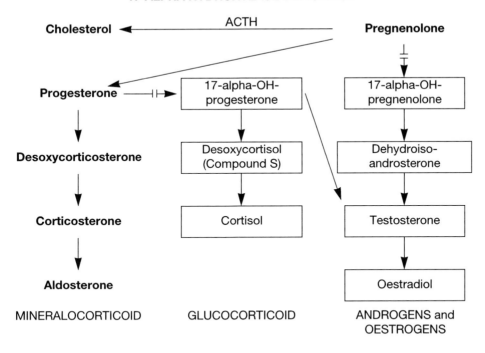

21-HYDROXYLASE DEFICIENCY

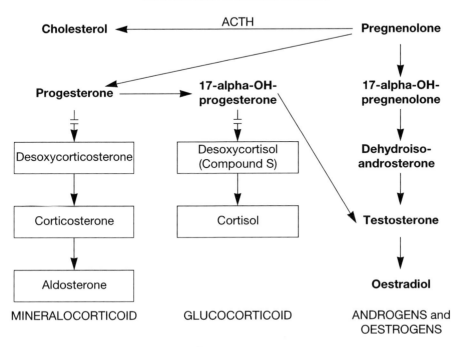

Fig. 15.1 *cont'd*

11-BETA HYDROXYLASE DEFICIENCY

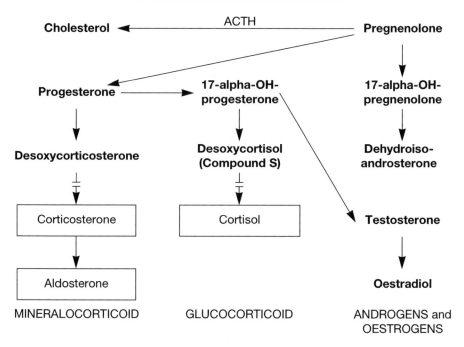

MINERALOCORTICOID   GLUCOCORTICOID   ANDROGENS and OESTROGENS

18-HYDROXYSTEROID DEFICIENCY

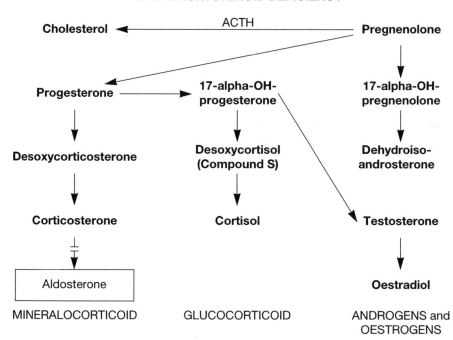

MINERALOCORTICOID   GLUCOCORTICOID   ANDROGENS and OESTROGENS

Fig. 15.1 *cont'd*

Dysmorphic appearances and the presence of pigmentation should be identified. Obviously, the presence of dehydration and electrolyte imbalance is extremely important.

INVESTIGATIONS

Blood tests should be performed to ascertain the child's chromosomal sex although this is not the final arbiter regarding the gender in which the child should be reared. Sodium, potassium and glucose levels will be abnormal in CAH. Plasma hormone profile will include testosterone and dihydrotestosterone levels and 17-hydroxyprogesterone levels.

Ultrasound of the pelvis will show whether or not a uterus is present, the uterus being more easily seen in the immediate neonatal period than in later childhood due to stimulation from maternal hormones. A recent study reported 94% sensitivity and 98% specificity in diagnosing the neonatal uterus using ultrasound (Kutteh *et al.*, 1995). Magnetic resonance imaging (MRI) will help identify the presence of intra-abdominal gonads (Gambino *et al.*, 1992) and other internal and external genitalia (Secof *et al.*, 1994). Depending on the degree of anomaly, a urogenital sinus X-ray may be performed.

If the child is to be reared as a male, androgen production and the ability of the genitalia to respond to the androgens is necessary. In order to assess the potential for androgen secretion, the testosterone response to HCG stimulation should be assessed (Berkowitz *et al.*, 1984).

The decision as to which gender a child should be reared in is a specialist one and beyond the scope of this book, but the general principles will be given. The important features are potential for sexual relationships and fertility. Thus, girls who are masculinised have potentially functioning ovaries and are usually raised as females although corrective surgery in the neonatal period and possibly also at puberty will be required to ensure a vagina of normal width for sexual intercourse. Girls with CAH are potentially fertile with good fertilty being reported in the non-salt-losing group (Mulaikal *et al.*, 1987).

In males who are undermasculinised, the decision is made on the potential for penile growth and for the penis to sustain an erection. This is likely to be poor in androgen insensitivity. Further, there is the additional problem that the testes are usually intra-abdominal and not usually correctable by surgery. This means that they will require to be removed because of the risk of malignancy. The decision is therefore often made to rear the child as a girl. The alternative is to have penile prostheses inserted at puberty and the long-term use of testosterone implants. Rearing the child with androgen insensitivity as a girl also requires the long-term use of female hormone replacement therapy (HRT) and she will also require either the use of vaginal dilators or possibly vaginal reconstructive surgery as well as gonadectomy because of the risk of malignancy. She will be infertile as she has no uterus.

Surgery for clitoridectomy in those for whom the decision has been made to rear the child as a girl, should be performed as soon as possible (see p. 93). Care must be taken to preserve the nerve supply to the glans (Hutson *et al.*, 1991). Follow-up studies have suggested a good result, both cosmetically and psychologically, in girls having clitoral reduction in childhood (Newman *et al.*, 1992).

There is debate as to when the best time for vaginal reconstructive surgery should be performed, most believing that it, too, should be carried out as soon as possible, usually at the time of clitoral reduction to allow the girl as little disruption in her life as possible later on. Some, however, believe that it is better to leave surgery until the girl is older when the tissues are larger and less friable. Leaving the surgery until adolescence allows the girl to have control over the decision. Obviously, support and counselling for the girl and her family are every bit as important as the surgical care (Goodall, 1991; see Personal View, 1994).

SEXUAL PRECOCITY

Precocious puberty in girls is defined as pubertal development before eight years of age. It may be described as 'central' (or true) where the stimulus of the hypothalamus causes premature activation of the hypothalamic-pituitary-ovarian axis. In these circumstances, the progression of puberty follows the normal pattern of puberty, only occurring at an earlier age. Sexual precocity (or pseudosexual precocity), in contrast, implies the development of secondary sexual features from sex steroids but not associated with central gonadotrophin production.

Central Precocious Puberty

The majority of central precocious puberty in girls is idiopathic, although improving imaging techniques such as computed tomography (CT) (Reith *et al.*, 1987) or MRI may show brain abnormalities not previously detected or suspected. Brain damage from hydrocephalus (with or without a neural tube defect), gonadotrophin producing tumours (particularly hamartomas), congenital anomalies, trauma (Sockalosky *et al.*, 1987) and infections may be followed by precocious puberty (Reith *et al.*, 1987; Kaplan and Grumbach, 1990; Juniper *et al.*, 1992). Hamartomas may cause precocious puberty at a very early age, not unusually in the early neonatal period, as their mechanism of action is to cause secretion of gonadotrophin releasing hormone (GnRH) as opposed to other intracranial lesions which damage those areas of the brain which suppress gonadotrophin release.

Precocious puberty is also associated with a wide variety of conditions such as neurofibromatosis, tuberose sclerosis, Silver's syndrome and primary hypothyroidism. Girls with breast development without an accompanying growth spurt or development of pubic hair are particularly likely to have hypothyroidism as an underlying pathology. In such circumstances, raised follicle stimulating hormone

(FSH) levels are found in association with the raised thyroid stimulating hormone (TSH) levels.

Pseudosexual Precocity

Pseudosexual precocity is much more unusual than central precocious puberty. It is characterised by the finding of raised sex hormone levels in the presence of pre-pubertal gonadotrophin levels. The most frequent cause in girls is a hormone-secreting ovarian tumour. By far the commonest of these are granulosa cell tumours, the others being arrhenoblastomas, which release androgens, or thecomas. Occasionally, adrenal tumours may produce oestrogen thus causing pubertal development.

Pubertal development independent of gonadotrophins may also occur in McCune–Albright syndrome. The aetiology of this syndrome is poorly understood but may represent a genetically determined signal transduction disorder. Mutations occurring in the G-protein binding system may stimulate production of the second messenger, cyclic adenyl monophosphate, in various tissues and endocrine glands causing autonomous hypersecretion of hormones. McCune–Albright syndrome is associated with polyostotic fibrous dysplasia of the bone, characteristic skin pigmentation, either in the form of café-au-lait spots or larger areas of pigmentation with a serrated edge known as 'coast of Maine' and endocrine hyperfunction. Gonadal overactivity is the commonest form seen, but thyroid, adrenal and pituitary overactivity have been described. Girls with McCune–Albright syndrome may have ovarian cysts, which may fluctuate in size, present on ultrasound examination (Mauras and Blizzard, 1986).

Gonadotrophin-secreting tumours are an extremely rare cause of precocious puberty as are iatrogenic causes due to ingestion of oestrogen-containing tablets, usually the oral contraceptive pill, or overusage of oestrogen creams.

Premature breast development is the most common presenting feature. A white, odourless vaginal discharge may be volunteered on direct questioning and, on occasions, blood spotting or menstrual bleeding may be present. The history, however, will usually confirm an preceding increase in growth rate compared with peers, along with mood and behavioural changes. The latter can cause practical difficulties in clinical assessment in an uncooperative, clinging child. History-taking should include questions about birth trauma; about any symptoms suggestive of a space-occupying lesion such as headaches, seizures or visual disturbances, and the possibility of oestrogen ingestion or use.

There may be clinical signs relating to the underlying brain abnormality as previously mentioned. Skin inspection may reveal the café-au-lait lesions and axillary skin freckling of neurofibromatosis, or the irregular 'coast of Maine' pigmented areas in McCune–Albright syndrome (Fig. 15.2).

A careful clinical assessment of height (including the use of growth charts), weight and pubertal signs is an important baseline evaluation as reassessment at intervals will document the tempo of this condition. The importance of this is obvious in girls on drug treatment, but, in practice, some girls with slow tempo

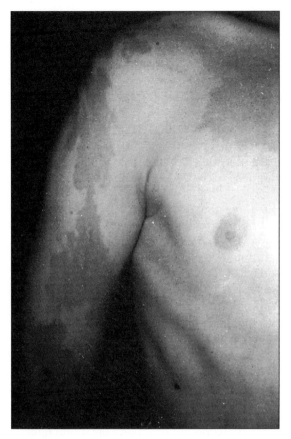

Fig. 15.2 'Coast of Maine' appearance of the skin of a child with McCune–Albright syndrome.

pubertal development and aged around nine years may require clinical support only rather than drug treatment.

Height and weight usually correlate in the higher centile lines or above and growth acceleration will be evident from previous measurements. Breast development to Tanner stage 2 or 3 is usual and there may be early pubic hair growth. The presence of facial hair, greasy hair and adult body odour would also suggest abnormal sex hormone production. Neurological examination, including fundoscopy and visual field examination should also be performed.

Investigations

Elevations of gonadotrophins may be clear cut on a random blood sample, although there is often considerable overlap with pre-pubertal values. In addition, the pulsatile release and circadian variation in gonadotrophin and sex hormone release means that a single estimation is rarely helpful. Abnormal levels, particularly of luteinising hormone (LH), may be seen after intravenous GnRH, with values often being three of four times the basal levels in girls with true central precocious puberty, contrasting with a very limited response seen in pre-puberty and in girls with pseudosexual precocity.

The demonstration of regular LH bursts, seen initially at night, on continuous sampling is conclusive evidence of central precocious puberty, although such techniques are not easily applicable to most patients. Oestradiol values in this context are often disappointingly low and at variance with the clinical features. This may reflect the lack of precision of present oestrogen assays at low levels. The finding of a high oestradiol level in the presence of pre-pubertal gonadotrophin levels is very suggestive of an oestrogen-secreting ovarian cyst.

Pelvic ultrasound may show enlarged ovaries with small follicular cysts as seen in normal puberty. The uterus is enlarged, with an adult shape and sometimes an increased endometrial thickness. A single ovarian cyst may be seen in those with McCune–Albright syndrome. Although the majority of cases of true central precocious puberty in girls are idiopathic, a cerebral lesion should be excluded by imaging using MRI in preference to CT scanning (Korneich *et al.*, 1995). MRI aided by the use of contrast medium, may also show an increase to adult size of the pituitary gland (Robben *et al.*, 1995). Skeletal maturation, as estimated by wrist X-ray, is advanced, except when the precocious puberty is related to hypothyroidism when it is retarded.

Treatment of True Central Precocious Puberty

The first decision to be made is whether or not the condition requires to be treated. The important factors to be considered are the girl's age, the speed of progression of puberty and her psychological response to it. Obviously pubertal development in a three year old requires treatment, but a girl aged seven with slowly developing puberty who is not undergoing teasing at school because of her breast development and who is well adjusted to her condition and well supported by her family may not require treatment.

In addition to the suppression of pubertal development, the objective of treatment is to minimise the compromise of adult height. Adult height may be compromised both due to premature closure of the epiphyses and because the pubertal growth spurt occurs at an earlier time on the childhood growth curve. Without treatment, this results in the paradox of a tall child becoming a short adult. A recent study suggested that stopping therapy prior to the age of twelve resulted in the girls having a greater height than those whose therapy was continued beyond the age of 12 (Boulgourdjian *et al.*, 1995).

An additional important factor in the management of these girls and their families, is the value of careful and repeated discussion about puberty mechanisms and the results of investigations. Emphasis should be given to the fact that the puberty process is abnormal in timing only and that treatment is designed to control hormone elevations only until the age when pubertal development is more acceptable. Psychological help is clearly of great value to some girls and their families and perhaps should be offered to all. This would provide an alternative forum and more time to discuss issues not covered in the Endocrine clinic. This aspect can be usefully addressed via an experienced endocrine nurse specialist working both in the clinic and the community. Liaison and informed discussion with school staff must not be overlooked. This should improve integration with peers and is particularly important until drug treatment becomes effective.

The most effective drug treatments at present are the long-acting analogues of GnRH (Comite *et al.*, 1981). These are available in various formulations, although no preparation is licensed for use in children and long-term experience in children is limited. GnRH analogues are given continuously either by nasal snuff, slow release implants or injections, and cause down regulation of the pituitary GnRH receptors thus reducing the release of LH and FSH. This causes a return to the pre-pubertal levels of hormone production. In turn, this results in a gradual reduction in height velocity and slowing of skeletal maturation and pubertal development. Breast size (although not the size of the areola) and other secondary sex characteristics are therefore also reduced. Ovarian size will also be decreased. Uterine size may not be decreased but the endometrial thickness will be. If the endometrium was greater than 4 mm before treatment, it is possible that the girl will experience a withdrawal bleed on starting GnRH treatment and she should be warned of this possibility. There will also be a reduction in body odour and acne as well as less moody or temperamental behaviour. The latter, however, may be multifactorial and may not always show a striking improvement on treatment.

The restoration of pre-pubertal LH and FSH profiles on nocturnal sampling or after intravenous GnRH would be the ultimate aim of treatment. However, in clinical practice, reliance is usually on random FSH, LH and oestradiol levels in conjunction with the clinical parameters. It has also been suggested that serial measurements of ovarian volume by ultrasound imaging may be helpful in monitoring response to therapy (Ambrosino *et al.*, 1994).

GnRH analogues are available as either nasal snuff (Buserelin or the longer acting Naferelin), as implants (Goserelin) or as a long-acting subcutaneous injection (Leuprorelin). There is some suggestion that the long-acting implants or injections are more effective (Shaw, 1988) but in any case they are probably, in practical terms, more appropriate for use in young girls. The French Leuprorelin Trial Group concluded that a dose of 3.75 mg subcutaneously every 28 days is sufficient to suppress LH levels in most children with central precocious puberty (Carel *et al.*, 1995). Our own experience would suggest that the use of local anaesthesia prior to the use of Goserelin can be very helpful in ensuring acceptance of treatment.

GnRH analogues have no consistent adverse reactions and normal ovarian and menstrual function has been reported following therapy (Jay *et al.*, 1992) although the number of girls treated remains small. The possibility of osteoporosis has been reported in adults (Fogelman, 1992) but does not seem to be a problem in children (Neely *et al.*, 1995). Pituitary activity recovers in about six weeks following the cessation of therapy. Other treatments that have been used include cyproterone acetate (Stanhope *et al.*, 1985), danazol and Depo–Provera.

Treatment of Pseudosexual Precocity

Treatment obviously depends on diagnosis of the underlying cause. Granulosa cell ovarian tumours should be removed but as they have a risk of recurrence follow-up with serum oestradiol levels is recommended. It is, however, essential that normal follicular cysts found in girls with central precocious puberty are recognised for what they are and not removed. In these circumstances, follow-up with ultrasound to ensure that the cysts regress is all that is required.

GnRH analogues can be used in the suppression of puberty associated with a hypothalamic hamartoma but is not appropriate for other forms of gonadotrophin-independent sexual precocity such as McCune–Albright syndrome. For such conditions treatment is with cyproterone acetate (Foster *et al.*, 1984).

Cyproterone acetate is an anti-androgen which works by suppression of gonadotrophin release. It also is reported to have some progestational activity (Stanhope *et al.*, 1985). Its main side effect is weight gain. An alternative treatment for non-gonadotrophin-dependent precocious puberty is the aromatase inhibitor, testolactone (Feuillon *et al.*, 1993). Reported side effects of this therapy are transient abdominal pain, headache and diarrhoea. Treatment with thyroxine is all that is required for the management of precocious puberty associated with hypothyroidism.

Most girls with precocious puberty have no subsequent problems in adulthood, although a minority have problems which has caused some authors to suggest that all girls treated for precocious puberty should be followed up to adulthood (Rosenfeld, 1994). There is no adverse effect on academic achievement and IQ. It is suggested that girls with precocious puberty tend to be sexually active somewhat earlier than their peers (Ehrhardt and Meyer-Bahburg, 1994).

PREMATURE THELARCHE AND PREMATURE ADRENARCHE

Premature thelarche is the term used to describe isolated breast development with no other signs of puberty. In its early stages it can be difficult to differentiate from the early stages of precocious puberty (Pescovitz *et al.*, 1988). The hormone profile is frequently normal for pre-puberty; there is a pre-pubertal response to GnRH infusion, there is no accompanying growth spurt and bone age is normal. No treatment is necessary although these girls should be followed up to ensure that precocious puberty does not occur.

Premature adrenarche is defined as being the growth of pubic or axillary hair before the age of eight. It is associated with early adrenal androgen secretion which, on assay, is found to be in the early pubertal range. Other investigations are normal. Other than ensuring that the appearance of pubic hair is not the first sign of late onset CAH, no treatment is necessary.

HIRSUTISM

Hirsutism is a very embarrassing problem for any woman but particularly so for a teenager. The condition is characterised by an increase in growth or distribution in terminal hair over the body and face.

The distribution of body and facial hair is age- and race-dependent. Hirsutism increases with age and is more common in some ethnic groups, such as those from the Indian sub-continent, or those from Mediterranean countries, whereas Oriental patients have a very low incidence.

Hair growth is dependent on androgens and so hirsutism is usually associated with either hyperandrogen states or an excessive hair follicle response to circulating androgens. Circulating free testosterone is converted by 5-alpha-reductase found in the hair follicle to dihydrotestosterone, which then acts on the follicle to stimulate hair growth and sebum production. Once terminal hair growth is stimulated in this way, less androgen is needed to maintain the growth.

Hirsutism may have the following causes:

- Racial
- Ovarian disorders
- Adrenal disorders
- Drugs
- Hypothyroidism
- Stress
- Idiopathic

A study on a group of 15–19-year-old adolescent girls reported that the cause was CAH in 3.4%, late onset adrenal hyperplasia in 24.1% and polycystic ovarian syndrome in 72.4% (Baron and Baron, 1993). A larger study, but dealing with a slightly older group of women (age 13–38 years), diagnosed polycystic ovarian syndrome in 53%, obesity in 18%, late onset adrenal hyperplasia in 2%, an ovarian tumour in 0.8% and 0.4% due to drugs or Cushing's syndrome. 25% of this study group were deemed to be idiopathic (Morgan *et al.*, 1994).

Obvious drugs associated with hirsutism are the androgen derivatives, either in the form of therapeutic drugs such as danazol, or in the form of anabolic steroids. Other drugs reported as being responsible for abnormal hair growth include phenytoin, corticosteroids and diazoxide. Stress has been reported to increase secretion of LH causing an increased release of androgens from the ovary. The diagnosis of idiopathic hirsutism is one of exclusion made as a result of repeated hormone profiles showing normal levels of both free and total circulating androgens in a patient with confirmed hirsutism and a normal menstrual cycle.

Ovarian and Adrenal Causes of Hirsutism

The major ovarian cause, and the commonest single cause, of hirsutism in adolescents is polycystic ovarian syndrome (PCO) (Hull, 1987). It is a disorder characterised by hyperandrogenism and insulin resistance (McKenna, 1988). Clinically, those with polycystic ovarian disease present with a variety of symptoms which may include all, or some, of the symptoms of obesity, oligomenorrhoea, anovulation and hirsutism. Obesity may not be such a prominent symptom in adolescents with PCO compared to adults (Gulekli *et al.*, 1993). Ultrasound imaging of the ovary will show a slightly enlarged ovary with thickened stroma and a row of small cysts arranged circumferentially in the cortex. Hormone profile shows an elevated LH level with an LH:FSH ratio greater than three and low sex hormone binding globulin (SHBG) levels.

As a result of the chronic hyperstimulation by LH, the ovary responds by releasing increased levels of androstenedione and testosterone. The combination of slightly elevated levels of testosterone and low SHBG levels result in a higher level of free testosterone causing hair follicle stimulation and excess hair growth.

The second major cause of hirsutism in adolescents is late onset CAH which is responsible for between 1 and 6% of cases (Azziz and Zacur, 1989). It is particularly prevalent among Ashkenazy Jews. As in the salt-losing form of CAH, the condition is an autosomal recessive one with the abnormality having been localised on chromosome 6. Those with the disorder usually present around the time of puberty with increasing hirsutism and irregular periods, although some remain asymptomatic. Screening for non-salt-losing CAH can be performed by measuring the early morning salivary 17-hydroxyprogesterone levels (Zerah *et al.*, 1987).

Other adrenal causes of hirsutism include acanthosis nigricans, Cushing's syndrome and adrenal tumours.

Management

Clinical history and examination

The important points when taking a history from a patient with hirsutism are the duration and development of the symptoms; the relationship of the onset of symptoms to the menarche and pubertal development; drug history; menstrual history; the presence or absence of other signs of hyperandrogenism including acne and weight gain and the presence or absence of signs of virilism. When examining the patient, the most important thing is to confirm that she does indeed have hirsutism. Some adolescent girls are so sensitive about any hair growth that they cannot be convinced that what they have is normal.

It is imperative that the amount of hair growth is quantified so that progression of the disease or its response to therapy can be assessed. The most widely used is that devised by Ferriman and Gallwey (1981) which was based on the findings on examination of 430 women aged between 15 and 74 years. A pictorial summary of their findings is shown in Fig. 15.3. Signs of virilism (see below) should also be looked for – their presence indicating the need for urgent evaluation of the patient. It is also important to assess pubertal development and to identify other signs of androgen excess.

Investigations

Whilst the diagnosis of hirsutism is made on clinical grounds by examination of the patient, investigations are necessary to identify the cause of the condition. Investigation is obviously by assessment of the hormone profile. Ideally, the hormone profile should be assessed first thing in the morning to overcome the problem of circadian release of hormones. In practice, however, this is not always possible. Hormone levels assessed include FSH and LH to assess the ovarian stimulation, androgen levels including testosterone, free testosterone and the specific adrenal androgen, dehydroepiandrosterone sulphate (DHEAS); SHBG to assess the degree of binding of the sex hormones present and 17-hydroxyprogesterone. LH and FSH levels should be assayed on Day 2 of the cycle if the girl is menstruating. Markedly elevated levels of testosterone and DHEAS are suggestive of either an adrenal tumour or of a 46XY karyotype discussed below. Cortisol, prolactin and thyroxine levels should also be measured. Ultrasound examination of the ovaries may also be helpful. Further specific tests

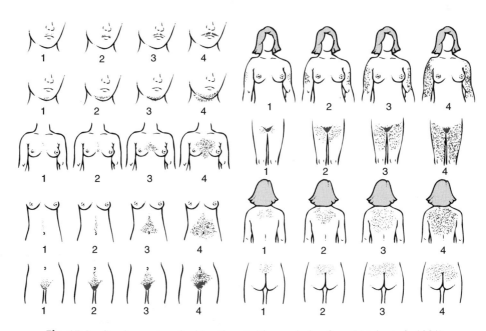

Fig. 15.3   Scoring system for hirsutism (with permission from Hatch *et al.*, 1981).

particularly of adrenal function will be required dependent on the results of these screening tests.

Treatment

Treatment of hirsutism should be started as soon as possible to maximise the chances of a successful response. Once the growth of terminal hair has been stimulated by androgens it can be difficult to stop. Treatment will obviously be dependent on cause. Late onset CAH is treated with either dexamethasone or prednisolone. Tumours obviously require treatment with surgery.

The main treatment of hirsutism secondary to PCO is with the anti-androgen, cyproterone acetate (Belisle and Love, 1986). Cyproterone acetate has to be given in conjunction with oestrogen, firstly to ensure regular menstruation, but also to prevent pregnancy as the anti-androgenic action of cyproterone acetate will interfere with the sexual differentiation of a male fetus. An additional benefit of the oestrogen therapy is that it causes an increase in SHBG levels, thus lowering the levels of free testosterone.

Treatment is given according to the reversed sequential regime of Hammerstein (1980) in which cyproterone acetate 100 mg is given from Day 5–14 of the cycle, along with ethinyl oestradiol 30–50 µg from Day 5–24. In practice this has now been adapted in most units to cyproterone acetate 50–100 mg daily from Day 5–14 along with ethinyl oestradiol 30 µg from Day 5–25 (Fraser *et al.*, 1983). The oestradiol is usually given in the form of a combined oral contraceptive pill, usually Dianette (ethinyl oestradiol 35 µg and cyproterone acetate 2 mg). The combination of cyproterone acetate and trans-dermal 17-beta-oestradiol has also been reported to produce good clinical results (Jasonni *et al.*, 1991). This dose of oestrogen is not contraceptive, however, so an alternative form of contraception will be required if the girl is sexually active.

Unfortunately, because of the low levels of androgens required to maintain the growth of terminal hair, response to treatment is slow. No changes in hair growth can be expected for a minimum of six months and improvement may not be clearly apparent for 24–36 months. Once remission has been achieved, a lower dose of cyproterone acetate, such as that in Dianette, may be sufficient to maintain it. Some workers have reported a satisfactory response to Dianette alone (Golland and Elstein, 1993). Side effects of cyproterone acetate are weight gain and tiredness. In addition, hepatotoxicity has been reported, although at higher doses than recommended above. Nevertheless, those starting on cyproterone acetate therapy should have liver function tests checked before starting therapy and at six month to one year intervals thereafter.

Spironolactone has also been used in the treatment of hirsutism. It has never been licensed for this indication in the United Kingdom, although widely used. Animal studies suggesting the possibility of carcinogenicity with high dose, long-term treatment has led to its use being discontinued for this indication. GnRH has also been successfully used in combination with the combined oral contraceptive pill (Falsetti and Pasinetti, 1994).

Along with medical management of hirsutism, there is obviously a need for cosmetic management, both while waiting for therapy to take effect and also as cyproterone acetate is not effective in all cases. The most helpful and frequently used technique is shaving, with plucking, waxing and depilatory creams also being used (Richards and Meharg, 1990). Electrolysis, although expensive, is also widely used.

VIRILISM

Virilism is much less common than hirsutism and is defined as the presence of clitoral hypertrophy (Fig. 15.4), hair recession or male pattern baldness, breast atrophy and deepening of the voice. Hirsutism is also usually present. Virilism is the result of excessive androgen production and is associated with more serious pathology. The causes of virilism are:

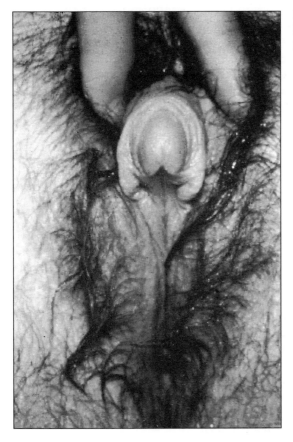

Fig. 15.4   Clitoral hypertrophy appearing in puberty in a teenage girl with partial androgen insensitivity.

- Androgen-producing ovarian tumour
- Adrenal tumour
- Some forms of XY female
- Congenital adrenal hyperplasia
- Cushing's syndrome
- Iatrogenic causes

The most common causes in adolescents are the appearance of virilisation in a 46XY girl at puberty or CAH. The most serious is obviously an adrenal or androgen-producing ovarian tumour.

The most common androgen-producing ovarian tumour is an arrhenoblastoma which is composed of Sertoli and Leydig cells or their precursors. The tumour may not be of sufficient size to be palpable on clinical examination and ultrasound examination of the pelvis should be performed. Cushing's syndrome is associated with virilism along with the other features of obesity, striae and moon face. It may be due to overactivity of the adrenal gland or due to an adrenal tumour – either benign or malignant. In addition to elevated androgen levels, elevated levels of ACTH will be found. If the elevation is due to overactivity of the adrenal gland, they will be suppressed by dexamethasone. The response of an adrenal tumour to dexamethasone varies. Most of them are suppressed but the highly malignant ones may not be.

The major cause of virilism in women with a 46XY karyotype is partial androgen insensitivity. The complete form of the disorder is associated with normal female phenotype and primary amenorrhoea and is considered on p. 142. The variability of expression of the partial form, however, results in a spectrum of abnormalities from mild clitoral hypertrophy to almost normal male phenotype. Most girls with partial androgen insensitivity will be diagnosed at birth with ambiguous genitalia (see above), but a minority will present at puberty when the testes begin to produce androgens. The diagnosis will be suggested by the karyotype.

Management

In addition to careful clinical examination to assess the degree of virilisation, examination of the genitalia should be carried out to assess if there has been virilisation *in utero* which will be identified by the presence of labio-scrotal fusion. This suggests androgen production *in utero* and therefore further suggests such diagnoses as partial androgen insensitivity.

Hormone profile should be performed including testosterone, androstenedione, DHA, cortisol (preferably measured in the morning and the evening to assess the extremes of the circadian rhythm), ACTH and 17-hydroxyprogesterone. A raised cortisol, particularly with the loss of the diurnal rhythm, requires a dexamethasone suppression test to be performed as mentioned above. Ultrasound of the ovaries and adrenal imaging should be performed as indicated by the hormonal investigations.

Treatment is again dependent on cause with surgery to remove tumours and the use of steroids to suppress androgen production in CAH.

GENERAL ENDOCRINE PROBLEMS

In addition to the specific endocrinological problems mentioned above, other general endocrine conditions can affect a girl's gynaecological health, particularly at puberty. Thyroid disorders are well recognised as causing problems with menstruation (Goldsmith *et al.*, 1952). Hyperthyroidism, in addition, has been reported as causing delayed menarche (Saxena *et al.*, 1964).

Diabetes mellitus is also associated with delayed puberty and menarche (Bergquist, 1954), seen in its extreme form in Mauriac syndrome – a syndrome related to over-insulinisation and characterised by hepatomegaly, truncal obesity, growth failure and delayed puberty. Delay in psychosexual development has also been reported in girls with insulin-dependent diabetes, with the delay being greater in girls who developed diabetes at an earlier age (Surridge *et al.*, 1984). In addition, diabetics often show changes in their insulin requirements around the time of menstruation (Pederson, 1982) and the onset of 'brittleness' in diabetic girls is often associated with puberty.

REFERENCES

Ambrosino MM, Hernanz-Schulman M, Genieser NB, Sklar CA, Fefferman NR, David R, 1994: Monitoring of girls undergoing medical therapy for precocious puberty. *Journal of Ultrasound Medicine* **13**, 501–508.

Azziz R, Zacur HA, 1989: 21-Hydroxylase deficiency in female hyperandrogenism: screening and diagnosis. *Journal of Clinical Endocrinology and Metabolism* **46**, 1011–1014.

Baron JJ, Baron J, 1993: Differential diagnosis of hirsutism in girls betwen 15–19 years old. *Ginekologica Polska* **64**, 267–269.

Belisle S, Love EJ, 1986: Clinical efficacy and safety of cyproterone acetate in severe hirsutism: results of a multicentred Canadian study. *Fertility and Sterility* **46**, 1015–1020.

Bergquist N, 1954: The gonadal function in female diabetics. *Acta Endocrinology Supplement (Copenhagen)* **19**, 3–20.

Berkowitz GB, Lee PA, Brown TR, Migeon CJ, 1984: Etiologic evaluation of male pseudhermaphrodism in infancy and childhood. *American Journal of Disease in Childhood* **138**, 755–759.

Boulgourdjian E, Escobar ME, Martinez A, Heinrich JJ, Bergada C, 1995: Bone age at discontinuation of medroxyprogesterone acetate therapy in girls with precocious puberty: effect on final height. *Hormonal Research* **44**, 12–16.

Carel JC, Lahlou N, Guazzarotti L, Joubert-Collin M, Roger M, Colle M, Chaussain JL, 1995: Treatment of central precocious puberty with depot leuprorelin. French Leuprorelin Trial Group. *European Journal of Endocrinology* **132**, 699–704.

Comite F, Cutler GB, Rivier J, Vale WW, Loriaux DL, Crowley WF, 1981: Short-term treatment of idiopathic precocious puberty with a long acting analogue of luteinizing hormone-releasing hormone. *New England Journal of Medicine* **305**, 1546–1550.

Ehrhardt AA, Meyer-Bahlburg HF, 1994: Psychosocial aspects of precocious puberty. *Hormonal Research* **41** (Suppl 2.), 30–35.

Falsetti L, Pasinetti E, 1994: Treatment of moderate and severe hirsutism by gonadotropin-releasing hormone agonists in women with polycystic ovary syndrome and idiopathic hirsutism. *Fertility and Sterility* **61**, 817–822.

Ferriman D, Gallwey JD, 1981: Clinical assessment of body hair growth in women. *Journal of Clinical Endocrinology and Metabolism* **140**, 1440–1447.

Feuillan PP, Jones J, Cutler GB, 1993: Long-term testolactone therapy for precocious puberty in girls with the McCune-Albright syndrome. *Journal of Clinical Endocrinology and Metabolism* **77**, 647–651.

Fogelman I, 1992: Gonadotropin-releasing hormone agonists and the skeleton. *Fertility and Sterility* **57**, 715–724.

Forest MG, Betuel H, David M, 1989: Prenatal treatment in congenital adrenal hyperplasia due to 21-hydroxylase deficiency: update 88 of the French Multicentric study. *Endocrine Research* **15**, 277–301.

Foster CM, Comite F, Pescovitz OH, Ross JL, Loriaux DL, Cutler GB, 1984: Variable response to a long acting agonist of LHRH in girls with McCune-Albright syndrome. *Journal of Clinical Endocrinology and Metabolism* **59**, 801–805.

Fraser IS, Shearman RP, Allen JK, McCarron G, 1983: Cyproterone acetate and the treatment of hirsutism. *Australian and New Zealand Journal of Obstetrics and Gynaecology* **23**, 93–98.

Gambino J, Caldwell B, Dietrich R, Walot I, Kangarloo H, 1992: Congenital disorders of sexual differentiation: MR findings. *American Journal of Roentgenology* **158**, 363–367.

Goldsmith RE, Sturgis SH, Lernan J *et al.*, 1952: The menstrual pattern in thyroid disease. *Journal of Clinical Endocrinology and Metabolism* **12**, 846–855.

Golland IM, Elstein ME, 1993: Results of an open one-year study with Diane-35 in women with polycystic ovarian syndrome. *Annals of the New York Academy of Science* **687**, 263–271.

Goodall J, 1991: Helping a child understand her own testicular feminisation. *Lancet* **337**, 33–35.

Gulekli B, Turhan NO, Senoz S, Kukner S, Oral H, Gokmen O, 1993: Endocrinological, ultrasonographic and clinical findings in adolescent and adult polycystic ovary patients: a comparative study. *Gynecology and Endocrinology* **7**, 273–277.

Hammerstein J, 1980: Possibilities and limits of endocrine therapy. In Hammerstein J, Lachnit-Fixson U, Neumann F, Plewig G (eds), *Androgenization in women*. Amsterdam: Excerpta Medica, 221–234.

Hatch R, Rosenfield RL, Kim MH, Tredway D, 1981: Hirsutism: implications, etiology and management. *American Journal of Obstetrics and Gynecology* **140**, 815–830.

Hull MGR, 1987: Epidemiology of infertility and polycystic ovarian disease: endocrinological and demographic studies. *Gynecology and Endocrinology* **1**, 235–245.

Hutson JM, Voigt RW, Kelly JM, *et al.*, 1991: Girth reduction clitoroplasty: a new technique with 15 years experience in 38 patients. *Pediatric Surgery International* **6**, 336–340.

Jasonni VM, Bulletti C, Naldi S, Di-Cosmo E, Cappucini F, Flamigni C, 1991: Treatment of hirsutism by an association of oral cyproterone acetate and transdermal 17 beta-estradiol. *Fertility and Sterility* **55**, 742–745.

Jay N, Mansfield MJ, Blizzard RM, Crowley WF, Schonfield D, Rhubin L, Boepple PA, (1992): Ovulation and menstrual function of adolescent girls with central precocious puberty after therapy with gonadotrophin releasing hormone agonists. *Journal of Clinical Endocrinology and Metabolism* **75**, 890–894.

Juniper MP, Wolf A, Hoffman G, Ma YJ, Ojeda SR, 1992: Effect of hypothalamic lesions that induce precocious puberty on the morphological and functional maturation of the luteinising hormone releasing hormone neuronal system. *Endocrinology* **131**, 787–798.

Kaplan SA, Grumbach MM, 1990: Clinical review 14. Pathophysiology and treatment of sexual precocity. *Journal of Clinical Endocrinology and Metabolism* **71**, 785–789.

Kornreich L, Horev G, Blaser S, Daneman D, Kauli R, Grunebaum M, 1995: Central precocious puberty: evaluation by neuroimaging. *Pediatric Radiology* **25**, 7–11.

Kutteh WH, Santos-Ramos R, Ermel LD, 1995: Accuracy of ultrasonic detection of the uterus in normal newborn infants: implications for infants with ambiguous genitalia. *Ultrasound Obstetics and Gynecology* **5**, 109–113.

Mauras N, Blizzard RM, 1986: The McCune-Albright syndrome. *Acta Endocrinologica Scandinavica* (Suppl.) **279**, 207–217.

McKenna TJ, 1988: Pathogenesis and treatment of polycystic ovarian syndrome. *New England Journal of Medicine* **318**, 558–562.

Meyers-Seifer CH, Charest NJ, 1992: Diagnosis and management of patient with ambiguous genitalia. *Seminars in Perinatology* **16**, 332–339.

Miller WL, 1991: Congenital adrenal hyperplasias. *Endocrinology and Metabolism Clinics of North America* **20**, 721–749.

Moran C, Tapia MC, Hernandez E, Vazquez G, Garcia-Hernandez E, Bermudez JA, 1994: Etiological review of hirsutism in 250 patients. *Archives of Medical Research* **25**, 311–314.

Mulaikal RM, Migeon CJ, Rock JA, 1987: Fertility rates in female patients with congenital adrenal hyperplasia due to 21-hydroxylase deficiency. *New England Journal of Medicine* **316**, 178–182.

Munden M, McEniff N, Mulvihill D, 1995: Sonographic investigation of female infants with inguinal masses. *Clinical Radiology* **50**, 696–698.

Neely EK, Bachrach LK, Hintz RL, Habiby RL, Slemenda CW, Feezle L, Pescovitz OH, 1995: Bone mineral density during the treatment of central precocious puberty. *Journal of Pediatrics* **127**, 819–822.

Newman K, Randolph J, Parson S, 1992: Functional results in young women having clitoral reconstruction as infants. *Pediatric Journal of Surgery* **27**, 180–183.

Pedersen LM, 1982: Clinical and hormonal characteristics in women with anovulation and insulin treated diabetes mellitus. *American Journal of Obstetrics and Gynecology* **143**, 876–882.

Personal view, 1994: Once a dark secret. *British Medical Journal* **308**, 542.

Pescovitz OH, Hence KD, Barnes KM, Loriaux DL, Cutler GB, 1988: Premature thelarche and central precocious puberty: the relationship between clinical presentation and the gonadotropin response to luteinizing hormone-releasing hormone. *Journal of Clinical Endocrinology and Metabolism* **67**, 474–479.

Reith KG, Comite F, Dwyer AJ, Nelson MJ, Pescovitz O, Shawker TH, Cutler GB, Loriaux DL, 1987: CT of cerebral abnormalities in precocious puberty. *American Journal of Roentgenology* **148**, 1231–1238.

Richards RN, Meharg G, 1990: Temporary hair removal in patients with hirsutism: a clinical study. *Cutis* **45**, 199–202.

Robben SG, Oostdijk W, Drop SL, Tanghe HL, Vielvoye GJ, Meradji M, 1995: Idiopathic isosexual central precocious puberty: magnetic resonance findings in 30 patients. *British Journal of Radiology* **68**, 34–38.

Rosenfeld RL, 1994: Normal and almost normal precocious variations in pubertal development, premature pubarche and premature thelarche revisited. *Hormonal Research* **41**, (Suppl 2.), 7–13.

Rowe MI, Lloyd DA, 1986: Inguinal hernia. In Welch KJ, Randolph JG, Ravitch MM, O'Neill JA, Rowe MJ (eds), *Pediatric Surgery*, 4th edn. Chicago, IL: Year Book Publishers, 779–793.

Saxena KM, Crawford JD, Talbot NB, 1964: Childhood thyrotoxicosis: a long term perspective. *British Medical Journal* **2**, 1153–1158.

Secaf E, Hricak H, Gooding CA, Ho VW, Gorczyca DP, Ringertz H, Conte FA, Kogan BA, Grumbach MM, 1994: Role of MRI in the evaluation of ambiguous genitalia. *Pediatric Radiology* **24**, 231–235.

Shaw RW, 1988: LHRH analogues in the treatment of endometriosis – comparative results with other treatments. *Clinical Obstetrics and Gynaecology* **2**, 659–675.

Simpson IL, 1987: Genetic control of sexual development. In Ratnam SS, Teoh E,

Anandakumar C (eds.), *Advances in fertility and sterility: releasing hormones and genetics and immunology in human reproduction, vol 3.* Proceedings of the 12th World Congress on Fertility and Sterility (Singapore 1986). Lancaster: Parthenon Press, 165–173.

Sockalosky JJ, Kriel RL, Krach LE, Sheehan M, 1987: Precocious puberty after traumatic brain injury. *Journal of Pediatrics* **110**, 373–377.

Stanhope R, Pringle J, Adams J, Jeffcoate SC, Brook CGD, 1985: Spontaneous gonadotrophin pulsatility in girls with central precocious puberty treated with cyproterone acetate. *Clinical Endocrinology* **23**, 547–553.

Surridge DHC, Erdahl DL, Lawson JS, Donald MW, Monga TN, Bird CE, Letemendia FJ, 1984: Psychiatric aspects of diabetes mellitus. *British Journal of Psychiatry* **145**, 169–176.

Zerah M, Pang S, New MI, 1987: Morning salivary 17-hydroxyprogesterone is a useful screening test for nonclassical 21-hydroxylase deficiency. *Journal of Clinical Endocrinology and Metabolism* **65**, 227–232.

PART V

SEX AND CONTRACEPTION

CHAPTER 16

Towards better sex education

ANNETTE LYONS ─────────────────────────────────

INTRODUCTION

Every aspect of health education is emotive but none gives rise to so much interest, controversy or personal opinion as the sensitive issue of sex education in schools. Ultimately in the United Kingdom school governing bodies have a legal responsibility to make, and keep up-to-date, a written statement of their policy on sex education which meets the needs of young people, satisfies parents and makes sense in the context of the wider society in which we live. Meeting the legal requirements and producing a written statement is the easy part; implementing and delivering effective sex education is a complex process.

Health education is not a core or foundation subject within the National Curriculum and as the Adviser for Health Education in the City of Liverpool I have felt at times, rather like a travelling sales representative 'selling' health education to schools with an already overcrowded curriculum. Elements of health education are identifiable within the National Curriculum programmes of study which means that, in practice, health education will be addressed to some extent by all schools. Unfortunately, much of this is factual knowledge, an important base but only one dimension of the learning process.

When formulating the Authority's strategy, I found it useful to map out all the dimensions involved in promoting 'better sex education' (Fig. 16.1). This diagram is simplistic; in reality each strand is inter-connected.

BACKGROUND

How do we encourage young people to take their health seriously when their own experience of being ill is coping with routine infections of everyday life? They are protected by means of vaccination from the more serious diseases, with the exception of the HIV virus, and have little direct experience of heart disease, cancer and strokes, still the major causes of ill-health in adult society. How do we encourage them to realise that these causes of ill-health are preventable and

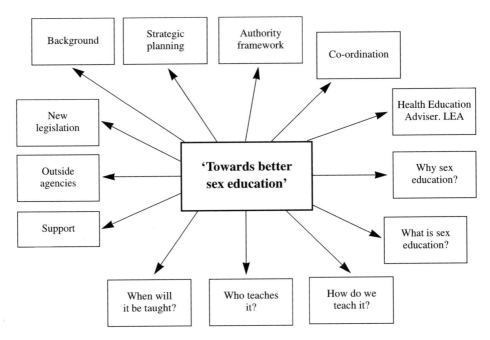

Fig. 16.1   Towards better sex education.

closely related to patterns of behaviour established very early on in life? This is the challenge of health education today; the task is not easy.

Health education is:

- not about shock horror stories,
- not about telling young people what they should or should not do,
- not about expensive media campaigns where health education is portrayed as a way of solving a series of crises affecting society, using messages such as icebergs, syringes, mortuaries etc; not always understood and often quickly forgotten.

Health education is about:

- Providing relevant information that does not assume ignorance, but builds on existing knowledge and experience and is relevant to young peoples' stage of development.
- Developing skills that will enable them to take control over their own lives.
- Promoting positive attitudes and values about health and the quality of life so that young people will make the right choices and develop healthy lifestyles.
- Above all, it is about promoting self-esteem so that young people have a sense of their own worth.

If a health education programme is to help young people make informed choices, establish a healthy lifestyle, build up a system of values, develop self-esteem and self-confidence, a balanced range of teaching methods is required. The active participation of young people in dealing with health issues is essential.

THE ROLE OF OUTSIDE AGENCIES IN THE PROCESS

In the United Kingdom, the Department for Education in 'Circular 5/94, Education Act 1993: Sex Education in Schools' (1994) states in paragraph 32,

> Teachers should take account of the range of expertise and other resources available to them, including the contribution which health authorities, other health service bodies, and health professionals – particularly doctors (including GPs) and school nurses – may be able to make.

I am presuming that in the main, readers of this publication will have a background in the medical profession and, therefore, are quite likely to become involved or be invited to become involved in sexual health work in schools. Consideration of your most appropriate and beneficial contribution to the process would therefore be an advantage.

Doreen Massey in '*School Sex Education – Why, What and How*' (1991) outlines eight features of what she describes as 'purposeful sex education', in any area of the curriculum:

1. It is developmental and appropriate to the age and stage of the pupil.
2. It puts forward factual knowledge and encourages exploration of the facts.
3. It needs to be taught several times in a number of different ways.
4. It examines opinions and concepts and encourages deliberation and discussion of a range of those options and concepts.
5. It encourages the development of personal and interpersonal skills.
6. It encourages awareness and respect of self and others.
7. It requires, as a prerequisite, some negotiation with pupils to establish what their starting point is, rather than assuming common levels and experiences.
8. It encourages reflection and responsibility.

STRATEGIC PLANNING

An overview of the process is shown in Fig. 16.2. These features can be achieved only if there is a co-ordinated approach at a strategic (Authority) and operational (school) level.

At an operational level the precise role of outside agencies (i.e. those with no specific and agreed remit to work in schools), needs to be clearly defined by governors, headteachers and the staff of a school following consultation with

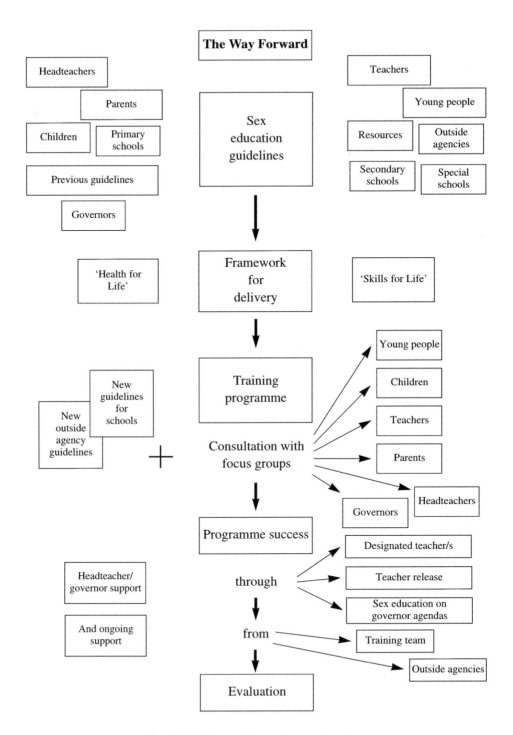

Fig 16.2   The way forward in sex education.

parents, pupils and the agencies themselves, and complemented with a planned programme to meet their needs. To achieve this, consideration of sex education needs to be given in the context of a whole school approach through the concept of the health promoting school.

There are three strands:

1. The taught health education curriculum.
2. School ethos.
3. Involvement of family and the wider community.

The taught health education curriculum requires the following:

- A flexible framework.
- To start with children's and young people's own perceptions of health.
- Show progression through a spiral curriculum.
- Use a variety of teaching and learning methods.
- To deliver as a subject, project, topic, cross-curricular activity etc.
- Co-ordination.

The school ethos requires consideration of:

- Policies which support the health education curriculum.
- The fostering and promotion of good relationships.
- The promotion of a clean, safe, stimulating environment.
- Shared values and beliefs promoting self-confidence and self-esteem.

The family and community requires consideration of:

- Family consultation and involvement.
- Community co-ordination.
- Community based work/projects.
- Drawing on the skills of the community.

I would like to consider some of the above issues a little further, none can be addressed in isolation; they are all inter-linked. I will begin by addressing the concept of starting with children's and young people's own perceptions of health. Although age appropriateness of any input is important, children and young people in schools should not be treated as a homogeneous group. There are differences of race, gender, socioeconomic status, sexual orientation, sexual experience, religion, levels of knowledge and understanding and home environment.

This has implications for all those involved in the delivery of sex education in schools as no two schools are alike. An understanding of the culture, the dynamics operating within the school together with a clear knowledge of the different needs of individual pupils is essential. Some effective methods of ensuring that such diversity is reflected in the sex education programme delivered. This requires:

- Involvement of a wide cross-section of pupils in the planning, delivery and evaluation of the programme.

- Involvement of parents in the planning and evaluation process.
- Planned and negotiated use of outside agencies, preferably to support teachers and governors.

It was decided to use focus groups of primary-aged children, secondary-aged young people, parents/governors and teachers/headteachers to inform the training programme at a strategic level.

A different format of working was required for each group, the parents/governors groups and the teacher/headteacher groups used a mixture of response sheets and large group discussion. The main focus was to find out about teachers' training needs regarding sex education policy and programme development and, to identify their planning procedure with particular reference to the involvement of young people and parents in this area. The focus for the parents/governors group was very much on policy development and planning sex education programmes.

The focus groups of young people took a different format not only from the above groups but between the age groups.

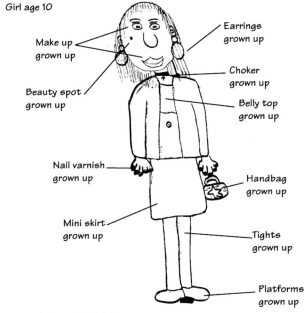

Girl age 10

Make up grown up

Beauty spot grown up

Earrings grown up

Choker grown up

Belly top grown up

Nail varnish grown up

Handbag grown up

Mini skirt grown up

Tights grown up

Platforms grown up

WHAT SHE IS FEELING
1. Do I look okay or am I overdressed?
2. What happens if my friends laugh at me?
3. Is my hair okay?
4. Is my makeup all smudged over my face?
5. Have I got a ladder in my tights?
6. Oh no has my skirt got caught up in my knickers?
7. What happens if I fall when I'm at the door?

Fig. 16.3(a)   Drawing by girl (aged 10).

The secondary-aged young people were asked the following questions which they were to discuss in groups:

What sex education have you had?
How was it done?
How do you feel about the sex education you have had so far?
What sort of sex education would you like (topics etc) and who do you wish to deliver them and how?

The primary-aged pupils were involved in a draw and write exercise, a method of finding out children's perceptions of health issues developed by the Primary School Project research team in Southampton. The following instructions were given:

On your paper I would like you to draw a girl or a boy of about your age getting ready to go out for the evening to a party, the youth club, a friend's house etc. The picture should show that the person is growing up. Write how the young person is feeling about growing up and draw anything they have with them which shows they are growing up. (Fig. 16.3a and b)

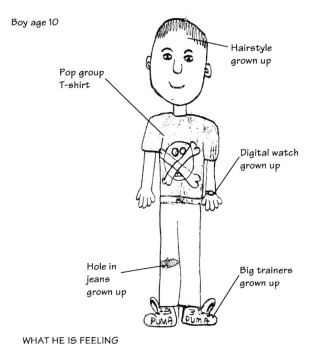

WHAT HE IS FEELING
1. Do I look cool?
2. Is my hairstyle okay or is it out of fashion now?
3. Have I got the right pop group T-shirt on?
4. Does the hole in my jeans make me look cool enough?

Fig. 16.3(b) Drawing by boy (aged 10).

Having completed that exercise the following instructions were given:

> Now, I would like you to show your person getting out of the bath or shower. How does this picture show they are growing up? How does the person in the picture you've drawn feel about their body changing and growing? (Fig. 16.4a and b)

No names were required on the drawings, the children were asked to indicate if they were a boy or girl and their age. In groups they were asked to discuss and record their responses to the following questions:

> Who do you want to talk to you about the physical changes happening to you? Have you any concerns or worries?

Although small scale, the data collected from the focus groups were extremely valuable. The following issues were highlighted:

- A need for teachers to receive support in writing and developing sex education policies and programmes, particularly with suggested curriculum for primary-aged pupils.

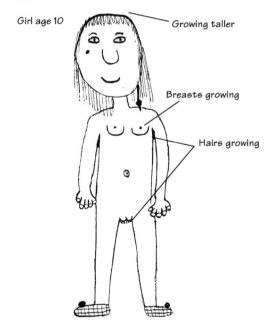

WHAT SHE IS FEELING
1. Nobody else has big breasts I wish I didn't have them
2. I wonder if I'm the only one with hair growing in strange places?
3. Nobody else wears a bra. I feel quite out of place.
4. Am I the only one with things happening to me?

Fig. 16.4(a)   Drawing by girl (aged 10).

- A need for improved communication between teachers, governors, parents, young people and other workers.
- A need and an expressed request by young people to be involved in the planning and needs assessment process.
- Acknowledgement that teachers are severely strained by their current workload, and must have support in order to deliver effectively and confidently.
- There is a need for teachers to receive clear guidance from headteachers and governors.
- There should be appropriate single sex work, an issue highlighted in every focus group. This has implications regarding the responsibility for delivery and methodology, and for ensuring that male teachers are involved. This can prove a major problem in many primary schools where sometimes the only male is the headteacher!
- Secondary-aged young people wanted to have the opportunity for one-to-one discussions with teachers and/or support workers such as school nurses. The young people involved did not feel that their confidentiality would be maintained. Schools should have clear guidance regarding confidentiality to ensure that young people's rights are respected and implemented, and which are available to all in the school.

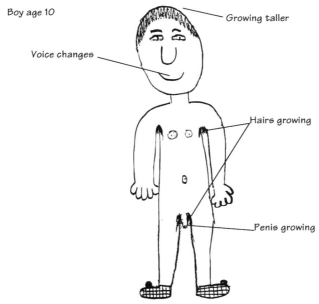

WHAT HE IS FEELING
1. I wonder if I'm the only one with hair growing in funny places?
2. I know we all grow taller but are everbody else's other bits growing?
3. My friend's voice is still the same but mine has changed. Do you think there's something wrong with me?

Fig. 16.4(b) Drawing by boy (aged 10).

- Primary-aged children felt very strongly that they wanted sex education to be delivered by their class teachers.
- Schools should respect young people's rights to receive factual information and be provided with the opportunity to explore a variety of different opinions as opposed to dogma.
- Finally, there is a strong need for training in the area of sexual health with ongoing support both inside and outside the classroom.

Any primary prevention health education initiative, be it at a national or local level, such as 'Towards better sex education' quite naturally places schools working with outside agencies at the focal point (Fig. 16.5). For prevention work to be effective it should be introduced at as early an age as possible; schools are, therefore, the perfect places on which to focus with their 'captured' audiences of children and young people.

Working in an inter-sectoral way is extremely beneficial for generating ideas, providing support, pooling resources, sharing out tasks, tackling health problems etc; but it is not without its problems. Each agency or organisation involved in health has its own targets, timescales, deadlines, agendas, pressures, expertise, method of working, priorities and personalities.

Many of the problems that do arise, stem from divergent professional perceptions of what constitutes good health education. I have, on occasions, been accused of being 'over-possessive' with regard to health education work in schools when I have opposed or challenged a proposed new initiative or practice. My response is always based on my professional expertise and commitment to working to a set of principles and established practice through which the Authority delivers health education. This is not always understood by others. A recent example was the publication by the Department of Health of the document 'The Health of the Nation'. My enthusiasm for this was quickly stifled as I found myself inundated with telephone calls and written correspondence from health professionals with posts of responsibility for what I describe as 'topics' such as cancer, coronary heart disease, drugs, HIV/AIDS etc, wishing to rush into schools to raise awareness and deal with the problem. For the past eight years I have moved schools on from 'topics' to a 'promoting healthy lifestyles approach'. I am totally opposed to addressing hundreds of young people in the hall for 45 minutes with what I call 'the let's tick it off we've covered it syndrome', educationally unsound and a complete waste of time.

Joking apart, schools need a comprehensive and established way of working through which all health concerns and issues can be successfully addressed, adopted and visibly supported by all agencies and support workers in the city. Crucial to improving the health of the future generation of Liverpool is honest, open and continued communication between all sectors regardless of how painful it becomes at times.

My role naturally involves supporting schools with curriculum development and providing in-service training with teachers, governors, parents and the wider

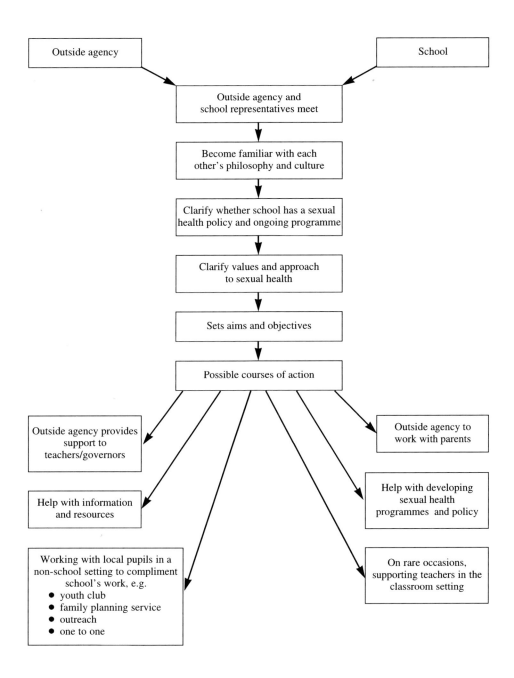

Fig. 16.5 Suggested process for outside agency and school staff to negotiate outside agency involvement in the sexual health programme (from Butler and Thompson, 1994).

community. Certainly with regard to sex education, I find myself answering a number of re-occurring questions such as:

>   Why teach sex education?
>   What is sex education?
>   How do we do it?
>   When should we do it?

and more recently,

>   What impact will the new legislation have?

WHY TEACH SEX EDUCATION?

There are many responses to this question, among others:

- The 1986 Education Act places responsibility for sex education with governors who have a legal obligation to 'make and keep up to date' a written statement of their policy. This should be drawn up following wide consultation with the headteacher, teachers, parents and representatives from the local school community. The Act also refers to sex education being ... 'given in such a manner as to encourage pupils to have due regard to moral considerations and family life.'
- The DFE Circular No. 5/94 (1994), 'Education Act 1993: Sex Education in Schools' explains the new legislation and also contains advice from the former Secretary of State for Education, on how he thinks aspects of the teaching of sex education should be dealt with.
- The provision of sex education at both primary and secondary school level is supported by all documentation from the DES, HMI and the NCC now the School Curriculum and Assessment Authority.
- HMI in 'Curriculum Matters 6' (1986) states, 'The importance of sexual relationships in our lives is such that sex education is a crucial part of preparing children for their lives now and in the future as adults and parents'.
- NCC Curriculum Guidance 5 (1990), outlines a spiral curriculum for sex education with learning to be achieved by ages 7, 11, 14 and 16, the four key stages of the National Curriculum.
- Research carried out by the Guttmacher Institute (1989) between 1982 and 1986 clearly indicated that the lowest teenage pregnancy rates were found in countries where, along with other factors, there were effective programmes of sex education.
- Research by Isobel Allen in 1987, indicated that 96% of parents questioned much preferred that sex education for their children took place in schools (Allen, 1987). Research with primary pupils in Liverpool in 1993, revealed that 100% of pupils questioned preferred to speak to their teachers in school about sexual health.
- Section 1 of the 1988 Education Reform Act (1990) places a statutory

responsibility upon schools to provide a broad and balanced curriculum which, 'promotes the spiritual, moral, cultural, mental and physical development of pupils at the school and of society; and prepares pupils for the opportunities, responsibilities and experiences of adult life.'

- National Curriculum Science includes the anatomy and physiology of reproduction, genetics etc. Much of this is factual knowledge, important but only one dimension of the learning process.
- Growing concern over the increased spread of HIV/AIDS, child sexual abuse and the increased number of teenage pregnancies and abortions make high quality sex education a necessity. The DFEE Circular No. 10/95 (1995) suggests that helping children protect themselves from abuse should be in the curriculum.
- In October 1991 the Children Act 1989 (1991) came into force emphasising the rights of children.
- The Department of Health publication, 'The Health of the Nation', recognises that sex education is vital in promoting sexual well-being and in reducing the rates of unwanted pregnancies.
- An international review of 19 studies on the effects of sex education in schools revealed that there was no increase in sexual activity in the young people exposed to sex education. In six studies, sex education led to either a delay in the onset of sexual activity or to a decrease in overall sexual activity. Two studies showed that access to counselling and contraceptive services did not encourage earlier or increased sexual activity (Baldo *et al.*, 1993). These findings are consistent with those of the 'Sexual Attitudes and Lifestyles' survey which revealed that those reporting formal school teaching as their main source of information on sex had the lowest rate of sexual activity before the age of 16 (Johnson *et al.*, 1994).
- The Sex Education Forum (1992) recommends that sex education should:

    (a) be an integral part of the learning process, beginning in childhood and continuing into adult life
    (b) for all children, young people and adults, including those with physical, learning or emotional difficulties
    (c) encourage exploration of values and moral issues, consideration of sexuality and personal relationships and the development of communication and decision-making skills
    (d) foster self-esteem, self-awareness, a sense of moral responsibility and the skills to avoid and resist unwanted sexual experience.

- In 1987, the Bishops' Conference document 'Laying the Foundations for Personal Relationships', outlined the requirement for all Catholic schools to have a developmental programme for education in personal relationships.
- Section 5 in the OFSTED handbook for schools states that schools are required to provide evidence of governors policy for sex education and details of cross curricular provision.

When addressing or training groups of parents, governors and teachers, I include in the 'why?' section a little time for personal reflection. I ask participants to take a few minutes to think back to the sex education they received in school from 4–18 years and focus on the three following questions:

What was it like for you?
Was it adequate?
Did it prepare you for adult life?

Following small group discussions, I open up the debate for a full group discussion. This usually reveals that no sex education was received in primary schools and the sex education experienced in secondary schools, 99 times out of 100, was of the nature of 'biological plumbing'.

In one training session with teachers from primary schools, one participant explained that she had received her secondary education at a Catholic grammar school. She went on to say that she would like to share her experience of a sex education session which had greatly troubled her.

It was a religious education lesson delivered by a Sister from the convent who was informing them of how to behave if they were at a party where 'boys' were present. Sister told her class that if they went to a party they should always take a telephone directory with them to be placed between them and the boy, should a relationship develop to the stage of considering sitting on a boy's knee.

No explanation as to the purpose was given and no-one was brash enough to ask why. As she spoke, I visualised myself going through the same experience when I was 14. I could still feel the panic inside me when I had heard this because at home we were not on the telephone! Where on earth was I going to get a telephone directory from? That evening I rushed home from school and while having our family evening meal, raised the issue of having a telephone installed for convenience. My mother's response as anticipated was to inform me that as they could not afford this piece of high technology I would have to use the local telephone box like everyone else in the family did. Ironically this stood outside our local church. I never discussed my concerns at home, but that experience had greatly troubled me and on reflection, had affected boy/girl relationships I had for some years to follow.

A number of other participants in the training session disclosed with relief similar experiences.

WHAT IS SEX EDUCATION?

'Sex education is not just about biological functions. The HMI document, Health Education 5–16 Curriculum Matters No. 6, 1986, states that:

In sex education, factual information about the physical aspects of sex, though important, is not more important than consideration of the qualities of the values, standards and the exercise of personal responsibility as they affect individuals and the community at large.

According to this view, sex education is about:

- Helping children and young people to make responsible decisions about the relationships they form with others.
- Encouraging children and young people to examine their own and other peoples' attitudes and values.
- Developing skills of assertiveness, communication and effective dialogue in relationships.
- Fostering self-esteem, positive self-image and confidence which are important aspects of decision-making behaviour, attitudes and relationships.
- Exploring feelings and attitudes such as love, anger, respect, sadness and grief.'

To teach sex education according to such a view obviously presents a great teaching challenge, particularly within the context of a structured health education programme. Such health behaviour, like sexual behaviour, is influenced by the young person's knowledge about health e.g. personal safety, growth and development, and how the body works and by the attitudes and values of the family, peer group, media and society in general. Health behaviour is also influenced by the skills that the young person has developed for decision-making and taking responsibility for his/her behaviour.

In order to achieve this, teachers must provide young people with the opportunity of working in groups, actively participating in discussion, role play and listening to other points of view. Positive attitudes will only be developed if teachers can establish a learning environment where respect, trust and confidentiality are secured. The drawing-up of ground rules is essential.

There are a great many opportunities for learning about aspects of sex education in drama, dance, art, music, humanities, science, english, RE and PE. In the primary phase, aspects of sex education can easily be integrated into topic or thematic work such as 'Growing and changing', 'Feelings and relationships', 'My healthy body', 'Lifestyles and culture' and 'Growing up'.

In the secondary phase, there are various ways of organising the delivery of sex education, viz. specialised team input within modules, in tutorials, through a chosen combination of subjects e.g. science, RE, english, or as a cross-curricular theme, where all subjects make a recognised contribution. Schools will adopt a model, or combination of models, to meet their needs and organisation. Whatever pattern is chosen, co-ordination by a member of staff with responsibility for health/sex education is crucial.

Not all teachers feel confident about dealing with certain areas of the sex education curriculum. The use of conscripts is not recommended! Schools can make internal arrangements such as team teaching and re-organisation of classes. They may also use the expertise of outside agencies to support staff.

The following outlines the content of the curriculum – knowledge, skills, attitudes and values based on the written recommendations of current documentation following the Education Reform Act 1988.

In Science at Key Stage 1, pupils aged 5–7 years should be taught:

- to name the main external parts of the human body;
- that humans move, feed, grow, use their senses and reproduce;
- that humans can produce babies and that these babies grow into children and then adults;
- to recognise similarities and differences between themselves and other pupils;
- that humans have senses which enable them to be aware of the world around them.

In Science at Key Stage 2, pupils aged 7–11 years should be taught:

- that there are life processes, including nutrition, movement, growth, and reproduction, common to animals, including humans;
- the main stages of the human life cycle.

In Science at Key Stage 3, pupils aged 11–14 years should be taught:

- the ways in which some cell types, including sperm, ova, are adapted to their functions;
- the human reproductive system, including the menstrual cycle, and fertilisation;
- how the fetus develops in the uterus, including the role of the placenta;
- about the physical and emotional changes that take place during adolescence;
- that bacteria and viruses can affect health.

In Science at Key Stage 4, pupils aged 14–16 years should be taught:

- that the nucleus contains chromosomes that carry the genes;
- the way in which hormonal control occurs, including the effects of insulin and sex hormones;
- some medical uses of hormones, including the control and promotion of fertility;
- the defence mechanisms of the body, including the role of the skin and blood;
- how variation may arise from both genetic and environmental causes;
- that sexual reproduction is a source of genetic variation while asexual reproduction produces clones;
- how gender is determined in humans;
- the basic principles of genetic engineering, cloning and selective breeding;
- that organ systems are adapted for their roles in life processes;
- that some diseases can be inherited;
- that the gene is a section of DNA.

   In Curriculum Guidance 5 it states that pupils at Key Stage 1 aged 5–7 should, with regard to sex education:

- know that humans develop at different rates and that human babies have special needs;
- be able to name parts of the body including the reproductive system and understand the concept of male and female;

- know about personal safety, e.g. know that individuals have rights over their own bodies and that there are differences between good and bad touches, begin to develop simple skills and practices which will maintain personal safety;
- appreciate ways in which people learn to live and work together: listening, discussing and sharing.

Pupils at Key Stage 2 aged 7–11 years should, with regard to sex education:

- begin to know about and have some understanding of the physical, emotional and social changes which take place at puberty;
- know the basic biology of human reproduction and understand some of the skills necessary for parenting;
- know that there are many different patterns of friendship; be able to talk about friends with important adults.

Pupils at Key Stage 3 aged 11–14 years should, with regard to sex education:

- recognise the importance of personal choice in managing relationships so that they do not present risks, e.g. to health, to personal safety;
- understand that organisms (including HIV) can be transmitted in many ways, in some cases sexually;
- discuss moral values and explore those held by different cultures and groups;
- understand the concept of stereotyping and identify its various forms;
- be aware of the range of sexual attitudes and behaviours in present day society;
- understand that people have the right not to be sexually active; recognise that parenthood is a matter of choice; know in broad outline the biological and social factors which influence sexual behaviour and their consequences.

Pupils at Key Stage 4 aged 14–16 years should, with regard to sex education:

- understand aspects of Britain's legislation relating to sexual behaviour;
- understand the biological aspects of reproduction;
- consider the advantages and disadvantages of various methods of family planning in terms of personal preference and social implications;
- recognise and be able to discuss sensitive issues such as conception, birth, HIV/AIDS, child rearing, abortion, and technological developments which involve consideration of attitudes, values, beliefs and morality;
- be aware of the need for preventative health care and know what this involves;
- be aware of the statutory and voluntary organisations which offer support in human relationships, e.g. Relate;
- be aware that feeling positive about sexuality and sexual activity is important in relationships;
- understand the changing nature of sexuality over time and its impact on lifestyle, e.g. the menopause;
- be aware of partnerships, marriage and divorce and the impact of loss, separation and bereavement;

- be able to discuss issues such as sexual harassment in terms of their effects on individuals.

Apart from the sex education element outlined above, there are obvious connections to some of the other elements, such as, family life education, safety education, personal hygiene, psychological aspects of health education and substance use and misuse.

In National Curriculum Guidance 8 – Education For Citizenship includes the theme family life. The area of study includes:

- the importance of the family for spiritual well-being, parenthood and child development, the fulfilment of emotional and physical needs;
- challenges facing family units, e.g. separation, divorce, domestic problems, single-parent families;
- family life-cycles, patterns of marriage and family structures and how these change;
- relationships and responsibilities, e.g. roles in the home, and legal responsibilities of parents and children;
- images of the family and marriage in the media.

Within the topic sex education there are issues which can be described as controversial such as contraception, homosexuality, sexual abuse and HIV/AIDS. All official documentation is in favour of the inclusion of these topics within the sex education programme in schools. A school which adopts the ostrich method – 'head in the sand' is leaving the young people in its establishment confused and at risk.

In 1985, Mrs Victoria Gillick brought a case against the DHSS, seeking to:

> try to establish that it was unlawful to give young persons under the age of 16 contraceptive advice and/or treatment without their parents' consent. The House of Lords ruled against her. (Sexual issues, the law and the teachers' responsibility. Assistant Masters and Mistresses Association, 1987.)

The AMMA booklet explains the matter as follows:

> The Gillick case makes clear that a teacher does not act unlawfully in giving information about contraception without parental consent – although he/she should act within the terms of the school's sex education policy.

Strong media attention and widespread public health campaigns have put AIDS into the language of even very young children. Some use it as a term of abuse in the playground, some worry unduly because of inaccurate and informal interpretation. Many young people exhibit misunderstanding and extreme prejudice. Schools are now required by law to include education about HIV/AIDS in their curriculum programmes. Schools can do much to counteract negative effects of informal learning.

The requirements to include HIV/AIDS education will of necessity include reference to homosexuals and bisexuals who are at risk because of certain sexual behaviours. Section 28 of the Local Government Bill Act, which was passed in 1988, caused much controversy and debate. Inevitably it gave many people, including teachers the belief that it was going to be illegal to talk about homosexuality in schools. This idea is erroneous and does not prevent objective discussion of the issue in the classroom.

The passing of the controversial Sex Education Amendment No. 62 to the Education Bill in July 1993 left me, for once, 'gob smacked' and that does not often happen! I could not believe that anything like this could happen given the level of Government commitment and support shown to date with regard to health. This was an enormous step backwards and didn't bear thinking about.

Unfortunately, it was not just a bad dream and the following changes came into effect from August 1994:

- Governors of maintained secondary schools are required to provide sex education (including education about HIV/AIDS and other STDs) to all registered pupils.
- Reference to HIV/AIDS, STDs and aspects of human sexual behaviour other than biological aspects from National Curriculum Science are removed.
- Parents are granted the right to withdraw pupils from all or part of sex education outside the National Curriculum in both primary and secondary schools.

The implications over the amendment raise a number of issues, in particular:

- How will cross curricular teaching be affected?
- What about confidentiality and contraceptive advice to under 16s?
- The parental right of withdrawal might be exploited by pressure groups and abusing parents.
- The Amendment is inconsistent with children's rights legislation such as the Children's Act, UN Convention and European Convention. I wonder how long it will be before a test legal case hits the tabloid press.

For schools this will mean in the primary sector that governors will continue to have the discretion to decide whether to provide sex education. Governors of maintained secondary schools will no longer be able to decide whether the school will provide sex education. This sex education must include education about HIV/AIDS and other STDs. The existence and implementation of school sex education policies will be monitored by OFSTED inspectors.

REFERENCES

Allen I, 1987: *Education in sex and personal relationships*, Policy Studies Institute.
Baldo M, Aggleston P, Slutkin G, 1993: *Does sex education lead to earlier or increased sexual activity in youth?*, WHO.

Butler K, Thompson Z, 1994: *Guidelines regarding outside agency and support workers involvement in sex education in Liverpool and South Sefton schools*, Liverpool and South Sefton Health Promotion Agency.

Department for Education, 1994: *Education Act 1993 – Sex Education in Schools, Circular 5/94*, HMSO.

Department for Education and Employment, 1995: *Protecting children from abuse: the role of the education service*, Circular No. 10/95, HMSO.

Department of Health, *The Children Act 1989*, HMSO, 1991.

Guttmacher Institute, 1989: *Pregnancy, conception and family planning services in industrial countries*, Yale University Press.

HEA Primary School Project, *Health for Life 1*, Nelson, 1989.

HMI, *Health education from 5–16, Curriculum matters 6*, HMSO, 1986.

Johnson *et al.* 1994: *Sexual attitudes and lifestyles*, Blackwell Scientific Publications.

Massey D, 1991: *School sex education, why, what, how,* 2nd edn, FPA.

National Curriculum Council, 1990: *Guidance 5 – Health education*, NCC, 1990.

National Curriculum Council, 1990: *Guidance 3 – The whole curriculum*, NCC, 1990.

Sex Education Forum, 1992: *A framework for school sex education*, National Children's Bureau.

TACADE, *Skills for Life*, TACADE, 1995.

BIBLIOGRAPHY

Allen, I. *Education in Sex and Personal Relationships*, Policy Studies Institute, 1987.

Butler, K., Thompson, Z. *Guidelines regarding outside agency and support workers involvement in sex education in Liverpool and South Sefton schools*, Liverpool and South Sefton Health Promotion Agency, 1994.

Department for Education and Employment, 1995: *Protecting children from abuse: the role of the education service*, Circular No. 10/95, HMSO.

Department for Education and Science, *HIV and AIDS: A Guide for the Education Service*, HMSO, 1991.

Department of Education, *Education Act 1993 – Sex Education in Schools, Circular No. 5/94*, HMSO, 1994.

Department of Health, *The Children Act 1989*, HMSO, 1991.

Department of Health, *The Health of the Nation Key Area Handbook: HIV/AIDS and Sexual Health*, HMSO, 1993.

Fraser, J. *Confidentiality in Secondary Schools: Ethical and Legal Issues*, Brook Advisory Centre, 1989.

HEA Primary School Project, *Health for Life 1*, Nelson, 1989.

HMI, *Health Education from 5–16, Curriculum Matters No. 6*, HMSO, 1986.

Liverpool Education Directorate, *Sex Education Guidelines for Primary Aged Children and Secondary Aged Young People in Liverpool Schools*, Liverpool City Council, 1997.

Lyons, A, *Health Education in Liverpool Schools*, Liverpool Healthy City 2000, 1992.

Massey, D, *School Sex Education, why, what, how,* 2nd edn, FPA, 1991.

National Curriculum Council, *Guidance 3 – The Whole Curriculum*, NCC, 1990.

National Curriculum Council, *Guidance 5 – Health Education*, NCC, 1990.

National Curriculum Council, *Guidance 8 – Education for Citizenship*, NCC, 1990.

Royal College of Gynaecologists, *Report of the Royal College of Gynaecologists Working Group on Unplanned Pregnancy*, RCOG, 1991.

Thomas Coram Research Unit, *Health Education and Young People: AIDS and other health related knowledge, Occasional Paper No. 9*, TCRI, 1991.

West, D. *Questionable Assumptions*, TES, 30.5.86.

CHAPTER 17

Teaching skills and the school nurse

MARION FERGUSON

Two of the main objectives of the Government's Health of the Nation strategy were to reduce teenage pregnancy by 50% by the year 2000, and to reduce the reported incidence of gonorrhoea by 20% by the year 1995.

How are we as School Nurses/Health Educators to achieve this? Sex education is now compulsory in maintained secondary schools in England and Wales; as a result of Section 241 of the 1993 Education Act. In response to this new legislation, the Department of Education have issued new guidance to schools on sex education (DFE 5/94).

This fact sheet:

- explains the implications of the changes to the provision of sex education in the 1993 Education Act;
- clarifies some of the advice given by the Department for Education. Circular 5/94;
- offers some practical and positive advice for those working in or with schools.

Single copies of this guidance can be obtained from the DFE on telephone number 0171 925 555, it is a must for anyone who intends delivering sex education.

WHAT ARE THE LEGAL REQUIREMENTS?

Section 241 of the 1993 Education Act, effective from August 1994.

- Requires governors of maintained secondary schools to provide sex education (including education about HIV/AIDs and other STDs to all registered pupils.
- Removes reference to AIDs, HIV, sexually transmitted diseases and aspects of human sexual behaviours other than biological aspects from the National Curriculum Science.

• Grants parents the right to withdraw pupils in all maintained primary and secondary schools from all or part of sex education outside the National Curriculum.

PRIMARY SCHOOLS

The situation for primary schools and middle deemed primary schools remains unchanged with the exception that parents are able to withdraw their children from all, or part of, sex education other than that specified in the National Curriculum. Governors continue to have responsibility to decide whether the school should provide sex education in addition to that in the National Curriculum (Science), to keep a written statement of this decision, and to develop a policy outlining where and how sex education will be provided. This policy should be made available to all parents and outside agencies, on request.

SECONDARY SCHOOLS

Governors of secondary schools no longer have the power to decide whether the school will provide sex education, but will continue to be required to develop a policy explaining how and where sex education will be taught and to make their policy available to parents.

SPECIAL SCHOOLS

In those special schools which cater exclusively for primary or for secondary age children, the responsibilities of governing bodies correspond to those of primary or secondary schools as outlined above. In all age special schools, the governing bodies will need to adopt separate arrangements for children under and over the age of 11 years corresponding to those applying to primary schools and secondary schools. In addition, the governors should ensure that their written policies explain any distinction they may have chosen to make between arrangements for children below the age of 11 and those above it.

WHAT IS THE APPROPRIATE ROLE OF A SCHOOL NURSE IN SEX EDUCATION?

The school nurse can play an important role in supporting school sex education in both primary and secondary schools.

- As a rule, their role should be complementary to that of the teacher. The contribution of the school nurse should not replace the school's responsibility to provide sex and relationships education.
- School nurses have a range of skills which can contribute to the schools sex education programme. Some school nurses have significant teaching and health promotion skills, others may be able to provide additional medical expertise. For example, as a health professional the school nurse can introduce pupils to the health services that are available to them within their community and help them to develop the confidence and skills necessary to make full use of them.
- The school nurse also has an important role within the school as a health professional, providing young people with individual advice about health-related issues and concerns.
- The school nurse can also play an important role acting as a link between school and parents, providing effective communication and liaising between schools and other relevant professionals such as health visitors, family planning doctors and nurses.
- Teachers responsible for PSE or sex education are able to consult and negotiate with the school nurse to help identify and clarify the role and contribution they can make to school sex education.

CONFIDENTIALITY

Like other professional groups (including teachers), a school nurse is able to give any pupil information about where they can receive confidential contraceptive and sexual health advice and treatment, including sexually transmitted diseases (STDs) and HIV. He/she is also able to give one to one counselling to a pupil on any health related matter and is obliged to respect that young persons' confidences, except where the welfare of the young person or someone other than the patient would otherwise be at risk, for example, in the case of suspected abuse. The duty of confidentiality owed to a person under 16 is as great as that owed to any other person.

As a health professional, school nurses are able to exercise their own professional judgement as to whether a young person has the maturity to consent to medical treatment (including contraceptive treatment) without parental consent. The criteria for making such a decision are based on the Gillick ruling and can be found in guidance issued jointly by the BMA, GMSC, HEA, Brook, FPA and RCGP. Any competent young person, regardless of age, can independently seek medical advice and give valid consent to treatment.

In spite of this, any young person under the age of 16 should be encouraged to confide in their mother if possible, or at least a reliable adult family member, if they feel they cannot comply with this request. On no account should any contraceptive medical treatment or advice be withheld.

Teachers should not promise confidentiality. A child does not have the right to expect that incidents in the class room will not be reported to his/her parents, and may not, in the absence of an express promise, assume that information conveyed outside that consent is private. No teacher could or should give such a promise.

MUST PARENTS BE INFORMED?

There is no basis in principle or authority for suggesting that there is any legal duty on a teacher or a head teacher to inform parents of matters which a child has confided to them. However, if the head teacher instructs staff to tell parents, failure to do so might be grounds for disciplinary action.

PARTICIPATING IN SCHOOL SEX EDUCATION

At some time in a school nurse's working life she will be asked to contribute to sex education. First feelings are usually ones of panic, but there are some questions you can ask yourself to help in your contribution.

Why? – are you responding to an incidence 'behind the bike sheds'?
Are you part of an ongoing Health Education programme? If so, where do you 'fit in'?
What is the pupils' prior knowledge?
What is the school's policy on Sex Education?

Make sure a teacher is going to sit in with you. Pupils are the schools responsibility not the responsibility of the visiting speaker.

PARENTAL CONSENT

Are the parents aware sessions are taking place?
Do they have any concerns or objectives?
Do they want any areas covered or left out?
Are there any cultural/religious factors to consider?

Be aware that there may be in the group young people who have been abused. These children often will 'switch off', or cause disruption by non-participation, or avoid the sessions altogether, or they may exhibit anxiety/emotional upset as a result of the session. A system of counselling/drop-in sessions may need to be offered.

Children/young people with learning difficulties e.g. learning/speech reading/writing difficulties, may well need additional input and back up to complement/reinforce the teaching session.

PREPARATION OF YOUR HEALTH EDUCATION SESSION

- Be clear about your aims and objectives.
- Be sure about the purpose of the session.
- How are you going to fulfil these?
- What resources/methods/videos are you going to use?

SOME PRACTICAL TIPS

The classroom

If possible ask to see the area to be used in advance. Check seating and layout. I prefer a U-shape. I can see all the pupils, help with written work and can move about within the U area.

> Check for comfort, is it too hot or too cold?
> Is it private, or like the M1 with people coming and going?
> Is it well lit?
> Is there enough room/plugs for overhead projector, video etc., if you intend using these aids?

Audience

Do not assume your audience has prior knowledge of the subject. Keep it simple, don't use medical terminology that they might not understand. If you do, make sure you have discussed what words you might use at the start of the session. Keep them interested by using your voice.

- Speak louder than usual, so people at the back can hear.
- Don't swallow your words, be aware of your diction.
- Vary tone and pitch, be dramatic and confident.
- Check difficult words are being understood.
- Over-emphasise when required to put over a particular point.
- Repeat key phrases.
- Use a fast delivery to stimulate the audience and a slow delivery to emphasise control.

Yourself

- Introduce yourself. Give them your name that you wish them to use.
- Be willing to listen and reply to questions/comments.
- Avoid putting your opinions forward, however strongly you feel.
- Acknowledge a variety of viewpoints.
- Be positive.

The session

- Create an interest from the beginning.
- Clearly present yourself/topic.
- Use brief anecdotes and humour.
- Make sure your knowledge of the subject is sound.
- Show confidence in any methods or resources you use.
- Good organisation and planning will make your session go smoothly.

Conclusion

- Make sure you leave time for questions – do not rush it.
- Go over aims and objectives – have you covered all these?
- What has the group learned?
- Evaluate the session.

    (a) Was it successful?
    (b) Does it need repeating?
    (c) Does it need changing?

USEFUL TEACHING METHODS

- Problem solving.
- What would you do if . . .?
- What might happen as a result of . . .?

Role play

- Act out situations.
- Saying no!
- Going on a date.
- Your boyfriend suggests you . . .?

Project work

Using a specific topic (can be group or individual work), for example, find out about young peoples lives in your area. The types of contraceptives used. For HIV and AIDs – who would you talk to/confide in?

Group Discussion

Divide into small groups, discuss given subjects, feed back to main group.

Handouts

Basic information which highlighted the areas you have covered.

Videos

There are many teaching packs, some containing videos which cover a variety of subjects. Don't rely on just one, use material from many, tailor aids to your group.

Brain storming

This is a good way of finding out the prior knowledge of the group and what words or vocabulary they use.

These can be put on a flip chart and hung round the room. Remember to remove these before you leave. The next room user might not appreciate this exercise.

Questionnaires

For both before and after – this is a good assessment tool to ascertain the prior knowledge of your group and what they might have learnt from your session.

Demonstrations

Show your audience how something works by:

- Using a condom.
- Packets of contraceptive pills.
- Various other methods of contraception.

Family planning nurses can usually be talked into providing condoms and packets of pills etc., for teaching purposes. Don't give out condoms, they usually end up being blown up and left around the school.

COUNSELLING/DROP-IN/FOLLOW-UP SESSIONS

This gives you the opportunity to reinforce your message by one to one talks. You might find that because you have instigated discussion in the rather taboo subject of sex you might have prompted someone to disclose sexual abuse to you. Be aware this might happen, and be clear about your local sexual abuse policy. The methods you use will be dependent upon what resources are available, how comfortable you feel using them, the learning capabilities of your group and the time factor. By varying the methods used during the session you are reinforcing the primary message, and more importantly keeping your audience awake and alert. The more active and participatory the group, the more information they will take in, and digest.

In conclusion, I must deal with the dreaded awkward questions that might be asked in a classroom setting.

1. Is this a genuine question or a wind-up to test you out?
2. Think. Is this what you would want your own child to discuss in this class at this age?
3. Would an answer be appropriate to the age and maturity of the group?
4. What is the thought behind this question i.e. hidden agenda?
5. Why does the pupil need to know this? Is the question in response to issues in the media at present, or is it a genuine need to understand something that requires a full explanation?

If the pupil is asking questions that are inappropriate for their age or they are using inappropriate language, there may be a case for investigating this further in private to exclude the possibility of abuse.

It may be better to stall and take advice about difficult questions rather than be caught unawares and answer inappropriately. In order to win confidence and trust, you have to be honest, but that doesn't mean you have to answer all questions as they are asked.

If these simple rules are followed, you should thoroughly enjoy working with young people and find they stimulate you to produce more imaginative ways to improve their learning.

KEY STAGES

What children should be taught at different ages.

KEY STAGE 1, 4–7 YEARS OLD

Sex Education

- Know that humans develop at different rates and that human babies have special needs.
- Be able to name parts of the body including the reproductive system and understand the concept of male and female.
- Know about personal safety, e.g. individuals have rights over their own bodies and that there are differences between good and bad touches, begin to develop simple skills and practices which will help maintain personal safety.
- Appreciate ways in which people learn to live and work together – listening, discussing, sharing.

KEY STAGE 2, 7–11 YEARS OLD

Sex Education

- Begin to know about, and have some understanding of, the physical, emotional and social changes which take place at puberty.
- Know the biology of human reproduction and understand some of the skills necessary for parenting.
- Know that there are many different patterns of friendship: be able to talk about friends with important adults.

KEY STAGE 3, 11–12 YEARS OLD

Sex Education

- Recognise the importance of personal choice in managing relationships so that they do not present risks, e.g. to health, to personal safety.
- Understand that organisms (including HIV) can be transmitted in many ways, in some cases sexually.
- Discuss moral values and explore those held by different cultures and groups.
- Understand the concept of stereotyping and identify its various forms.
- Be aware of the range of sexual attitudes and behaviours in present day society.
- Understand that people have the right not to be sexually active, recognise that parenthood is a matter of choice, know in broad outline the biological and social factors which influence sexual behaviour and their consequences.

KEY STAGE 4, 13–16 YEARS OLD

- Understand aspects of Great Britain's legislation relating to sexual behaviour.
- Understand the biological aspects of reproduction.
- Consider the advantages and disadvantages of various methods of family planning in terms of personal preference and social implications.
- Recognise and be able to discuss sensitive and controversial issues such as contraception, birth, HIV/AIDs, child rearing, abortion, technological developments, which involve consideration of attitudes, values, beliefs and morality.
- Be aware of the need for preventative health care and know what this involves.
- Be aware of the availability of statutory and voluntary organisations which offer support in human relationships, e.g. Relate.

- Be aware of feeling positive about sexuality and sexual activity is important in relationships, understand the changing nature of sexuality over time and its impact on lifestyles, e.g. menopause.
- Be aware of partnerships, marriage, and divorce, the impact of loss, separation and bereavement.
- Be able to discuss issues such as sexual harassment in terms of their effects on individuals.

APPENDIX 1

LESSON PLAN

Name ....

Date .... **Time** .... **From** .... **To** ....

Location

Name of course

Number in group

Topic

Aims
(To make students aware of)

Objectives
(Students should know by the end of lesson)

Resources needed

APPENDIX 2

A summary: some models for planning health education in schools for 4–13-year-olds.

Health education as a one off/or incidental can be:	
DANGER **HEALTH EDUCATION** **MAY NEVER HAPPEN**	Immediate and relevant In response to the unexpected or children's changing interests Response to other needs, concerns and pressures
Health education as a separate, regular slot can:	
DANGER **HEALTH EDUCATION** **COULD BE ISOLATED**	Be planned for systematically Make use of specialist talents Make use of outside support and resources Be in the form of visits and visitors
Health education as a strand in a topic (presupposes the allocation of topic time):	
DANGER **HEALTH MESSAGE** **COULD BE MANIPULATED**	Can be integrated and integrative Children see health education in the context of other subjects and topics
Health education as a central theme of a topic (presupposes the allocation of topic time):	

DANGER
HEALTH MESSAGES COULD
BE LOST OR DILUTED
	Can show the children the relevance of health
	  education to other subject areas
	Specific health messages can be planned to fit
	  'where children are'
	Can be planned to fit in with current needs and
	  pressures

Health education located in one or two specific subject areas can be:	

DANGER
THIS COULD NARROW THE
MEANING OF HEALTH
EDUCATION
	Planned for progression and therefore seem easier
	  to evaluate
	The starting point for staff discussion and a wider
	  cross-curricular approach

Health education across the curriculum can be:	

DANGER
HEALTH EDUCATION CAN BE
PUSHED OUT BY OTHER
PRESSURES
	Planned into a wider or narrow range of ideas,
	  taking account of children's development
	Flexible and adaptable to the needs of the health
	  education topic itself
	Health messages can become part of the
	  children's total activity without being contrived

APPENDIX 3

WHERE TO GO FOR HELP AND ADVICE, USEFUL ADDRESSES AND PHONE NUMBERS

Pregnancy and Contraception

1. Youth Advisory Centres.

2. In some places there are Family Planning Services for young people. Look under Family Planning in the telephone book. These provide confidential advice and information and will supply contraceptives free of charge.

3. Brook Advisory Centres,
   233 Tottenham Court Road,
   London
   W1P 9AE.

   Tel: 0171 580 2991

   Confidential help and advice for young people (under 26) on personal relationships, contraception, abortion and pregnancy. Services are free. For details of your local service contact the above number.

   Brook Helpline   Tel: 0171 617 8000
   Recorded information on the above subjects. Calls charged at normal rates; cheaper after 6.00 pm.

4. British Pregnancy Advisory Service (BPAS)   Tel: 0121 455 7333 (Helpline)
   Monday–Friday   8.00 am–8.00 pm
   Saturday   9.00 am–3.00 pm
   Sunday   10.00 am–2.00 pm

   Pregnancy Advisory Service (PAS),
   11–13, Charlotte Street,
   London
   W1P 1HD

   Tel: 0171 637 8962

Counselling

1. Childline,
   Freepost 1111,
   London N1 0BR

   Tel: 0800 1111
   A free telephone counselling service for young people in trouble or danger.

2.   National Society for the Prevention of Cruelty to Children (NSPCC)   Tel: 0800 800500
     A free 24 h telephone helpline for young people offering help and advice.

3.   SPOD (Association to Aid the Sexual and Personal Relationships of People with a Disability),

     286 Camden Road,
     London
     N7 0BJ

     Tel: 0171 607 8851

4.   Friend   Tel: 0171 837 3337 between 7.30 pm and 10.30 pm (London Friend).

     A national advice and counselling service for anyone who is, or who thinks they might be gay.

5.   Lesbian and Gay Switchboard   Tel: 0171 837 7324
     Phone and help service providing information on all aspects of gay and lesbian life. Ring this number for local switchboard.

6.   Who Cares Trust,
     City Bridge House,
     235–245, Goswell Road,
     London
     EC1V 7JD

     Tel: 0171 833 9047

     Welcome calls and letters from young people in care who need advice on issues ranging from education and employment to health. The Trust publish a quarterly magazine *Who Cares?*

Medical Concerns

1.   National AIDs Helpline   Tel: 0800 567123
     A national service offering free and confidential advice and information about HIV and AIDs – 24 h a day, 7 days a week. Calls are not itemised on bills.

2.   Terence Higgins Trust,
     52–54 Grays Inn Road,
     London WC1X 8JU

     Tel: 0171 242 1010 (helpline)
     Giving advice and information about HIV and AIDs. Open from 3.00 pm to 10.00 pm.

3.   Body Positive,
     51b Pilbeach Gardens,
     London
     SE1 0EE

     Tel: 0171 373 9124 (helpline)
          0171 835 1045 (HIV Self-help Group)

Sexually Transmitted Diseases

Ring local hospital and ask for GUM clinic.
Herpes Association Helpline   Tel: 0171 609 9061
Offering information about herpes.

Assault

Rape Crisis Centre,
PO Box 69,
London
WC1X 9NJ

Tel: 0171 837 1600 (London Rape Crisis Centre)

For girls and women – to find out the local number, ring above or look under Rape in telephone book.

BIBLIOGRAPHY

Sex Education Matters, quarterly newsletter of the Sex Education Forum.
Education Act 1993, *Sex Education in Schools*, Circular Number 5/94.
HEC Primary Schools Project/University of Southampton 1986.
Judy Whitmarsh RGN PGCE Cert Couns. Manchester Metropolitan University.
Communicating Sex Education to Young People. Andrea Selkirk Unit Manager Dewi Jones,
   RLCH Alder Hey.

CHAPTER 18

Contraception

MEERA KISHEN AND JENNIFER HOPWOOD ⎯⎯⎯⎯⎯⎯⎯⎯

INTRODUCTION

Adolescence is the process of psychological and cognitive growth and development that transforms dependent children into self-sufficient adults. The World Health Organisation defines adolescence as the period between the ages of 10 and 19 years, characterised by a series of physiological, anatomical and psychological changes to which young people need to adjust within a changing socio-cultural environment. Today's adolescents attain physical maturity much earlier than in previous generations and, as this is not necessarily accompanied by a parallel development in psycho-social maturity, they may experience difficulty in adjusting to this stage in their life in general and in dealing with their sexuality in particular. From a sociological and cultural point of view, sexual maturation has always been part of the individual's initiation into adulthood with rights and responsibilities, gaining the right to raise a family and acquiring the responsibility to care for and maintain a family. However, sexuality could force adolescents into the role of adulthood before they are ready to do so by its potential ability to result in pregnancy and unplanned parenthood.

Throughout the world, sexual activity among adolescents is changing. Young people now start sexual activity at a younger age and have more sexual partners during their lifetime. This has resulted in the need for services that enable them to protect themselves against the risks of unplanned pregnancy and sexually transmitted diseases (STD) (Cohen, 1989). Though their needs are much the same as those of adults, adolescents have a very different perception of health-care systems and are more reluctant to access the services provided by them. They are also sensitive to negative attitudes about premarital sex prevalent in society. Being dependent legally, and often emotionally and financially too, on their parents or guardians, they find it difficult to acknowledge openly their contraceptive needs. When first relationships are established, they often face dilemmas of what to do or not to do, and may even have concerns regarding sexual orientation, rape or abuse. Service provided in a clinical setting may address the practicalities of contraception and safer sex advice but ignore these very important aspects of a young person's needs. Sexual health and contraception for young people must be addressed within the wider context of their general health and well being to be of real value to them in their passage into adulthood.

BACKGROUND INFORMATION

The use of contraception by teenagers has lagged behind the changes in their sexual behaviour. The rate of sexual activity among adolescents in developed countries differs significantly. Studies from United Kingdom report a varying proportion of sexually active teenagers (Farrell, 1978; Bowie and Ford, 1989). However, most agree that the proportion rises with age and while a substantial proportion of 16 year olds may have had sexual intercourse, perhaps only half of these use contraception regularly (Zabin *et al.*, 1979). A detailed study into the sexual and contraceptive lifestyles of young women in England (Ford, 1992) found a diverse pattern in terms of age of first intercourse, number of sexual partners and attitudes to the timing of sexual intercourse within relationships. The overall pattern of sexual culture among young people in Britain is one in which premarital sex is accepted and practised. The findings in this study indicate an early age at first intercourse occurring in about 50% of 16 year olds, 67% of 17 year olds and over 80% of 18 year olds. Although most sexual intercourse took place within 'steady relationships' within the context of serial monogamy there was a significant level of partner change within these relationships. In view of the fact that contraceptive usage among sexually active adolescents is poor, and that they are likely to have a higher number of lifetime partners compared to those starting sexual activity later in life, these findings highlight the serious risks for their sexual health.

The risk of pregnancy among adolescents is high. A large study from the United States found that 22% of all teenage premarital pregnancies occurred during the first month of sexual activity and 50% during the first 6 months (Jones *et al.*, 1985). The Guttmacher Institute in 1986 published an international study of adolescent pregnancy and childbearing in 37 developed countries (Jones *et al.*, 1985). It concluded that the startling differences in teenage pregnancy rates in different countries were mainly related to the variation in the effectiveness with which young people used contraception. It also showed that the background to better contraceptive use in teenagers was easily accessible, user-friendly, confidential and free contraceptive services coupled with appropriate sex education programmes in schools. A greater degree of openness about sexuality in society also facilitated the uptake of contraceptive services by young people. The Guttmacher study further compared in depth the situation in 6 western countries with similar cultural and economic background and similar patterns of adolescent sexual activity. Among the 6 countries – United States, Canada, France, United Kingdom, the Netherlands and Sweden – the United States had the highest teenage pregnancy rate, being 2–3 times higher than Canada, France, United Kingdom and Sweden, and 7 times higher than the Netherlands. (Table 18.1).

Table 18.1   Comparison of pregnancy rates for teenage women.
The Guttmacher Report (Jones *et al.* 1985).

Country	Rate per 1000 women aged 15–19 years
United States	96
England and Wales	45
France	43
Canada	44
Sweden	35
The Netherlands	14

Provision of school-based sex education and contraceptive services targeted at young people often raise moral and ethical concerns in society. It is common belief that providing sex education to young school children who may not yet be sexually active may encourage earlier sexual activity. This assertion has been refuted by a number of studies (Zelnik and Kim, 1982; Hofman, 1984) and, in fact, in the United Kingdom there are now attempts to enhance sex education in schools as part of strategies designed to reduce unplanned teenage pregnancy (see Department of Health Handbook, 1993). Sexual activity among young people is spontaneous and can not be fitted into any specific schedule. Hence, they need to be fully aware of the implications of sexual activity and contraceptive availability long before they actually become sexually active. Increasing access to contraceptive services for the young has not resulted in increasing promiscuity as suggested before (Strasburger, 1989).

LEGAL ASPECTS

If the young person seeking contraceptive advice is under 16 years of age, concerns may arise about the legality of providing contraception to a minor without parental consent. Sexual intercourse before the age of consent is a violation of the law in the United Kingdom. However, prosecutions are rare if the young people concerned are of a similar age. It is the recommendation of the Royal College of Obstetricians and Gynaecologists of Great Britain that 'The health professional has a responsibility to help the young person to understand the implications of sexual activity and the value of confiding in his/her parents. However it is also important to appreciate that the developing sexuality of young people creates a barrier between them and their parents that is part of the process of growing up. A trained responsible outsider may be a more effective source of counselling than the parents' (see RCOG Report 1989).

If an under 16 year old presents for contraception, some discussion needs to take place between him/her and the professional about the advantages of delaying intercourse. If this is not received as appropriate message or if sexual activity is already established and the young person intends to continue sexual activity, then contraceptive advice at this stage is surely in the best interests of the individual. When a parent does not accompany the young person, the suggestion that parents may be involved should be made. The most common reason for adolescents not confiding in their parents is because they assume that their parents would be angry or disappointed if they knew they were sexually active. Yet there are parents who, despite their initial discomfort, would appreciate the chance to discuss sexual activity or even contraception with their children. However, if young people are not receptive to the suggestion of including parents in the discussions, their choice should be respected unconditionally. They are, in their own way, taking adult responsibilities and making adult decisions in their lives. Involvement of parents is a sensitive issue and should be handled carefully.

In England and Wales, the legal situation for the prescribing physician has been eminently clarified following the famous 'Gillick case' (Gillick and West Norfolk, 1985) and has been set out in the Department of Health's Memorandum of Guidance (DHSS HC(FP) 86). This states that it is good medical practice to proceed to prescribe a medical contraceptive without parental knowledge and consent if:

1. The girl, although under 16 years of age, will understand the doctor's advice.
2. She cannot be persuaded to inform her parents or allow the doctor to inform them.
3. She is very likely to begin or to continue having sexual intercourse with or without contraceptive treatment.
4. Her physical or mental health or both are likely to suffer unless she receives contraceptive advice or treatment.
5. Her best interests require the doctor to proceed without parental consent.

At all times the young woman must have complete assurance of confidentiality. Ethical and legal considerations may also arise when providing contraceptive advice for mentally handicapped adolescents. The Universal Declaration of Human Rights (1948) stated and the Declaration of Teheran (1968) reiterated that every person of 'full age' has the right to have children and 'found a family' (Gike-Henner, 1989). Partly on this basis, many jurisdictions have rejected non-consensual sterilisation of the severely mentally handicapped as being discriminatory and unethical unless performed to safeguard the health and welfare of the handicapped person. However, it can be debated whether the severely handicapped meet the precondition for such a right (Zabin and Clark, 1981). Some methods of contraception which seem appropriate for these people may also be considered intrusive e.g. intrauterine contraceptive device (IUCD), implants. Consideration of these matters by those involved in the care of young disabled people will hopefully allow ethically appropriate decisions to be made for each individual.

SERVICE DELIVERY

Of the estimated 52 000 sexually active 15 year old females in England in 1991, only just over a third visited family planning clinics. One of their major reasons for delaying contraception is the fear of discovery of their sexual activity by their parents (Winter and Breckenmaker, 1991). Because of their fears of adult disapproval, adolescents need to feel confident that the healthcare systems they access will respect their confidentiality. A supportive and encouraging environment is required whereby not only the necessary clinical services but counselling on contraceptive and other related issues can also be provided. Informal 'youth clinics' rather than formal medical sessions have been shown to be more popular among young people.

The service must provide what the adolescent population needs. Sexual activity among young people is often unplanned and hence unprotected. The most common reason to seek help is the immediate fear of possible pregnancy. In fact some girls are already pregnant when they first access contraceptive services. Sympathetic counselling at this point can assist the young person enormously in making difficult decisions regarding continuation of the pregnancy or termination. A good relationships built at this contact may lead to more effective an contraceptive usage by the young person and hopefully planned pregnancies in future.

Pregnancy testing and emergency contraceptive services are an essential component of any clinical service for young people. Unnecessary vaginal examinations which do not contribute to meeting with the individual's needs must be withheld at initial consultations. Routine smears and pelvic examinations can be deferred until several months of contraceptive use. A non-judgemental approach and a capacity for empathy on the part of the provider is essential in gaining the trust of adolescents. A good relationship established at the first contact often provides an opportunity to discuss whether or not someone wishes to continue sexual activity and offer counselling on the risks of early intercourse which may lead to changes in behaviour. In such a setting it may even be possible for a young person to reveal other problems they may be experiencing such as rape or abuse. Links with services that offer support in such issues are valuable to any youth clinic and need to be developed.

Teenagers are often not easy patients. Their anxiety and nervousness frequently translates into non-communication and even abrasive behaviour. All health professionals involved in providing services for adolescents must acquire the ability to look beyond such attitudes and concentrate on the positive aspects of the young person's behaviour. Because adolescents have a less developed future orientation, they may place greater emphasis on the immediate contraceptive needs rather than the remote risks associated with sexual activity. Such distorted risk perception is not unique to them but is, perhaps, more common at their stage of cognitive development when they tend to believe in the myth that disasters such as an unplanned pregnancy will somehow not befall them.

Young people from certain cultural and religious backgrounds may experience difficulty in coming to terms with parental expectations and peer group pressures they experience in society. Immigrant parents from traditional societies are often shocked by Western values and find them a threat to their cultural integrity. This makes communication about sexual matters with their children very difficult. These young people often desperately need an unbiased atmosphere to help them work through their own values and reach decisions which may have a profound impact on their lives.

Disabled young people often face problems in accessing information and services related to their sexual needs. Many able bodied adults, including health professionals, fail to recognise that the disabled have the same sexual feelings and needs as them. Sensitivity to their needs is of paramount importance in the planning and provision of services to adolescents.

Services should be accessible, preferably near to schools or youth clubs. Clinics should be open at times when it would be most easy for young people to attend without attracting the attention of adults i.e. following close on end of school, or coinciding with youth club times. Saturday services in town centre locations have also proved to be popular with young people as clinic visits can often be combined with a shopping trip into town with friends. It is essential to ensure that the services are advertised in places where they usually obtain information such as school common rooms, leisure centres, youth clubs, libraries and youth magazines. It is important that young people should find it easy to know where and when these clinics are held. Access to telephone information regarding availability and location of services is often useful in helping them reach these services.

COUNSELLING FOR CONTRACEPTIVE USE

All young people requesting contraceptive services need to be given information on the complete range available to them to allow a fully informed choice. When dealing with adolescents, it is especially important for this information to be provided in a manner which is easy to understand and assimilate. Visual aids are very useful in demonstrating how the various contraceptive methods work and how they should be used. Discussion in explicit and concrete terms is likely to have a greater impact than abstract descriptions of contraceptive use. Adolescents also differ from adults in the way they tolerate side effects of various contraceptive methods. They are also more likely to discontinue their method of contraception if problems develop. Hence it is worthwhile spending more time on compliance related issues at the initial consultation and encouraging early follow-up visits whenever they have any concerns about side effects. It has been demonstrated that continuation with contraceptive methods is better if there has been initial discussion and reassurance about possible side effects (Winter and Breckenmaker, 1991). Written information in addition to verbal instruction is useful especially in early stages of contraceptive usage. However, it must not be forgotten that 'print is evidence!'. Adolescents who wish to keep contraceptive visits secret will not want to take home lots of leaflets. Wallet cards carrying essential information are more likely to be retained and may need to be designed for use specially in adolescent services. Providing adequate time is an important factor in ensuring that the services offered truly do meet the young person's needs.

Counselling in contraceptive issues should ideally encompass many aspects of their concept of contraceptive use. They may have feelings of guilt or embarrassment, difficulties in negotiating the sexual relationship with their partner, fears of side effects associated with the contraceptive they choose, as well as problems grasping the technicalities of contraceptive use. It is also important for health professionals to be aware of the fact that some may actually want a pregnancy, which they may perceive as their route to financial independence, respect or simply gaining attention. They may actually profess great difficulty in using contraception effectively. Such youngsters are often ill informed and unrealistic, tending to underestimate the demands of parenthood at great personal cost to themselves subsequently. Experienced counsellors can explore these feelings with their young clients and hopefully bring realisation of the true life of a teenage parent to them.

CONTRACEPTIVE CHOICES FOR ADOLESCENTS

When presented with the 'contraceptive menu' in an easily understandable version, young people should be able to choose appropriate contraception for themselves taking into account the particular risks of early sexual activity they feel relevant and important to them. Though the combined oral contraceptive pill is the most popular choice, the increasing risk of STDs has increased the interest in barrier methods either on their own or in addition to the pill. Whatever contraceptive method they choose, it must be easy to use, safe, reliable and easily obtained.

Condoms

Condoms fit all the above requirements and are a convenient option for sexually active adolescents. They serve the dual purpose of preventing pregnancy and reducing the risk of STDs. However, the effectiveness of condoms is influenced by a number of factors – the cost, or else access to, free supplies; the unplanned nature of teenage sexual activity; alcohol and drug use; and risk-taking behaviour among adolescents due to their 'cognitive immaturity'.

Many young people report difficulties in condom use, often resulting in a request for emergency contraception. This may also be linked to lack of instruction provided to young men on the use of condoms. Most contraceptive services still fail to attract young men who are in as much need of contraceptive education as their female partners. Adequate instruction in condom use is as essential to its successful use as is a 'pill teach' for correct oral contraceptive use.

The female condom is now available as another option in barrier contraception controlled by women. They are available over the counter and so are easily accessible. However, their high cost puts them beyond the reach of most adolescents. They are made of polyurethane which is much stronger than the latex used to make male condoms and less likely to break during intercourse. They also require a fair degree of instruction for correct and successful use.

Oral contraception

The combined oral contraceptive pill is often the method of choice for a teenager who requires an effective, non-intercourse related convenient method of contraception. Additional benefits of the combined pill such as lighter, regular, pain free periods also make it much more attractive to young girls. The main disadvantage of the pill to an adolescent in health terms is its inability to afford protection against acquiring STDs. When sexual activity starts early, with the established pattern of 'serial monogamy', the young adolescent is at greater risk of acquiring infections such as chlamydia which may result in damage to their reproductive health. The contraceptive benefits of the pill need to be balanced against the lack of protection against STD risk. Ideally, the combined use of condoms along with the pill ('double dutch method') should be recommended to all adolescents.

The pharmacological considerations for oral contraceptive use in the teenager are the same as for a woman in her early 20s. There is no evidence that a daily dose of 30 to 50 µg of ethinyl oestradiol to post-pubertal girls has any effect on epiphyseal closure. Menstruation normally commences when adult height and weight have been achieved.

Proper pill usage may be a problem for people with erratic lifestyles and the possible need to conceal it from parents. Prescribing the pill should include not only instructions on when to start it and how to take them correctly but also address finding ways of remembering to take them regularly. Some young people may find the stop–start associated with the pill free week most difficult to handle. They often have the erroneous impression that the start and the end of the packet are not risky in terms of pregnancy, mentally equating the pill cycle to the normal menstrual cycle. They may require educating in the differences between the two especially in terms of fertility risk. In view of the greater risk of ovulation associated with the lengthening of the pill free interval, it may be useful to recommend the every day version with 7 dummy pills to provide continuity in the pill taking routine. There is no evidence to show that the heavily marketed 'phasic pills' offer any advantage in terms of reducing side effects or risks to young pill users. In fact for young people in the early stages of mastering the routine of pill taking, the more complicated instructions associated with their use may cause more problems in compliance. Phasic pills in addition do not offer the advantage of being able simply to run 2 packets consecutively if ever the young girl wished to avoid a period at an inopportune time such as examination or during holidays. This practice is also of value in helping a young girl prone to epilepsy avoid period associated attacks. On the whole the phasic pills have little to recommend over the standard low dose monophasic preparations in use today.

Breakthrough bleeding with pill usage may well be due to poor compliance among adolescents. However, if persistent, it must not be forgotten that endometritis or cervicitis due to infections such as chlamydia could be a potential cause. It may be necessary to review the pill-taking history carefully and recommend appropriate examination and tests rather than a random change of the pill in the hope that one may eventually solve the problem. It must also not be forgotten that many teenagers require treatment for conditions such as acne and reduced pill absorption due to antibiotic therapy could result in loss of cycle control. They need to be educated clearly on the need for additional contraceptive protection when taking drugs which may interfere with pill absorption and efficacy. Long-term antibiotic therapy has risk of reduced pill efficacy only at the start and end of therapy when there is a sudden alteration in the gut flora. The beneficial effect of an oestrogen dominant contraceptive pill may obviate the need for antibiotic treatment of acne. Powerful hepatic enzyme inducers such as rifampicin and grieseofulvin reduce efficacy of oral contraceptives, not only during the duration of treatment, but for up to 4 weeks after stopping the drug.

Other beneficial effects of combined oral contraception such as reduction in pelvic inflammatory disease, premenstrual tension, endometriosis, ovarian and endometrial cancer and ectopic pregnancy are often totally unknown to adolescents. It may be helpful at initial consultation to point out the benefits of the combined pill to them as this may allay anxiety and hopefully improve compliance.

Combined oral contraceptive use remains a risk factor for developing deep vein thrombosis in teenagers following major surgery associated with immobilisation (Winter and Breckenmaker, 1991). As oral contraceptive usage often is concealed from parents by young people, it is important to elicit this information in private at assessment for any impending major surgery. It is recommended that those undergoing major surgery should discontinue combined oral contraceptives for at least 4 weeks before and after the surgery and attendant immobilisation. In such circumstances, progestogen only contraceptives are a safe option. Information about this alternative and where to obtain replacement contraception must be provided before stopping the combined pill. However, surgical procedures not associated with subsequent immobilisation such as tonsillectomy and dental surgery do not pose a similar risk and the pill may be safely continued up to and immediately after surgery.

Progestogen only pills (mini pills) have a higher failure rate than combined pills as they exert their contraceptive effect mainly through cervical mucus changes. Ovulation suppression occurs in only up to 50% of cycles in 'mini pill' users. The margin of safety for delayed pills is also narrower as compared to the combined pill – three compared to 12 hours. This may increase the problems in pill compliance thus contributing to higher user failure rates with the mini pill.

They are also associated with poor cycle control. Irregular bleeding causes undue concern and often results in discontinuation of pill use among adolescents. Hence progestogen only pills are not recommended as first choice for young people. However, they can be advocated to young breast-feeding mothers.

Emergency contraception

As mentioned earlier, emergency contraception has a very important place in the contraceptive services for adolescents. The need for emergency contraception is often the commonest reason for them to make first contact with a clinic service. They are likely to experience unplanned and unprotected sexual activity. They are often reluctant to obtain contraceptive supplies prior to first sexual experience in the belief that 'it won't happen to me!'. Those who have become sexually active may need a backup to condom use. It can not be emphasised enough that where young people are concerned *at all possible opportunities* emergency contraception should be discussed or information given. This will not only help the young person concerned, but will have a community effect among the young population, helping many more avoid an unplanned pregnancy.

The most frequent method of emergency contraception used by adolescents is the hormonal 'Yuzpe' regime. This involves administration of combined pills containing 100 µg of ethinyl oestradiol within 72 hours of a single risk episode to be followed by a similar, second dose 12 hours after the first. It has a failure rate of 2 to 5% depending on the time of administration in the menstrual cycle. It has very few contraindications for its use and side effects are mainly nausea and vomiting due to the high oestrogen content. The time of administration can be easily adjusted to follow meal times and the convenience of the young person to minimise the incidence of side effects and improve compliance with the second dose. A follow-up visit 3 weeks following administration of post-coital contraception is offered to exclude a possible failure of the method. In addition, this visit provides an ideal opportunity to offer counselling for future contraceptive needs. In the adolescent, failure of the Yuzpe method may sometimes be due to unacknowledged episodes of previous unprotected sex in that cycle. This needs to be borne in mind while counselling a young person and often explanation of the use of the interuterine contraceptive device (IUCD) for post-coital contraception may lead to more openness and therefore better efficacy of post-coital contraception.

Other Hormonal Methods

Injectable progestogens

Depot medroxyprogesterone acetate (Depo provera) is used most frequently worldwide. Norethisterone oenanthate (Noristerat) is another injectable contraceptive available in the United Kingdom. They are administered by deep intramuscular injection, Depo provera in doses of 150 mg at 12 weekly intervals and Noristerat 200 mg at 8 weekly intervals. They provide very effective contraception by ovulation suppression and have an additional effect on cervical mucus and the endometrium. They are convenient in that administration is not related to sexual intercourse and their longer duration of action reduces the need to remember a daily routine for administration. The great advantage perceived by many young people is the secrecy afforded by the method. The main problem with injectable progestogens is cycle irregularity and amenorrhoea associated with their use. However, with detailed counselling and ongoing support, some young girls find the eventual amenorrhoea associated with Depo provera use quite acceptable. The delay in return of fertility following discontinuation of its use poses very little problem for the adolescent who has plenty of time to establish her family. There are no significant health risks associated with long-term use of this method by adolescents.

Subdermal implants

Norplant consists of 6 silastic capsules containing 36 mg of Levonorgestrel released at a steady rate over a 5 year period providing good contraceptive protection. The main advantage of this method over injectable progestogens is the rapid return of fertility following their removal. The major advantage of this method for the adolescent is that it takes away the compliance factor completely for 5 years. However, this should not result in the restricted use of implants in only those young people deemed non-compliant e.g. those requiring terminations, but it should be offered as part of the 'contraceptive menu'. Though this method is licensed for use in women aged 18–40 years, there are no medical reasons for not offering it to younger women. Insertion and removal of the implants require a minor surgical procedure. Detailed counselling and careful patient selection are important factors in ensuring successful continuation of the method over the 5 year period. Irregular menstrual bleeding is the main side effect related to its use and is the commonest reason for requests for early removal. In a study of Norplant users in Baltimore (Blumenthal, 1993), it was noted that adolescents returned to the clinic for more 'problem' visits than adults during the early follow-up period though this difference disappeared by 6 months. Effective ongoing support is a key factor in the success of any contraceptive method and more so in long-acting methods such as implants.

Intrauterine Contraceptive Devices

The ideal IUCD user is a parous woman in a monogamous relationship with a low risk of acquiring STDs whatever her age. The sexual activity pattern of an adolescent often makes the IUCD an unsuitable choice of contraception; the practice of serial monogamy among young people increases the risk of acquiring STDs and then the presence of an IUCD increases the risk of developing pelvic inflammatory disease and subsequent tubal infertility. Many teenage girls suffer from heavy painful periods, which is likely to be made worse by IUCD use. However, the frameless copper intrauterine implant 'Gynefix' overcomes the problem of dysmenorrhoea and spontaneous expulsion in nulligravid women – should their sexual activity pattern make them suitable for consideration of an intrauterine method of contraception. Another disadvantage is that, young being highly fertile, the use of IUCD may be associated with higher failure rates for the method in this group.

An IUCD may be offered as a post-coital contraceptive to those seeking help after the 72 hours limit for the hormonal method. It is effective at preventing a pregnancy if inserted within 5 days of unprotected intercourse or up to corrected day 19 of a 28 day cycle in the event of multiple episodes of unprotected intercourse in the first half of the cycle. Even if unsuitable as an ongoing contraceptive for an adolescent, it can be used to prevent pregnancy in that cycle and removed at the onset of a period by which time alternative contraception can be established.

Other Methods

Diaphragms

Proper and consistent use of the diaphragm requires a high degree of motivation and skill which may be lacking in many teenagers. The diaphragm is ideal in many ways for a sexually active adolescent by the protection it affords to the cervix and being available for use only when needed providing instant contraception like the condom. However, it may not be very convenient for a young person to find suitable facility/privacy for insertion prior to intercourse and for washing and storage. It may be difficult to maintain secrecy with such a method.

Spermicides

Spermicides are usually easy to obtain and can be bought over the counter in many countries. They also have some protective effect against some STDs but they are not an equal alternative for condoms. When used alone they have low contraceptive effectiveness and therefore are not to be recommended for use by young people without the accompanying use of condoms or diaphragms.

Withdrawal

Withdrawal is widely used among adolescents especially during early intercourse. Though it is not an effective method of contraception, it may be the only method available at the time of need. It is important not to condemn it totally, as that would result in some making no attempt at contraception at all in the absence of access to contraceptive supplies. Instead it might be helpful to educate young people about the limitations of the method so that they themselves realise the benefit of using the more effective methods available to them.

Natural methods

Adolescents often have irregular menstrual cycles which make rhythm or calender methods unreliable. Sympto-thermal methods are also difficult to use and often unsuited to their needs. These methods requiring periodic abstinence are difficult for young people to comply with. However, they should be educated about the fertile times in their normal cycle. General fertility awareness helps people understand the way in which many contraceptive methods work and will enable them to use the methods more effectively.

Permanent methods

These are rarely ever considered in this age group except in medically indicated circumstances.

SUMMARY

If our goal is to provide acceptable effective contraceptive services for our adolescent population, we need to ensure that the services are user-friendly, providing not only the whole range of services for the sexually active young but also paying attention to their special needs. In order to change risk behaviour among adolescents, efforts should be directed to educating them before sexual debut occurs and attitudes are formed. Provision of such services should enable adolescents to grow into adults with self-esteem and the ability to enjoy healthy personal and sexual relationships in their lives.

REFERENCES

Blumenthal P, 1993: Preliminary experience with Norplant in an inner city population. Presented at: *Long-acting progestins: management of bleeding disturbances*, Durham, NC.

Bowie C, Ford N, 1989: Sexual behaviour of young people and the risk of HIV infection. *Journal of Epidemiology and Community Health* **43**, 61–65.

Cohen SJ, 1983: Intentional teenage pregnancies. *Journal of School Health* March, 210–211.

Department of Health, 1993: *The Health of the Nation. Key area handbook: HIV/AIDS and sexual health*. London: DOH.

Eike-Henner W, Kluge, 1989: *Ethical problems in reproductive medicine*, 12–15.

Farrell C, 1978: *My mother said*. London: Routledge and Kegan Paul.

Ford N, 1992: The sexual and contraceptive lifestyles of young people. *British Journal of Family Planning* **18**, 52–55.

Gillick V. Wisbech and West Norfolk AHA, 1985: 3 AII ER402HL.

Hofman AD, 1984: Contraception in adolescence; a review. I. Psychosocial aspects. *Bulletin WHO* **62/1**, 151–62.

Jones EF, Forrest JD, Goldman N, *et al.* 1985: *Determinants and policy implications: teenage pregnancy in developed countries*. New York, NY: Alan Guttmacher Institute.

Royal College of Obstetricians and Gynaecologists, 1991: Report of the RCOG working party on unplanned pregnancy. London: RCOG.

Strasburge VC, 1989: Adolescent sexuality and the media. *Pediatric Clinics of North America* **36/3**, 747–773.

Winter L, Breckenmaker LC, 1991: Tailoring family planning services to the special needs of adolescents. *Family Planning Perspectives*; **23**, 24–30.

Zabin L, Clark S, 1981: Why they delay: A study of teenage family planning clinic patients. *Family Planning Perspectives* **13**, 205–217.

Zabin LS, Kanter JF, Zelnik M, 1979: The risks of adolescent pregnancy in the first months of intercourse. *Family Planning Perspectives* **11**(4), 215–222.

Zelnik M, Kim YJ, 1982: Sex education and its association with teenage sexual activity, pregnancy and contraceptive use. *Family Planning Perspectives* **14**, 117–126.

PART VI

CHILD SEXUAL ABUSE

CHAPTER 19

Medical aspects

W JOAN ROBSON AND ELIZABETH M MOLYNEUX ─────────

INTRODUCTION

Child sexual abuse is any use of a child for adult sexual gratification (Bamford and Roberts, 1989). The working party of the Standing Medical Advisory Committee in their guidelines for doctors on the diagnosis of child sexual abuse and in the document *Child Abuse Working Together* adopt the definition by Schechter and Roberge (1976) and promoted by Kempe and Kempe. This states that sexual abuse is:

> The involvement of dependent, developmentally immature children and adolescents in sexual activities they do not truly comprehend, to which they are unable to give informed consent; or which violates social taboos or family roles (see Diagnosis of Child Sexual Abuse, 1988; Child Abuse – Working Together, 1988).

This definition is not all inclusive; not all children are developmentally or physically immature, not all are unable to comprehend sexual activities, nor do all children refuse consent. In Great Britain, sexual relationships between adults and children under 16 years of age are regarded as always and inherently abusive, whether forced or unforced, violent or gentle. Sexual relationships between children are regarded as sometimes abusive, dependent on the age difference, type of abuse and relationship. In this situation, the line between 'normal' sexual experimentation and sexual abuse is sometimes hard to draw. Sexual abuse includes attempts at, or commission of, vaginal, anal or oral intercourse; fingering, the introduction of objects into anal or vaginal orifices; the fondling of children's genitalia and involvement of children in pornography (see Diagnosis of Child Sexual Abuse, 1988).

McCleod and Saraga (1981) argue that any definition of child sexual abuse should contain three elements; the betrayal of trust and responsibility, the abuse of power, and the inability of children to consent.

CLASSIFICATION

Kempe and Kempe (1984) offer the following categorisation of child sexual abuse:

1. Incest – sexual activity between close blood relatives.
2. Paedophilia – the adult preference for pre-pubertal children as sex objects.
3. Exhibitionism – genital exposure by an adult.
4. Molestation – such as fondling, touching, kissing and masturbation.
5. Sexual intercourse – oro-genital (fellatio and cunnilingus), anogenital (buggery), or penile vaginal contact.
6. Rape – sexual intercourse or attempted intercourse without consent of the victim.
7. Sexual sadism – sexual gratification obtained by the infliction of physical injury.
8. Child pornography – the production and distribution of books, films, videos or audio tapes, involving minors in sexual acts.
9. Child prostitution – the involvement of children in sexual activity for profit.

INCIDENCE

Child sexual abuse (CSA) is not new, but was largely unreported in Great Britain until the late 1970s. In 1987, in Cleveland, during 5 months' 121 children from 57 families, were diagnosed by two paediatricians to have been sexually abused (see Cleveland Report, 1987). This episode generated enormous publicity through the media, resulting in heightened public awareness of the problem. Information on frequency of CSA has been derived from police prosecutions, investigations by professionals, population studies and telephone helplines. In America, it has been estimated that one in ten of the adult population as a whole has been sexually abused (Hobbs *et al.*, 1991). In Great Britain, an overall abuse rate of 93 per 1000 has been quoted (Baker and Duncan, 1985). In 1992, 38 600 children in England were on the Child Protection Register, 31% of whom were adolescents. 17% of the children were registered under the category of sexual abuse (see Child Protection Registers, 1993).

Sexual abuse is often within the family and is kept secret. The true figure for its incidence is unknown.

THE ABUSER

Some children are abused by strangers, but in the vast majority of cases the abuser is known to the child. The abuser is usually male, though recently there have been increased reports of female perpetrators (Finkelhor and Williams, 1988). The abuser is frequently a member of the family household, or a trusted and close friend of the family or of the child, such as a baby sitter, teacher or family friend.

In the annual Home Office figures for 1989, of all offenders cautioned or found guilty of sexual offences, 32% were under the age of 21 and 17% were under the age of 16 years (see National Childrens Home Factfile, 1993).

Hengeller (1989) found that 36% of CSA cases involved a juvenile perpetrator. In a recent study of sexual abuse investigations in Liverpool (1989–90) Horne *et al.* (1991) found that 34.4% of allegations involved children or young persons abusing other children or young persons. In London, where 28% of cases of sexual abuse involved a perpetrator under the age of 18, in 15% of those cases (4.2% of cases overall) the perpetrator was female (See National Childrens Home Factfile, 1993).

   There are no distinguishing features of adults who abuse children. CSA is perpetrated by individuals from all social classes and all cultural backgrounds. There are greater risks in families where an adult or person is already known to have abused a child, where the use of alcohol or drugs is uncontrolled, or where there is little sexual gratification within the adult partnership of the household.

THE ABUSED

Children of all ages and either sex are abused, but the vast majority of abused children are girls. The incidence in males increased from 7% in 1979 to 11% in 1983 in a study from the USA, indicating that boys too are at considerable risk of sexual abuse (Spencer and Dunklee, 1986).

PRESENTATION

Sexual abuse may present to the clinician in a wide variety of ways:

- The child may have described abusive behaviour.
- Social Services or the police may request a medical evaluation on a child as part of an investigation.
- Carers may recognise abnormal sexualised behaviour in a child.
- There may be behavioural difficulties with deliberate self-harm (particularly self-inflicted cuts), personality changes, eating disorders, learning difficulties, sleeping difficulties, promiscuity, drug or alcohol abuse, truancy, stealing or temper tantrums.
- There may be vague, generalised physical complaints, especially of abdominal pain, in an adolescent girl. There may be frequent visits to the doctor or hospital with minor complaints and a reluctance to go home.
- Encopresis or a relapse of bed wetting may occur.
- Localised problems may occur such as vaginal bleeding, a discharge, soreness or recurrent urinary tract infections or a STD.
- The child may be pregnant and refuse to say who the father is.
- In cases of undisclosed abuse, local complications may be found on examination – e.g. perianal or vulvar and vaginal warts; hymenal or anal tears; bruising or swelling of the genitalia and perianal skin.

THE DIAGNOSTIC PROCESS IN SEXUAL ABUSE

Medical examination is only a part of the investigation in suspected sexual abuse. A coordinated, considered discreet approach is needed by medical staff, police and social workers. It requires sharing of information, mutual trust and confidence. The medical examination can usually be planned and arranged. Only in episodes of acute sexual abuse, where forensic evidence must be sought as soon as possible, is there urgency in carrying out the medical examination.

Where To Investigate

A child should be interviewed and examined in a place where (s)he feels unthreatened, which is not identified with guilt or punishment. A police station is therefore not a suitable setting. There may be a specially designed suite set aside for such investigations, in a hospital or in the community, in a general practice or a clinic where the child feels safe. Ideally, video facilities for interviewing, interview rooms, an examination room, a bathroom and a kitchen should be available.

The History from the Parents

If the parent has alleged that the child has been abused, a careful history should be taken of the allegation, with as much background into family relationships and circumstances as possible.

The History from the Child

The child's description of abuse is vital. This history needs to be taken with great expertise and sensitivity. It should be carried out by an interviewer trained in child abuse investigation. This is usually a social worker and a woman police officer from the child protection team dealing with the allegation. If the interview is recorded on video, it will be evidence for court and must therefore be legally acceptable, both in the manner in which it is undertaken and in its storage (see Home Office Memorandum, 1988).

Who Should Examine?

The child should be examined by someone experienced in the diagnosis of child abuse and in examining and talking with children. It is preferable that the examination be carried out by two doctors together. This may be two paediatricians or a paediatrician and a police surgeon. This gives the opportunity for two opinions and should prevent any re-investigation and re-examination of a child. Signs change so quickly in the genital area with acute injury healing rapidly, it is important that opinions are given at a combined examination rather than sequentially. Repeated examinations are abusive to a child.

Any doctor who deals with children should be aware of the possibility of sexual abuse and refer to the expert in the area if appropriate. The main responsibility of the referring doctor is to keep an accurate record of what was said and what is known. There is rarely a need for immediate detailed clinical examination.

Why Examine?

Where there is a history of possible injury, or where forensic evidence may be available, examination is essential. In many cases of alleged sexual abuse there are no positive physical findings. However, the examination is important to exclude injury, to confirm to the parents and to the child the lack of physical harm and to reassure the child of her or his genital and anal normality.

Permission for Examination

In *Working Together under The Children Act 1989* (1991), it is made clear that a child must give permission for a medical examination. In addition, if the child is under 16 years, someone with parental responsibility must give consent. If the child is unable to give permission (e.g. is severely handicapped or immature) and unable to understand what is being requested, parental permission only will be obtained. However, if a parent demands an examination and the child refuses, then the child's wishes must be accepted.

Confidentiality

Doctors are rightly concerned to maintain confidentiality towards their patients. However, the over-riding principle in child protection work is to protect the child and secure the best possible outcome for him or her. The needs of the child must always be regarded as of first importance, as her age and vulnerability render her powerless to protect her own interest.

> The present GMC guidance published in May 1993, states *where a doctor believes that the patient may be the victim of abuse or neglect, the patient's interests are paramount and will usually require a doctor to disclose information to an appropriate responsible person or officer of a statutory agency* (see Diagnosis of Child Sexual Abuse, 1988; Working Together under The Children Act, 1989, 1991; Child Protection Registers, 1993).

THE MEDICAL HISTORY AND EXAMINATION

History

If a full interview has been carried out by members of the Child Protection Team, the doctors should be informed of their findings before they see the child and her carers. They should then talk to the child with any adult or adults that the child chooses to be present. A full medical, family and social history is taken. It may be necessary to ask some specific points relating to the alleged abuse which would help in the examination. In the medical history it is of particular importance to note any history of allergy or skin disorder which could lead to genital soreness, any history of vaginal discharge, with or without itchiness, any previous urinary tract infection and any history of bowel disorder (in particular constipation or bleeding per rectum). A note should be made of any medications the child is on, or any chronic disorder the child suffers from. In a girl the menstrual history is important, noting the age of menarche, the regularity of periods and the date of the last period. A note should be made of whether or not internal sanitary protection is used. A girl should be asked if she has had or has any boyfriends and if so whether she has had intercourse in the past and if so, how long ago. Specific details of the alleged abuse, when volunteered, should be written in the words of the child.

Examination

It is important to reassure a child, respect his or her anxiety, explain what is going to happen and that it will not be painful. The child should choose who remains in the room during examination. An adolescent may prefer to have no accompanying adult present. It is convenient to have a room which can be divided by a curtain so that the examination can be carried out in private, but if required a parent or professional carer can be present but out of view.

Make a full and thorough examination. This includes height and weight. It is unnecessary and embarrassing for a girl or boy to be naked and feel exposed during this process. It is kinder to examine parts of the body sequentially, covering up each area as the examination is completed. Examine the abdomen and external genitalia with the child covered by a sheet and lying on an examination couch. By judiciously moving the sheet, embarrassment is reduced and yet good exposure can be ensured. It is important to have a good light source preferably with a magnifying lens and a colposcope. (Some doctors prefer to examine children in the knee-chest position. Although this gives a better view of the vaginal walls and sometimes of the hymenal edge, some children dislike the position.) Look carefully for evidence of physical injury, such as grip marks to arms and legs, love bites, or pinches to any part of the body, including the breasts. Oral injury and soft palate trauma may occur with oral intercourse. Note the degree of sexual maturity.

When examining the genitalia, identify the anatomy (see Fig. 19.1), look for evidence of redness, swelling, bruising, lacerations or discharge. Look carefully

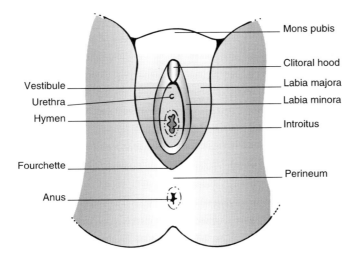

Fig. 19.1 Diagram of post-pubertal female external genitalia.

for scars, especially on the posterior fourchette and the hymen. Note the hymenal shape and thickness, orifice size and contour.

The hymenal edge may be better viewed with the aid of Glaister rods. It may be necessary to do a digital vaginal examination although in young, non-sexually active girls, consideration should be given to performing this under a general anaesthetic. Be gentle, using one finger and only introducing a second, if the first examination is not painful. Note how 'roomy' or otherwise the vagina feels.

The perianal region is examined with the child curled up in the left lateral position. Note the anal tone and appearance. The perianal skin should be healthy. It is sometimes dusky in colour, but this is a normal finding. The perianal veins encircle the anus and are especially prominent in a semicircle towards the back when the rectum is full or there is a history of constipation. Reflex anal dilatation should be looked for and noted (see p. 362). Anal fissures (Fig. 19.2), skin tags, swelling, bruising, soreness, lacerations or scratches should be sought. If an examination is very painful by virtue of the degree of injury sustained, then an assessment may require a general anaesthetic, but this is seldom necessary.

Findings

External genitalia – girls

Redness

Redness of the vestibule and vulvar area is a non-specific finding. It is present whenever there is local irritation, such as scratching (e.g. in a child with threadworms), sensitivity to bubble bath, enuresis and poor personal hygiene. Redness

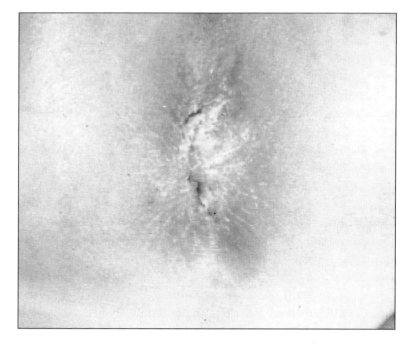

Fig. 19.2 Anal fissure.

of the skin may accompany a discharge in a child with local bacterial infection (see p. 108). Bright red painful erythema of the vulval area can occur with a streptococcal infection. *Herpes simplex* infections produce painful blisters on a red base see p. Bruising may be caused by recent abuse from rubbing or injury (Fig. 19.3) McCann found that 25% of pre-pubertal girls have non-specific redness of the vestibule (McCann *et al.*, 1990).

Swelling

Like redness, swelling is a non-specific sign and may accompany any local infection or irritation.

Injury

Bruising in the vulvar area may be accidental or inflicted. Accidental straddle injuries usually cause bruising and injury over bony areas (Fig. 19.4), such as pubic bones and the anterior part of the vulva, whereas sexual abuse with attempted or forced penetration causes injury to the posterior fourchette (often in the midline posteriorly) with or without hymenal tears. Accidental injury may be accompanied by grazes to the inner leg and are usually more prominent to one side, suggesting a fall astride a hard surface (Pierce and Robson, 1993). Abuse may be accompanied by grip marks to the thighs in an attempt to abduct the legs.

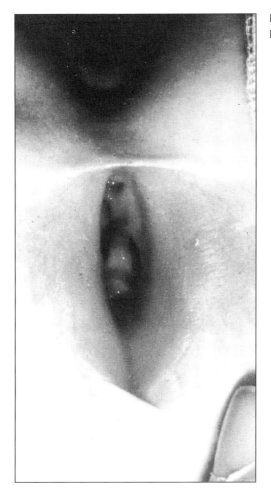

Fig. 19.3 Redness of the vulvar orifice produced by fondling.

Discharge

Leucorrhoea is normal during and after puberty. A frank purulent discharge implies infection or the presence of a foreign body in the vagina. A bloody discharge suggests the presence of a foreign body or a malignancy and warrants examination under anaesthetic. Threadworms with scratching and secondary infection may cause a discharge. Candidiasis gives a creamy, itchy discharge. A firm diagnosis will require swabs for microscopy, culture and sensitivity. The presence of gonococcal infection suggests sexual abuse. Chlamydial infections can be transmitted by hand, but abuse must be considered.

Hymen

The hymen may be thin and narrow or thick and fleshy with folds. The hymen tends to be more fleshy with increasing sexual maturity. It may have a circular

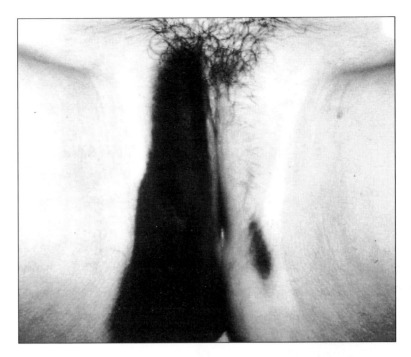

Fig. 19.4   Extensive vulvar bruising due to straddle injury.

shape or be crescentic with an absent anterior margin. The hymenal edge may be sharp or rolled and little mounds or projections may be present on the edge. McCann looked at 114 pre-pubertal girls with no history of sexual abuse and found 34% had mounds, 33% projections and 18.5% septal remants. The mounds tend to be between 11 and 1 o'clock on the hymen. Hymenal septi were rare (2.5%) but bands (usually bilateral) were common. Vaginal ridges and rugae could be seen in 90% of cases (McCann *et al.*, 1990). Notches were present in 6%. Hymenal irregularity is not uncommon but deep V notches to the base of the hymen or absence of the hymenal wall posteriorly suggests scarring and previous injury (Fig. 19.5). The orifice size varies according to the method by which examination is done (the labia separated or traction applied) and the position (the child prone or in knee–chest position) and as the vagina is a muscular tube the hymen can 'wink', i.e. open and close, while watched. Too much emphasis should not be placed solely on hymenal opening measurements.

If a girl alleges sexual abuse with full penetration, it may be necessary to do a digital examination of the vagina. One finger should be introduced into the vagina and a second only if the first causes no pain. The ease with which the examination can be carried out should be reported and the roominess of the vagina should be noted. A capacious vagina suggests repeated vaginal penetration and is compatible with frequent sexual intercourse or insertion of other objects.

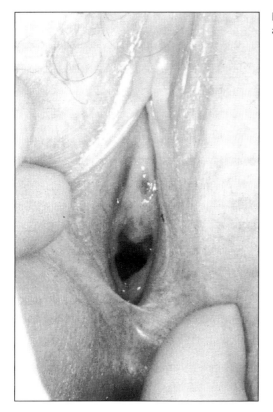

Fig. 19.5 Deep 'V' notches in the hymen as a result of sexual abuse.

Posterior fourchette

The posterior fourchette is stretched and injured in forced penetrative vaginal intercourse. The injury sustained is usually in the midline. This heals quickly and leaves a linear scar. However, if vaginal entry has been unforced the posterior fourchette may stretch without tearing and subsequent scarring.

Anus

Anal tone may be affected by the presence of faeces in the rectum, a history of chronic constipation or abuse. Hypertrophy of the external sphincter has been described in repeated anal sexual abuse, giving the 'tyre sign' (Bamfird and Kiff, 1987). Anal scars and skin tags are markers for old injury to the anal verge and are more common in sexually abused children than non-abused children, but are not a reliable sign of abuse. Anal fissures are associated with bowel disorders or abuse and medical reasons for anal abnormalities must be excluded. The anal orifice when dilated is circular and smooth. A very irregular orifice (not to be confused with the presence of anal ampullae) suggests chronic injury. Fresh multiple anal fissures with swelling of the perianal verge and soiling and incontinence are found in recent forced, aggressive anal sexual intercourse, but, 'if the act has been performed carefully, or if the passive agent is habituated, no signs may be found as the anus can undergo considerable distension without injury if it is dilated slowly' (Gordon *et al.*, 1988).

Perianal skin and veins

Perianal skin may be dusky in colour. This is a normal variant. Bruising in this area, especially on the anal verge is unusual in accidental injury. Perianal veins appear distended and full when the rectum is full. If the buttocks are separated and the veins observed for a minute or more, they are seen to distend gradually. This is more prominent in the posterior half of the circle of veins surrounding the anus. In chronic anal sexual abuse the veins may be prominent and one of the last signs to disappear when abuse ceases (Hobbs and Wynne, 1993).

Reflex anal dilatation

This test is carried out by separating the buttocks and observing the anus for about 30 seconds. The anus will gradually open as the external sphincter relaxes. In true reflex anal dilatation the internal sphincter also relaxes so that the rectal mucosa is visible. The normal anus can dilate to about 2 cm with a round orifice. This 'reflex' is present in a higher proportion of sexually abused children than non-abused children, but alone it has a poor discriminator value in the diagnosis of anal abuse in children. Its presence may add weight to other positive evidence of abuse.

Warts

These may be transmitted by sexual contact or by hand. It is important to know who has hand or genital warts in the home. They may be spread by self contact if the child has warts on their own hands. Perianal warts and vulval warts may be transmitted in this way. Warts on the hymen suggest sexual contact and the presence of warts on the genitalia of the suspected or alleged offender is significant. The type of wart virus may help to differentiate the cause and possible mode of transmission.

Pregnancy

This is the one single positive physical finding that confirms sexual intercourse.

Forensic examination

This includes the taking of specimens for medico-legal purposes. The labelling, packaging, transport and manner of taking specimens is important for legal credibility. This is outside the scope of this Chapter.

DIFFERENTIAL DIAGNOSIS

Some alternative causes for various physical findings have already been given. Skin disorders, such as lichen sclerosis or psoriasis which are confined to the genital area, can bleed and may be mistaken for sexual abuse. The presence of a skin disease does not exclude sexual abuse, but the natural history of the dermatological disorder must be understood. Causes of vaginal irritation, such as bubble bath, threadworms, simple infections, thrush, must be considered. Diabetes and urinary tract infections should be excluded. Bowel disorders must be considered in any child with abnormal anal findings. The possibility of accidental injury must be considered.

EXPLANATION TO THE CHILD

After the examination, discuss the findings with the examinee and accompanying person, if the child agrees. If there are no positive findings, explain that this does not mean that a history of touching or indecent assault is disbelieved. Reassure the child that their genitalia and anal area is entirely normal and ask if they have any questions for you and give them the opportunity to come back and discuss any problems at a later date should they need to do so.

TREATMENT

If there is any possibility of pregnancy the morning after pill should be prescribed (see p. 343). Two tablets are swallowed in front of the doctor and two 12 hours later. If the pills are vomited, a repeat dose must be given.

SEXUALLY TRANSMITTED DISEASES (see Chapter 10)

Clinical findings may suggest the presence of an STD and appropriate bacteriological and viral swabs must be taken. Many girls and boys will be anxious about the likelihood of having contracted HIV infection. All these patients should be referred to an STD specialist who can investigate, treat and counsel as necessary.

Acute injury may occasionally require examination and treatment under general anaesthetic, but this is rare. Any infection that is found will need treatment.

RECORDS

Keep detailed, contemporaneous, complete and careful notes. Diagrams are very helpful in demonstrating genital findings and physical injuries. Any descriptions of alleged abuse by the child should be quoted in full, using his or her vocabulary. Note his or her emotional state. Record negative as well as positive physical findings. A police statement or social services report will probably have to be based on these notes. The child and carer should be aware of this.

REFERRAL

Some girls or boys will benefit from referral to a counsellor, psychologist, or psychiatrist. If a child has a STD or is pregnant, appropriate referrals must be made for her physical welfare. After some injuries, it is clinically necessary to review the child and note healing. This review is an opportunity for further discussion and reassurance.

CASE CONFERENCE

A case conference is called when the child is considered to be at ongoing risk of further abuse. In many areas a conference is held following all cases of abuse. It is essential in intrafamilial abuse. It is important that the doctor should attend a case conference, as important decisions concerning the child's welfare are made and the medical input into this decision is valuable. A typed medical report should be taken to the case conference or sent to the conference before it is held.

REFERENCES

Baker AW, Duncan SP, 1985: Child sexual abuse – a study in prevalence in Great Britain. *Child Abuse and Neglect* **9**, 457–488.

Bamfird F, Kiff ES, 1987: Child sexual abuse (letter). *Lancet*, **ii**, 1396.

Bamford F, Roberts R, 1989: Child sexual abuse – I. In Meadows R (ed.), *ABC of child abuse*, London: British Medical Journal, 29–30.

Child Abuse Studies Unit, Polytechnic North London 1993. Quoted in *National Childrens Home factfile: British children in need 1993*. London: NCH, 59.

Child Abuse–Working Together, 1988: DHSS Guidance issued under HC(88) 38/LAC(88)10. London: HMSO.

Child Protection Registers 1993: In *National Childrens Home factfile. British children in need 1993*. London: NCH, 54–55.

Child protection: Medical responsibilities, 1993: Draft guidance produced by a joint working party of the Department of Health, British Medical Association and Conference of Medical Royal Colleges. London: Department of Health.

Children and young people who sexually abuse other children, 1993. In *National Childrens Home factfile: British children in need 1993*. London: NCH, 59.

Diagnosis of child sexual abuse: guidance for doctors, 1988: Prepared by the Standing Medical Advisory Committee for the Secretaries of State and Social Services and Wales. London: HMSO, 1, Appendix B, 34–36.

Finkelhor D, Williams LM, 1988: Perpetrators in nursery crimes. In Finkelhor D, Williams LM (eds), *Sexual abuse in day care*. London: Sage, 57.

Gordon I, Shapiro HA, Berson SD, 1988: *Forensic medicine: a guide to principles*. London: Churchill Livingstone, 361.

Hobbs CJ, Wynne JM, 1993: The evaluation of child sexual abuse. In Hobbs J, Wynne JM (eds), *Clinical paediatrics – child abuse*. London: Bailliere Tindall.

Hobbs CJ, Wynne JM, Hanks HGI, 1991: Sexual abuse. *Current Paediatrics* **1**, 157–165.

Home Office (in conjunction with Department of Health), 1992: Memorandom of good practice. On video recorded interviews with child witnesses for criminal proceedings. And Appendix B. Criminal Justice Act 1988 Section 32a. London: HMSO.

Horne L, Glasgow D, Cox A, Calam R, 1991: Sexual abuse of children by children. *The Journal of Child Law* September–December, 147–151.

Kempe RS, Kempe CH, 1984: *Sexual abuse of children and adolescents*. New York: Freeman.

Macleod M, Saraga E, 1981: Challenging the orthodoxy: towards a feminist theory and practise. In *Feminist review: family secrets – child sexual abuse* no. 28.

McCann J, Wells R, Simon M, Voris J, 1990: Genital findings in prepubertal girls selected for non abuse. *Pediatrics* **86**, 428–439.

Pierce AM, Robson WR, 1993: Genital injuries in girls – accidental or not? *Pediatric Surgery International* **8**, 239–243.

Report of the Inquiry into Child Abuse in Cleveland 1987, 1988. London: HMSO.

Schecter MD, Roberge L, 1976: Sexual exploitation. In Helfer RE, Kempe CH (eds), *Child abuse and neglect: the family and the community*. Cambridge MA: Ballinger.

Spencer MJ, Dunklee P, 1986: Sexual abuse of boys. *Pediatrics* **78**, 133–138.

Working Together Under the Children Act 1989, 1991: 3.2, 3.12, 3.15. London: HMSO, 9–12; Appendix 2: 1.4, 63.

CHAPTER 20

Emotional aspects

SAM WARNER ————————————————————————

Children who have been sexually abused can suffer from a range of emotional consequences and much discussion in recent years has focused around attempts to develop a model which can encapsulate the effects. This has proved difficult, primarily because most studies have found that the impact of sexual abuse produces many effects, rather than a core symptomatology (Kendall-Tackett *et al.*, 1993).

One model which I have found useful in understanding the different aspects associated with being sexually abused is the Traumagenic Dynamics model proposed by Finkelhor and Browne (1985). Using this model, I want to look at some of the issues for sexually abused children in order to highlight the specific emotional consequences. I will then address some factors which may mediate the effects of sexual abuse. Finally, I want to look at some of the ways children communicate their emotional distress. The conclusions I draw, and the interpretations I make, are based on my experience as a clinician working with sexually abused children and adolescents.[1]

APPLYING THE MODEL

Finkelhor and Browne (1985) suggest four main dynamics that may account for the range of effects of sexual abuse. These are:

1. powerlessness
2. betrayal
3. stigmatisation
4. traumatic sexualisation.

I will address each of these dynamics in turn, highlighting the specific issues involved and relating them to the likely emotional consequences found in sexually abused children.

---

[1] Throughout the chapter I refer to the abused child as 'she', as this is a textbook on adolescent gynaecology. However, the majority of comments apply equally to boys.

Powerlessness

Most definitions of child sexual abuse (CSA) emphasise the abuse of power as being a key element in understanding the experience of sexual abuse (Macloed and Saraga, 1987). When a child is sexually abused her body is violated. The child's wishes are disregarded and overridden. The child has no choice and no control over what happens to her. The child constantly lives with threat: the threat that it may happen again and that she or the people she loves may be hurt if she does not do as the abuser demands. The physical experience of powerlessness translates into a number of key emotional issues.

Anxiety and fear

Being vulnerable and unable to protect oneself leaves the child with increased levels of fear and anxiety. This is the case whether or not any actual threats were made by the abuser. Sexual abuse can take place in seconds, so the fear of being re-abused may be present for the child whenever she is in situations where the abuser may be present. This may be an almost permanent emotional state for the child who is sexually abused in her own home, which is commonly where most sexual abuse occurs. Anticipatory anxiety is associated with returning to the place where abuse occurs and then waiting for the inevitable.

Fear and anxiety may be further exacerbated by additional threats of harm to the child and others. These may be real or imagined. Children are still largely brought up to obey adults, particularly those adults who have direct control over their lives, such as parents and teachers. Such perceived threats may induce as much fear and anxiety as actual threats by the abuser. Actual threats may include the removal of positives, such as love; as well as the addition of negatives, such as pain. Threats to the self may lose their potency as the child becomes accustomed to being hurt. Consequently, threats are often levelled against people and things the child loves, such as carers, siblings, family pets and toys. Interestingly, these may provide catalysts for disclosing abuse. For example, it is not uncommon for a child to tell when a sibling reaches the same age as the abused child was at the onset of abuse.

Fear and anxiety regarding the abuse may generalise to all situations and people associated with being abused. For example, children may show fear of all bathrooms, if this is where abuse normally happened. Girls often become fearful of all men and become anxious when men are around.

Depression and helplessness

As the child learns that she has no control over what happens to her body and that her wishes and needs have no status, a profound sense of helplessness can be internalised. Sexually abused children often talk about 'trying to get it right'. As the child strives to understand why she is being abused and hurt, often by someone she loves, she looks for the things she may have done wrong in the belief that if only she could be 'good', it would not happen. As it is never the child's fault she can never 'get it right'. She comes to learn that whatever she does has no effect. In her attempt to rationalise the abuse she may come to believe that she is 'bad'. These dual feelings of helplessness and badness can often lead to depression and sadness.

Helplessness may be further reinforced after disclosure via the investigative process, which affords the child very little control. Feelings of sadness may be compounded with grief as the child experiences the loss of the good relationship with, and the expectation of care from, the abuser.

Psychological splitting

For the child who has been sexually abused the world can become split into abusers and victims. As the child internalises her helplessness in relation to the abuser, she can come to perceive herself as a victim in all situations. This may lead to further abuse as she both fails to protect herself ('whatever I do has no effect, so I cannot avoid it') and accepts any negative consequences ('I deserve it'). Adopting a victim role can also affect the child's ability to deal with emotional difficulties after detection. This is because a child who remains a victim cannot actively take part in her recovery. Her coping style is psychologically damaging, because from this perspective there is no hope in a better future; simply the expectation of more of the same.

Conversely, some children reject the victim role in favour of their only perceived alternative which is becoming abusive towards others, either physically and/or sexually. This is because the child's main experience of control is of the abuser and so control and power come to mean abuse. This appears to be less common in girls and may be related to societal expectations of the role of women as carers and non-aggressors.

Another corollary of splitting is that of idealisation, whereby the child invests those people who do not abuse with all things good. Minor transgression can have a profound psychological impact on the child, engendering renewed fear and anxiety that the idealised person is now a potential abuser. In order to defend against such feelings, children sometimes refuse to accept information which tarnishes the idealised image.

Finally, the child may split off parts of herself which are psychologically unbearable. If the child has internalised that it is 'bad' children who are sexually abused, she may attempt to split off from this aspect of her personality. Each time she is sexually abused is a confirmation of her 'badness'. Defending against feelings of despair and depression associated with being wholly bad may result in the child denying that the abuse is happening to her. In its most extreme form this has been characterised as 'multiple-personality disorder'.

Dissociation

Another consequence of being powerless, which is related to splitting, is dissociation. One way children can cope with being sexually abused is by psychologically removing themselves from the situation. The child may have no control over what happens to her body, but can project her mind elsewhere. For example, children may visualise themselves on the ceiling or doing some favoured activity. Again this can become generalised to other stressful situations and is characterised by concentration problems, 'day-dreaming', emotional distancing and inappropriate affect.

Psychological defences such as splitting and dissociation can be so powerful that the child can actually 'forget' the sexual abuse, when it is not occurring or after it has stopped. However, the memory is not lost from the mind entirely, only from conscious thought. Hence feelings of free-floating anxiety, fear and depression will persist and the trauma may be re-experienced via intrusive thoughts, nightmares and sudden feelings.

Betrayal

There are two main features of betrayal which have an emotional impact on the child. These are the betrayal of her need to be protected and the betrayal of her need not to be harmed.

Betrayal may be most keenly felt by the child who has been abused by someone with whom she has a close relationship, such as a father or brother. As Finkelhor (1987) notes, feelings of betrayal will be affected by how much the child perceived the abuser to be a good carer prior to the abuse. Thus, there may be less sense of betrayal by an abuser who was never caring. Many abusers will have demonstrated some prior care. It is easier to gain access to children and to draw children in, if initially the abuser appears to be caring.

Loss

The experience of being sexually abused can leave the child with severe feelings of loss. She has lost the carer who has become the abuser. She may also feel that she has lost relationships with other people round her, such as her mother and siblings. This loss may be compounded by the abuser who often attempts to isolate the child from other family and peers, in order to decrease the likelihood of detection. Loss of and betrayal by others may be particularly intense where the child believes others to know about the abuse and not to act. Loss adds to the child's feelings of depression and sadness. This sadness will be further intensified as the child compares herself to her peers and becomes aware of the loss of her childhood.

Rejection and alienation

When a child has been betrayed by one adult, she may still search for care and protection from another. In doing this children often become extremely dependent and 'clingy'. This may result in the non-abusing carer pulling away because of her (or his) own feelings of being smothered. This can increase the child's feelings of rejection and alienation, which have already been initiated by the abuser's betrayal.

Mistrust

To some degree, all abused children will experience a lowering of trust in others. For some children there can also be a lowering of trust in themselves and their ability to make judgements and a commensurate decrease in their self-confidence. The child may learn to mistrust her judgements when someone she perceived as caring has subsequently abused her. The child can also be left with very confused feelings and related cognitive distortions where the abuser has repeatedly told her that she enjoys the abuse and where her body has responded to sexual stimulation. Experiences of abuse can therefore affect a child's actual and perceived ability to make judgements.

Anger and hostility

A common response to betrayal is anger and hostility. However, anger is an extremely powerful emotion and the abused child often copes with it by sub-merging and denying it. The child may feel that her anger is so great that if she showed some of it she would lose control and her anger would destroy the people around her. At the very least, she may believe that if the people around her witnessed her anger they would reject her, something she is already sensi-tive to.

As with all submerged emotions, expression will be given to them elsewhere. If they are well defended against, indiscriminate expression of hostility and aggression can be experienced as particularly frightening, because they have no obvious source. Alternatively, many abused children, especially girls, turn their anger inwards, directing it against themselves through self-harming behaviour. Anger with the self is often compounded by self-blame for not stopping the abuse. Although the major source of betrayal is the abuser, it may be too fright-ening to direct there. This is another key reason why anger will be directed else-where at 'safer' targets. For example, the abused child may initially express hostility towards the non-abusing carer and professionals, rather than the actual abuser.

Stigmatisation

This refers to the way the child's self-concept is attacked through the experience of being sexually abused. The negative messages which surround the abuse, and which are reinforced by the abuser and directed towards the child, become inter-nalised. Children learn about themselves and their place in the world through the relationships they have. As such, if a child's main relationship has been abusive, she may come to learn that she is bad and worthless. This dynamic is particularly powerful for the child who has been abused from an early age and has had little chance to develop a resilient positive self-image and where the child has been denied access to other good relationships through which positive aspects of the self could be experienced and internalised.

Guilt

Most children who have been sexually abused will be left with some feelings of guilt. A child who feels responsible for the abuse is much less likely to tell and so the abuser will encourage the child to blame herself. This has the additional purpose of reducing the abuser's own internal inhibitors against abusing. He can persuade himself that the child wanted sexual contact by sexualising the child's need for love and affection. Many abusers 'groom' children for later abuse by starting with non-sexual contact, such as hugs, which the child enjoys. Such gradual onset can compound the child's feelings of guilt as she will be unsure of when the actual abuse started and may indeed continue to gain some enjoyment from the physical closeness and affection, if this is still part of it.

As the abuse continues and the child comes to know that it is wrong, her guilt may be exacerbated because of feelings that she should have stopped it earlier. Most children by the age of nine or ten will have a clear understanding of the prohibitions against sexual abuse. This may happen earlier and is related to the developmental level of the child and her access to other sources of information outside of the family, such as school and television.

Guilt feelings are especially engendered where the child has been made to be an active participator in the abuse. This includes activities in which the child has been made to perform sexual acts on the abuser or other children, the child has been sexually stimulated and experienced orgasms or where the child has been made to seek out the abuser. The reasons why the child does this becomes secondary to the actual activity. For example, one girl talked about going to her abuser's bedroom because she could not bear the wait for the inevitable abuse. She carried an enormous amount of guilt for this long after the abuse had stopped.

Wider systems and society can confirm the child's guilt. Very often the result of telling about abuse is the break-up of the family, for which the child may feel responsible and also blamed. The child may experience direct blame from other adults, in comments such as, 'she was no angel'. Media images and texts which infantilise women's sexuality and sexualize children's can further attenuate the guilt feelings of the child. Additionally, society often demands an unequivocal response from the child regarding the abuser. This may not be possible, when the child often both loves the abuser and hates the abuse. All these things serve to disable the child with guilt.

NEGATIVE SELF-IMAGE AND LOWERED SELF-ESTEEM

As the child learns that sexual abuse is regarded as dirty and wrong, these aspects may become internalised by the child as integral parts of her. Unless she is able to split these parts off, this will have a deleterious effect on her self-image. The secretiveness which surrounds sexual abuse further attests to its (and her) dirtiness.

The physical side of sexual abuse is often accompanied by verbal abuse by the abuser, whereby the child may be told that she is 'dirty' or a 'slag'. These are words that she will also hear from her peers in the playground at school, which are applied to promiscuous girls. Wider society reinforces these messages with its emphasis on female virginity and its condemnation of girls who are sexually active. The child will recognise herself in these descriptions and internalise the accompanying sense of badness and with it lowered self-esteem. Each time the child is re-abused, her badness is reinforced and her lowered self-worth and negative self-concept reconfirmed and strengthened.

Differentness

In her attempts to understand why she is being abused the child may also come to see herself as a freak, somehow different from other children. Differentness may be internalised as another negative component of her personality, thus adding to her feelings of isolation and alienation. The child who believes she is somehow a freak may withdraw from relationships for fear of contaminating others or in the belief that others will reject her anyway. This may be further reinforced by the abuser isolating the child from other family members and friends.

Unclear boundaries

The repeated attacks on the child's self-concept and the very real experiences of having her body invaded can leave the child with some confusion about where she stops and others begin. This is particularly the case where abuse has started at a very early age (under five years), when the child is just beginning to develop an understanding of the world as separate and independent of her. However, for all abused children, it remains important for those around them to set very clear, explicit boundaries if they are going to be able to experience some sense of safety.

Traumatic Sexualisation

Children typically show interest in their own and other people's bodies. Children under five years will giggle over 'bottom' jokes. Whilst there may be scant understanding, older children up to the age of about twelve will be curious about sex, joke about sex and play sexually exploratory games with peers, such as 'doctors and nurses'. Sexual relationships begin in earnest in adolescence.

When a child has been sexually abused, her normal sexual development is traumatised. The development of her sexual identity and feelings are distorted by inappropriate sexual attention which is beyond her control and which is developmentally incongruent. This can lead to a number of effects.

Sexual identity

Experiences of sexual abuse can lead to some confusion over sexual identity in late puberty, but more commonly in adolescence, when it becomes of paramount importance. Because of adverse sexual experiences with men, some girls may question their heterosexual identity. It should be stated, however, that for some girls becoming a lesbian is a positive choice in favour of women, not simply a rejection of men.

The older child can experience a numbing of sexual feelings, because of negative associations with sex and sometimes feel 'asexual'. She may feel that her sexual identity, like the rest of herself, is rotten and corrupting and be unable to positively reconcile herself with her sexual self. In order to defend against these attacks on her self-concept, she may deny her sexuality altogether.

Inappropriate sexual feelings and behaviour

Inappropriate sexual feelings can be manifest in a number of ways. At the most simple, a child's sense of what is appropriate sexual behaviour can become distorted through the process of being sexually abused. Sometimes children come to confuse sex with receiving and giving care and affection. This can lead to a child offering herself sexually to peers and adults in the belief that this is the only way closeness and affection can be achieved. This can have additional problems for adolescent girls who, as noted early, are heavily stigmatised for being sexually active.

Another problem sometimes encountered is with the abused child becoming inappropriately sexualized to younger children herself. This can lead the child to being sexually abusive to other children. More commonly, girls carry the anxiety and fear that they will sexually abuse others, when there is very little chance that they will. This anxiety is provoked by societal myths that all sexual abusers have been sexually abused themselves. Most girls who have been sexually abused are not sexually abusive towards others.

Fear of sexual intimacy

Obviously, because of the negative associations with sex, some abused girls can experience difficulties in adolescence in having sexual relationships with peers. The girl may feel that she cannot enter into any close relationship because of the fear that she will be further abused or that she would be unable to stop the relationship progressing to activities with which she feels uncomfortable. Her fear may be so great the she cannot enter into any intimate relationships at all, particularly where she has learned that intimacy equals sex equals abuse.

MEDIATING FACTORS

Some children come through experiences of sexual abuse with very few or none of the emotional difficulties which I have described, while others are severely affected. I have given some indication of why some differences may be found. Additionally, there are a number of other factors which have been suggested as having particular importance in mediating the effects of sexual abuse. These factors do not impact in isolation and their effect can only be considered as part of the whole experience of abuse. There are two general areas which should be considered. The first area relates to features of the abusive experience and the second area relates to issues following disclosure.

FEATURES OF THE ABUSE

There is some evidence to suggest that increased severity of abuse, in terms of anal, oral and/or vaginal penetration, is associated with increased symptomatology (Kendall-Tackett *et al.*, 1993). Abuse which is frequent and continues for a sustained period of time is also associated with greater emotional disturbance (Kendall-Tackett *et al.*, 1993).

It has also been suggested that sexual abuse which has ritualistic and/or sadistic features is associated with more severe emotional disturbance (Kelly and Scott, 1991). However, as satanic abuse is only a relatively new area of concern and discussion, the specific issues and consequences need exploring.

It is important that artificial hierarchies of distress created for abused children are not solely based on features of the abuse without reference to other factors. There is a danger that children's distress can be minimised because they do not appear to have suffered severely. Clinicians should always remain mindful of what the child is actually presenting with and not be led by what the child 'should' be feeling. This is especially so as many children initially only reveal a limited amount of information about their abuse. It may be many years before they reveal the full story.

AFTER THE CHILD HAS TOLD

The single most important factor that can ameliorate the effects of abuse is that the child is believed. The child may have been told by the abuser that she will not be believed and her fear will be that this will be true. If a child is not believed then her sense of betrayal, worthlessness and isolation is increased. I would also argue that, for the very few children who make false accusations of sexual abuse, understanding should still be proffered. This is because such accusations are usually an indication of other areas of distress and upset for the child which need addressing.

Sometimes the child's story may change. This may be for a variety of reasons. For example, the child may minimise the abuse in order to protect the abuser and/or the non-abusing carer or she may tell professionals what she thinks they want to hear. Sometimes children will initially describe a single event so that should the consequences of telling become too painful she can retract her story. Detailed descriptions are harder to deny later. Children again should not be condemned for this but reassured that they have a right to live without abuse and that they will continue to be listened to when they feel able to tell again.

Involvement in criminal proceedings can have a deleterious emotional effect on the child, where the child must face the abuser in court and where there is a long delay between initial investigations and trial. There is some provision for younger children to give evidence at court through a video link, so that they do not have to be physically present in the same room as their abuser. Emotionally, the child lives in a state of limbo until the trial is completed. She also cannot let go of her anxiety while ever she lives with the fear of facing her abuser again. She may also experience the medical examination and the necessity to repeat her story to a wide number of professionals as abusive.

Another important issue following disclosure of abuse is family support. In particular, mothers who are supportive of their children can greatly help in their recovery. It is crucial therefore that mothers are supported at this time. They will have their own issues to address relating to their feelings about the abuse and the possible relationships they have lost as a result of this (particularly where the abuser was a partner) and sometimes resurfacing of unresolved issues relating to their own abuse as a child. It is common for such feelings to re-emerge when a woman discovers that her child has been sexually abused. Often the best support professionals can offer an abused child is to empower the mother to care for and protect her child in the future.

COMMUNICATING EMOTIONAL DISTRESS

It is often difficult for adults to hear children tell about sexual abuse because of the pain engendered, particularly where the adult knows the child. Many children never directly tell about the abuse because of the pressure exerted on them by abusers to keep them silent and compliant. There is a need to be aware of the various ways children communicate, consciously and unconsciously, distress through their behaviour.

Inappropriate sexual behaviour and knowledge is the most obvious feature associated with sexual abuse. Judgements about this should be made with reference to the developmental level of the child. A child may attempt to tell indirectly about her abuse through her play, drawing and writing. The older child may tell stories about a friend who has been sexually abused in order to gain information about the likely consequence of breaking her own silence. The younger child may talk about 'monsters' not because she is deliberately disguising her abuser, but because she has no other words to describe what is happening to her. Additionally, abusers often use innocuous words to describe sexual acts, such as 'lollipops' instead of fellatio, so that should a younger child 'tell', she would not necessarily be heard.

The child may become overcompliant with adults; always seeking to please. She may also appear to be wary and suspicious. This may be accompanied by anxious clinging to the (non-abusing) caretaker. Abused children often regress to an earlier stage of development. This indicates both a desire to return to a time prior to the abuse and also the wish to be cared for as a child and not as an adult sexual partner. This may be demonstrated both in terms of behaviour and speech. A particularly eloquent communication is where the child starts bed-wetting after previously being dry.

The child may demonstrate her fear of particular adults and places by a number of methods. The younger child may become tearful and distressed or throw a tantrum. The older child may actively avoid particular adults or places. For example, she may start staying out late. As stated previously, this fear and resultant avoidance behaviour may generalise to similar places and people. Ultimately the child may try to escape. For the older child this may include psychological escape through drug and alcohol abuse or physical escape by withdrawing or running away.

Related to this is the potential for self-harm. Low self-esteem coupled with a limited ability to control the external world can lead to high incidences of deliberate self-harm, a disregard for personal welfare and eating disorders, such as bulimia and anorexia nervosa.

Submerged feelings may be expressed through nightmares and night terrors. During the day 'inexplicable' outbursts of anger may be noted or high levels of irritability and low tolerance of even minor stressors. The child may also appear to have low levels of concentration and a tendency to switch off or day-dream.

The child may engage in 'attention-seeking' behaviour, in an attempt to motivate adults to ask why she is behaving in this way. Behavioural problems such as lying, stealing and acting out at school may be observed. Sometimes the child may make repeated presentations to the G.P. or hospital casualty department. Girls sometimes fear that the abuse has caused them permanent harm and may need medical reassurance that they can still conceive, for example. Additionally, sometimes girls harbour fantasies that any gynaecological problems they may have are directly related to the abuse and are consequently 'their fault'. Again, there is a need for reassurance that they are not to blame.

These behaviours will persist until someone hears the child. They will continue until the issues have been resolved and the threat of abuse has receded. The abuser may continue to exert an influence over the child many years after the abuse has stopped. This is because the psychological power the abuser has over the child does not necessarily recede once the physical threat is removed.

The difference between normal and abnormal stages of development are often small and may be affected by other issues such as learning difficulties. Additionally, some of the emotions and behaviour may indicate other stressors in the child's life or have an organic basis. Caution should be exercised in over-interpreting single behaviours. Real and sudden changes in behaviour should be looked for, although this may not be evident when sexual abuse has been happening for some time and the onset has been gradual. Finally, when making judgements about a child's behaviour reference should be made to the child's individual personality, her specific cultural and religious background and other life events which may have affected her behaviour.

SUMMARY

Children who have been sexually abused can suffer from a wide range of emotional consequences which can last into and throughout adulthood. Indeed, these emotions will persist until the issues are resolved, which may be a long time after the actual abuse ends. They may even be exacerbated if the process of telling is further abusive. In order to survive, abused children mobilise a number of defence mechanisms and coping strategies. These give an indication of children's strength and ability to survive. Some children may need more internal resources than others, depending on the circumstances, the actions of potential carers/protectors and features of the abuse. Whilst children may be too frightened to tell directly about their abuse, emotional distress will be communicated, both consciously and unconsciously, through their behaviour. Unfortunately, because this communication is indirect it may not be heard. There is, therefore, a need to be sensitive to all children we come into contact with. In a clinical context, this means giving girls as much power and control as is possible in relation to medical procedures. This should include setting clear boundaries, by making the process explicit, offering a choice regarding the gender of the medic (if at all possible), and discussing potential difficulties involved with medical procedures, such as undressing, prior to the event. This may not mean that a silenced child will immediately speak, but she will have had at least one experience of being heard and treated with respect and knowing that her body is her own and that she matters.

REFERENCES

Finkelhor D, 1987: The trauma of sexual abuse: Two models. *Journal of Interpersonal Violence* **2** (4), 348–366.

Finkelhor D, Browne A, 1985: The traumatic impact of child sexual abuse: A conceptualisation. *American Journal of Orthopsychiatry* **55** (4), 530–541.

Kelly E, Scott S, 1991: Demons, devils and denial. *Trouble and Strife* **22**, 33–35.

Kendall-Tackett KA, Meyers Williams L, Finkelhor D, 1993: The impact of sexual abuse on children: A review and synthesis of recent empirical studies. *Psychological Bulletin* **113** (1), 164–180.

Macloed M, Saraga E, 1987: Child sexual abuse: Towards a Feminist professional practice. *Polytechnic of North London Press* **66**.

PART VII

TEENAGE PREGNANCY

CHAPTER 21

Medical aspects

ANNE S GARDEN ————————————————————————

INTRODUCTION

Teenage pregnancy is recognised as being a major social and medical problem. Its importance is acknowledged by the government in the United Kingdom and the reduction in the teenage pregnancy rate is a priority area in the White Paper, 'Health of the Nation'. Media coverage of 'gym-slip pregnancies' has raised national awareness.

Traditionally, pregnancy occurring in teenage girls, particularly those under 16 years of age, has been considered high risk for both the mother and her child. However, as will be discussed in the following chapters, much of the risk is related to the social environment and emotional disturbance of girls who become pregnant at an early age and their families. It is, therefore, important when considering the problems associated with teenage pregnancies that the culture of the society, the socioeconomic status of the girl and her family within that society, and the society's attitude to pregnancy in young teenagers are all considered. In Shakespeare's *Romeo and Juliet*, Juliet is not yet 14 years old at the time of her fatal attempted elopement and her mother had been younger than Juliet when she conceived her. The unhappy outcome of this situation was not due to a poor socioeconomic status – and pregnancy in early adolescence was obviously considered acceptable in that society.

Additional factors such as the opportunity to continue schooling, the provision of sex education and the availability and uptake of family planning services are all important. In this respect, much of the research around teenage pregnancy has originated from developing countries or from deprived ethnic minority groups within developed countries and may not be relevant to our society.

A survey of teenage mothers and their partners in the United Kingdom (Simms and Smith, 1986) found that four fifths were from lower socioeconomic groups and that the incidence of smoking was twice that of their peers. In addition, a study from the United States showed a higher incidence of drug and alcohol abuse among pregnant adolescents (Kokotailo and Adger, 1991). These factors are determinants of low birth weight, premature labour, sudden infant death syndrome and other complications attributed to teenage pregnancy.

This Chapter will concentrate on the obstetric aspects of pregnancy in teenagers under the age of 18. There is evidence that pregnancies occurring in older teenagers of 18 and 19 have outcomes similar to women aged 20–24 years (Adelson *et al.*, 1992) and are not, therefore, considered an at-risk group. This is probably due to the better social and economic circumstances found in the older teenage group.

ANTENATAL PROBLEMS

The vast majority of pregnancies in girls under the age of 16 are unplanned. Antenatal clinic attendance is therefore often poor (Bury, 1985). Delay in recognising that she is pregnant, compounded by unwillingness to confide in parents, results in many teenagers presenting in the second or even the third trimester before booking for antenatal care. Late booking, in conjunction with an irregular menstrual cycle which occurs more commonly in younger age groups, causes difficulty in dating the pregnancy accurately by clinical means. Ultrasound scan estimation of gestation after 20 weeks' gestation is less reliable than those performed before this time due to variation in fetal growth, so accurate dating of the pregnancy, an essential basic of antenatal care, is difficult. Teenagers are further inhibited from attending antenatal clinics as they report that attending clinics with older women is both 'humiliating and boring'. This may mean that pregnancy complications experienced by these girls, such as growth retardation and pregnancy induced hypertension, are not detected until later in the pregnancy when the complication may be more serious. Special arrangements for teenagers to attend clinics and classes has been found to improve attendance (Black, 1986).

Inaccuracies in the estimation of gestation also leads to problems in interpreting the results of serum screening for Trisomy 21. One study from the United States (Philips *et al.*, 1993) reported that, whereas in the adult population with a 'positive' serum screening result, 52.5% had it explained by ultrasound recalculation of their gestational age, in the adolescent population, the figure was 65.1%.

Specific antenatal problems reported among teenagers are an increased incidence of pregnancy induced hypertension, premature labour, low birth weight babies and anaemia.

Pregnancy induced hypertension

Konje *et al.* (1992) in their group of pregnant teenagers from Hull reported an incidence of gestational hypertension and pre-eclampsia of 18.5% compared with 13.8% in the control population aged 20–24. Higher incidences have also been reported in other studies (Utian, 1967; McIntosh, 1984). Pregnancy induced hypertension is more common among women from the lower social classes and the reported increase among pregnant teenagers may be related, at least in part, to their social class rather than their age. The workers from Hull also suggested that anxiety and fright may cause a false increase in blood pressure, although this is probably not a major factor and certainly would not be a factor in proteinuric hypertension.

Management of pregnancy induced hypertension in teenagers is the same as in adults with monitoring of the blood pressure, renal function and other indices of maternal and fetal well-being with delivery at term or earlier if deterioration in either is detected. There is a suggestion that fulminating pre-eclampsia may occur very rapidly in this young age group and so close monitoring is essential. Day unit assessment may not be appropriate due to poor compliance, or difficulty in arranging transport, and so in-patient monitoring may be required. Because the numbers are small, it is not possible to obtain figures for maternal or perinatal mortality associated with pregnancy induced hypertension in the under-18s. There is no increased incidence, however, in either of these indices in teenagers under 20.

Premature Labour

Because of the difficulties in accurate assessment of gestation already mentioned, the increased incidence of premature labour reported in earlier studies (Osbourne *et al.*, 1981) may be spurious and the result of wrong dates. The more recent study by Konje *et al.* (1992) found no increased incidence of premature labour. A study of teenagers in Malta who delivered between 1983 and 1986, however, reported an increase incidence of premature labour which was responsible for the increased perinatal mortality and morbidity which they reported in this age group (Savona-Ventura and Grech, 1990). A more recent American study of pregnant 11–15 year olds compared to older groups (Sattin *et al.*, 1994) also found a significant increase in the numbers of babies born with a birth weight of under 1500 g, with subsequent admission to the Special Care Nursery, which they attributed to prematurity. Low social class and smoking are both confounding variables when considering the incidence of premature labour in this age group.

In most patients, the cause of premature labour is unknown. Among the known causes, the most common is vaginal infection. One study of women identified as having chlamydial infection in the first trimester of pregnancy (Martin *et al.*, 1982), found that 81% of those infected were under 20 years of age while only 15% of the non-infected women were in this age group. It may be, therefore, that the reported increase in premature delivery in adolescents is related to the increased incidence of infection.

Another American study reported that preterm delivery was associated with poor weight gain in late pregnancy in adolescents (Hediger *et al.*, 1989).

Low Birth Weight

Low birth weight is defined as weight at delivery less than 2500 g. This may be due to either prematurity or intrauterine growth retardation and, unfortunately, it is not clear in many of the early studies on teenage pregnancy which cause they are considering.

In addition to the social factors known to be associated with intrauterine growth retardation, factors such as cigarette smoking, drug usage and social class, nutritional factors are also important and particularly pertinent in this age group.

Adolescents have higher baseline nutritional requirements than adult women (Heald and Jacobson, 1980) and teenage diets, in general, are not generally famous for their balanced intake of nutrients! Scholl *et al.* (1991) found that those adolescents who had poor weight gain in pregnancy had a lower intake of protein and carbohydrate than those with normal weight gain. There was no direct effect, however, on birth weight. Hediger *et al.* (1989) found that adolescents with a low weight gain in the first half of pregnancy had a significantly increased risk of having an infant that was small for its gestational age. One study on the effect of dietary supplementation given to black, underprivileged adolescents in the United States showed an average increase in birth weight of 157 g in the study group as a whole, and an increase of 269 g for those adolescents under the age of 16 (Paige *et al.*, 1981) suggesting that, in this group, poor nutrition is, partly at least, a cause of low birth weight. An evaluation of the John Hopkins Adolescent Pregnancy Program, which included intensive psychosocial support and patient education, showed that the incidence of low birth weight in the group attending the Program was lower than those who were looked after by the same staff but were not enrolled in the program (Hardy *et al.*, 1987). No reason for this increase in birth weight was suggested. Those attending the Program also had fewer pregnancy complications and a lower perinatal mortality.

Anaemia

Anaemia was found in 34.9% of pregnant teenagers compared to 13.8% of the controls in the study by Konje *et al.* (1992). An increased incidence of iron deficiency anaemia in pregnant teenagers had previously been reported by many other workers (Osbourne *et al.*, 1981; Khwaja *et al.*, 1986) and is probably due to poor dietary habits and nutrition. It may be also associated with the heavy periods often experienced by adolescents soon after the menarche. One study (Osbourne *et al.*, 1981) also suggested that the higher incidence of late booking for antenatal care in this age group resulted in late diagnosis of anaemia, with less time available subsequently for therapy. Treatment is with dietary advice and oral iron supplementation.

LABOUR

While many general practitioners and even paediatricians may be involved in looking after a teenage girl during the course of her pregnancy, care in labour will be the responsibility of midwives and obstetricians. However, as it is important that those looking after a girl in early pregnancy are aware of the likely outcome of labour and the post-natal period, these factors will also be considered in this Chapter.

The traditionally held view that labour in young women is high risk because of the small size of their pelvis is not confirmed by research studies. Russell (1983), describing his practice in Newcastle, reported a spontaneous delivery rate of 74% in girls under 16 years of age, compared with 78% in older teenagers. The Caesarian section rates were 4% and 7%, respectively. Similarly, the Hull study (Konje *et al.*, 1992), reported a spontaneous delivery rate of 78.8% in the young teenagers, compared to 80.5% in the older control group. The Caesarian section rate was 6.3% compared to 11.3%. There was, however, an increased forceps delivery rate in the teenage group (11.6% compared to 4.9%) which the authors suggested may be due to fright or lack of co-operation. Another possible cause is the probable increased uptake of epidural anaesthesia by young teenagers who are apprehensive about the pain of labour. A vaginal delivery rate of 86% was reported in both the 11–15 and the 16–19 year age groups compared to 82% in those over 20 years of age in a recent American study (Sattin *et al.*, 1994). The Caesarian section rate for dystocia in the two younger groups was 6% compared to 8% in the older group. The results quoted from the American study were all statistically significant. Zhang and Chan (1991), reporting from Australia, found that teenagers were less likely to have either an induction of labour or a Caesarian section.

There are no data either to suggest that labour is prolonged in teenagers. Jovanovic (1972), in an early study, found that 2.1% of the teenagers had a labour which lasted over 24 hours compared with 2.3% of controls. Bradford and Giles (1989) from Australia, while reporting no difference in operative and spontaneous delivery rates between teenagers and controls found that the teenagers had significantly shorter labours.

From these studies therefore, it would appear that labour for the teenager is not the high risk event that it has gained the reputation for. It is important, however, to remember that young teenage girls are very frightened about going into labour. The need for appropriate parentcraft classes, preferably arranged specifically for teenagers, to prepare them for labour cannot be over-emphasised. It is also essential that these girls are accompanied in labour by a relative or friend of their choice who can provide reassurance.

There are no data, either, to suggest that young teenage mothers have a poor perinatal outcome. The mean birth weight in the study from Hull (Konje *et al.*, 1992) was 3414 g for the teenage group and 3431 g for the older control group. The perinatal mortality in the study group was 13.6/1000 compared to 15.7/1000 for the control group. The earlier study (Osbourne *et al.*, 1981) from Glasgow also showed a lower perinatal mortality in the teenage group of 18.2/1000 compared to 25.9/1000 for the controls. The Glasgow study, however, considered an older teenage group of 19 years and under. If the study group was subdivided into those who were or became married during the pregnancy and those who remained single, there was a significant difference in perinatal mortality of 9.1/1000 among the married group compared to 32.6/1000 in the never married group confirming that factors such as social support are more significant than the chronological age of the mother. The married teenagers, however, were also older. The main causes of perinatal death among teenage mothers in the Glasgow study were low birth weight, antepartum haemorrhage and fetal abnormality.

POST-NATAL

Osbourne *et al.* (1981) found no increased incidence of post-natal complications among the teenagers in their study. In contrast, Konje *et al.* (1992) found an increased incidence of primary post-partum haemorrhage among the young teenage group. They made no suggestions as to why this happened. There was no association with an increased duration of labour, increased size of the baby or increased use of epidural anaesthesia.

As is mentioned in the later chapter (p. 406), psychological problems are more common among pregnant teenagers than in the older population. An increased incidence of deliberate self-harm, including both suicide and attempted suicide, has been reported among pregnant teenagers (Appleby, 1991). There does not, however, appear to be an overall increase in post-natal psychiatric illness in this group.

Attendance for post-natal examination and contraceptive advice does not seem to be a problem in those units where teenage girls have been well looked after during their pregnancy. Klein (1974) reporting from her unit in Atlanta, found that 86% of girls returned for their post-natal examination and 97% of them accepted a method of contraception.

The situation is not so satisfactory outside special clinics, particularly when considering breast-feeding. Only 14% of teenage mothers, compared to an already low population incidence of 30–35%, in Liverpool breast-fed their babies (Gregg, 1989). The author reports that although the majority of teenagers realised that breast-feeding was healthier than bottle feeding, a high percentage said they would be prevented from doing so because of embarassment. This is obviously another area where a focussed and sympathetic education programme would be of great benefit to both mother and child.

THERAPEUTIC ABORTION IN TEENAGERS

A high percentage of teenage pregnancies end in therapeutic abortion. Termination of pregnancy was the single most common reason for hospital admission for girls aged 15 and 16 years in the Oxford region during the years 1979–86 (Henderson *et al.*, 1993). This is obviously not unexpected as such pregnancies are almost invariably unplanned and usually unwanted. Bury (1985) in her study reports that approximately one third of the pregnancies in her series were terminated while the later study of Kronje *et al.* (1992) found that 59.6% of pregnant teenagers had a termination of pregnancy. This increase is probably due to the greater availability of abortion services, the greater acceptance of abortion by the public and also, rather paradoxically, by the increased acceptance of unmarried mothers allowing girls to acknowledge their pregnancy earlier and so attend for consideration for abortion earlier in their pregnancy.

The uptake of abortion services, however, is not just related to their availability. The social and educational expectations of the teenager has a big influence. A study from Dundee (Smith, 1993) showed that two-thirds of the teenage pregnancies from the affluent areas ended in abortion compared with one in four from the deprived areas. Parental expectations and pressure obviously also has a role.

When counselling a teenager about abortion, therefore, it is particularly important to ensure that the decision being discussed is that of the girl as opposed to the one her parents want. It is wise to both interview the girl on her own and to interview her parents independently, in addition to discussing the matter together. It is also important to make some assessment of her mental state. This is particularly important in the light of a study by Maskey (1991) which reported that a quarter of the pregnant teenagers in his study had a probable psychiatric disorder on the General Health Questionnaire (see also p. 411). Failure by health professionals to recognise and deal with this and other pressures on the girl will have long-term sequelae.

The procedure of performing the abortion will of course depend on the gestation of pregnancy. Suction aspiration of the pregnancy, usually under general anaesthetic, will be the route employed for pregnancies of less than 12 weeks gestation; while later pregnancies will be terminated by the induction of labour by prostaglandin analogues. Unfortunately, due to the social background outlined earlier, a high percentage of young teenagers present for consideration of abortion at a gestation too late for suction aspiration to be considered (Russell, 1983).

It is important to prevent damage to the cervix while carrying out the dilatation prior to suction aspiration in girls of this age group, as laceration may lead to short-term problems of haemorrhage and long-term problems of cervical incompetence and recurrent pregnancy loss. The Medical Advisory Committee of the International Planned Parenthood Federation has recommended that either prostaglandin therapy or a laminaria tent be used prior to suction aspiration in first trimester abortion (see Editorial, *IPPF Medical Bulletin*, 1984). In the United Kingdom, the method of choice is usually the prostaglandin analogue, gemeprost.

The use of medical methods of termination of pregnancy using progesterone receptor blockers, such as mifepristone, in conjunction with prostaglandins has not been specifically researched in teenagers. The lack of need of a general anaesthetic is of undoubted advantage but the risk of bleeding at home, particularly if her parents are unaware of the pregnancy, may be unacceptable.

Given appropriate care, there is no evidence that termination of pregnancy carries any increased risk in teenagers than in the general population.

SUMMARY

Many of the problems commonly reported to occur during pregnancy in girls under the age of 18 are probably related to the social circumstances of the girl rather than her age (Lee and Corpuz, 1988). Pregnancy complications in this group will require attention to factors such as nutrition, smoking and clinic attendance as much as to medical aspects of her care. There is a need also for appropriate education in pregnancy and advice and support for labour and child care.

Pregnancy care for teenagers, including these broader aspects of care, are best provided through special teenage pregnancy clinics with dedicated midwifery staff and where input can be provided by all those who can provide educational and social support.

REFERENCES

Adelson PL, Frommer MS, Pym MA, Rubin GL, 1992: Teenage pregnancy and fertility in New South Wales: an examination of fertility trends, abortion and birth outcomes. *Australian Journal of Public Health* **16**, 238–244.

Appleby L, 1991: Suicide during pregnancy and in the first postnatal year. *British Medical Journal* **302**, 137–140.

Black D, 1986: Schoolgirl mothers. *British Medical Journal* **293**, 1047.

Bradford JA, Giles WB, 1989: Teenage pregnancy in Western Sydney. *Australian and New Zealand Journal of Obstetrics and Gynecology* **29**, 1–4.

Bury JK, 1985: Teenage pregnancy. *British Journal of Obstetrics and Gynaecology* **92**, 1081–1085.

Editorial, 1984: *IPPF Medical Bulletin* **18**, 2–4.

Gregg JEM, 1989: Attitudes of teenagers in Liverpool to breast feeding. *British Medical Journal* **299**, 147–148.

Gutierrez Y, King JC, 1993: Nutrition during teenage pregnancy. *Pediatric Annals* **22**, 99–108.

Hardy JB, King TM, Repke JT, 1987: The John Hopkins Adolescent Pregnancy Program: an evaluation. *Obstetrics and Gynecology* **69**, 300–306.

Heald FP, Jacobson MS, 1980: Nutritional needs of the pregnant adolescent. *Pediatric Annals* **9**, 95–99.

Hediger ML, Scholl TO, Belsky DH, Ances IG, Salmon RW, 1989: Patterns of weight gain in adolescent pregnancy: effects on birth weight and preterm delivery. *Obstetrics and Gynecology* **74**, 6–12.

Henderson J, Goldacre M, Yeates D, 1993: Use of hospital inpatient care in adolescence. *Archives of Disease in Childhood* **69**, 559–563.

Jovanovic D, 1972: Pathology of pregnancy and labour in adolescent patients. *Journal of Reproductive Medicine* **9**, 61–66.

Khwaja SS, Al-Sibai MH, Al-Suleimar AS, El-Zibdeh MY, 1986: Obstetric implications of pregnancy in adolescence. *Acta Obstetrica Gynaecologica Scandinavica* **65**, 57–61.

Klein L, 1974: Early teenage pregnancy, contraception, and repeat pregnancy. *American Journal of Obstetrics and Gynecology* **120**, 249–256.

Kokotailo PK, Adger H, 1991: Substance abuse by pregnant adolescents. *Clinical Perinatology* **18**, 125–138.

Konje JC, Palmer A, Watson A, Hay DM, Imrie A, 1992: Early teenage pregnancies in Hull. *British Journal of Obstetrics and Gynaecology* **99**, 969–973.

Lee KS, Corpuz M, 1988: Teenage pregnancy: trend and impact on rates of low birth weight and fetal, maternal, and neonatal mortality in the United States. *Clinical Perinatology* **15**, 929–942.

Martin DH, Koutsky L, Eschenbach DA, Daling JR, Alexander ER, Benedett JR, Holmes KK, 1982: Prematurity and perinatal mortality in pregnancies complicated by maternal chlamydia trachomatis infections. *JAMA* **247**, 1585–1588.

Maskey S, 1991: Teenage pregnancy: doubts, uncertainties and psychiatric disturbance. *Journal of the Royal Society of Medicine* **84**, 723–725.

McIntosh N, 1984: Baby of a schoolgirl. *Archives of Disease in Childhood* **59**, 915–917.

Osbourne GK, Howat RCL, Jordan MM, 1981: The obstetric outcome of teenage pregnancy. *British Journal of Obstetrics and Gynaecology* **88**, 215–221.

Paige DM, Cordano A, Mellits ED, Baertl JM, Davis L, 1981: Nutritional supplementation of pregnant adolescents. *Journal of Adolescent Health Care* **1**, 261–267.

Philips OP, Shulman LP, Elias S, Simpson JL, 1993: Maternal serum screening for fetal Down syndrome using alpha-fetoprotein, human chorionic gonadotrophin, and unconjugated estriol in adolescents. *Adolescent Pediatrics and Gynaecology* **6**, 91–94.

Russell JK, 1983: School pregnancies – medical, social and educational considerations. *British Journal of Hospital Medicine* **29**, 159–166.

Satin AJ, Leveno KJ, Sherman ML, Reedy NJ, Lowe TW, McIntire DD, 1994: Maternal youth and pregnancy outcomes: Middle school versus high school groups compared with women beyond the teen years. *American Journal of Obstetrics and Gynecology* **171**, 184–187.

Savona-Ventura C, Grech ES, 1990: Risks in pregnant teenagers. *International Journal of Gynaecology and Obstetrics* **32**, 7–13.

Scholl TO, Hediger ML, Khoo CS, Healey MF, Rawson NL, 1991: Maternal weight gain, diet and infant birth weight: correlations during adolescent pregnancy. *Journal of Clinical Epidemiology* **44**, 423–428.

Simms M, Smith C, 1986: *Teenage mothers and their partners*. Research report no 15. London: HMSO.

Smith T, 1993: Influence of socioeconomic factors on attaining targets for reducing teenage pregnancies. *British Medical Journal* **306**, 1232–1235.

Utian WH, 1967: Obstetric implications of pregnancy in primigravidas aged 16 years or less. *British Medical Journal* **2**, 734–736.

Zhang B, Chan A, 1991: Teenage pregnancy in South Australia, 1986–1988. *Australian and New Zealand Obstetrics and Gynaecology* **31**, 291–298.

CHAPTER 22

Social aspects

M ALISON CLARKE

INTRODUCTION

Statistical evidence indicates that pregnant schoolgirls comprise only a very small part of the overall figures for all teenage pregnancies. They are, however, a very important group. While sharing a number of common aspects with older teenagers, they also have specific factors which are different and need to be highlighted. They are potentially a very vulnerable group because they are still dependent on society to support them (Clark, 1989). As the numbers are so small nationally, it has meant that professionals rarely see more than a few in their working lifetime, unless they have a particular specialism in this field (Coyne, 1986). This has meant that schoolgirl mothers have had a low profile in terms of empirical research.

The term 'Schoolgirl pregnancy' is a relatively new definition to describe young teenage pregnancy. Very young women have always become pregnant, albeit in small numbers, but what has changed over time, is how our society has viewed this phenomenon and how it has subsequently dealt with it. Historically, young women were not required to receive an education but were expected to marry at an early age. The role of women altered with the introduction of compulsory education for all under the age of 16 years and the assumption that they will endeavour to enter the labour market. Early parenthood has now become a 'problem' (Birch, 1991). The raising of the school-leaving age from 15 to 16 years, brought a sharp focus on young teenage pregnancy. This was not so clearly evident before, as most early teenage pregnancy occurs when the girls are approximately 15–16 years old.

The consequence of schoolgirl pregnancy is viewed as more of a problem in social rather than in medical terms. In Western society, the teenage years are seen as a time for learning skills and developing knowledge to secure a good future. Early pregnancy is seen as a factor which would adversely affect the outcome and would therefore be undesirable (see Factsheet 5a, 1992). Childhood and adulthood are seen as separate stages of our life cycle with a period of adolescence between the two. This time is seen as a period of physical, social and emotional development and as a transition from childhood to adulthood. It is when young people establish a form of personal and social identity, but as Sharpe (1987) points out, when this includes sexual identity, our society 'condemns and denies' its existence. The adolescent period is not well defined and it is not clear when it ends (Phoenix, 1991). There is also a mismatch between biological maturity and social maturity, with social maturity being reached at a later stage (Phoenix, 1991). In Western society, adolescents are still seen as children despite their move towards adulthood. Longer compulsory education and the need for greater numbers of academic and professional qualifications have kept teenagers dependent on parents for longer periods (Phoenix, 1991). All these factors mean that the effect of a pregnancy on a younger teenager has wider reaching implications for herself, her baby, their immediate family and society's response than the effect on an older teenager in the same position (Sharpe, 1987). The young girls who attend the Arbour Project in Liverpool (a unit for pregnant schoolgirls and schoolgirl mothers funded by the local authority and managed by Personal Service Society – a voluntary agency) have to deal with their own personal development, society's response to their situation and the contradictory position of their social and legal status.

Although the research indicates that there has been increase in sexual activity (Christopher, 1980; Factsheet 5a, 5b, 1992) there has not been a corresponding up-surge in births and terminations or pregnancy. From the Office of Population Census and Surveys (F.M. Series 10–20; A.B. Series 10–18), information on abortion rates and birth rates, it can be noted that from 1983 onwards, the trend for the numbers of pregnancies by maternal age 11–15 years has remained fairly static. When adding 16-year-old girls to this group the trend, while more undulating, displays only a slight upward trend. The abortion trends for the same period and groups defined by maternal age, have continued to fall (see Tables 22.1, 22.2 and Fig. 22.1). It can be concluded that although the uptake of contraception is not as high as it needs to be, it is increasing slowly, particularly for girls under 16 years of age. The 'Brook Advisory Annual Report' (1991/1992) stated that the number of under 16s attending family planning clinics had gone up by 12% the previous year.

Table 22.1 Births (live and still), by maternal age in England and Wales

Age (years)	Year									
	1983	1984	1985	1986	1987	1988	1989	1990	1991	1992
11–15 *	1249	1323	1402	1366	1305	1261	1317	1306	1426	1314
11–15 •	17	10	7	13	10	12	6	5	9	—
11–16 *	5279	5424	5833	5669	5703	5755	5556	5472	5566	—
11–16 •	43	45	36	48	41	48	27	22	39	—

* Live births; • still births.
Figures compiled from statistics taken from Birth statistics, F.M. Series Nos. 10–20 (Tables 3.2) OPCS (HMSO) and Mersey Regional Health Authority – Information Unit (Table B4).

Table 22.2   Abortions by maternal age in England and Wales

Age (years)	Year									
	1983	1984	1985	1986	1987	1988	1989	1990	1991	1992
11–15	4087	4158	4002	3984	3765	3568	3383	3422	3158	2999
11–16	—	10 960	10 650	10 069	10 016	10 081	9344	8977	8098	—

Figures compiled from statistics taken from Abortion statistics A.B. Series Nos 10–18 (Tables 5) OPCS (HMSO) and Mersey Regional Health Authority – Information Unit (Table B11).

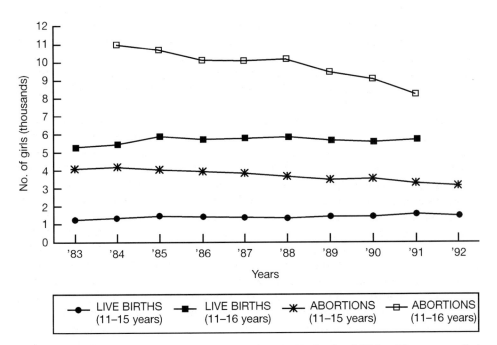

Fig. 22.1   Live births and abortions by maternal age in England and Wales. Figures compiled from statistics taken from birth (FM Series) and abortion (AB Series) Statistics – OPCS (HMSO) and Mersey Regional Health Authority – Information Unit.

   In Great Britain, for every one girl who continues with a pregnancy approximately two have the pregnancy terminated (Coyne, 1986). This is not surprising as the research indicates that nearly all schoolgirl pregnancies are unplanned (Konje *et al.*, 1992). It is important, however, to clarify that not all unplanned pregnancies are unwanted (Dawson, 1994). Of those who do continue, most want the baby they are carrying. It is generally thought that girls who terminate pregnancies tend to be those considering themselves to have academic aspirations and a promising career (Hudson and Ineichen, 1991). Very few opt for adoption

(De'Ath, 1984). In Birch's study (1991) only 2% of babies were given up for adoption. The research indicates that the girls who decide to continue are more likely to come from areas of socioeconomic deprivation. Birch found in her study that only one in four girls in Camberwell chose to terminate the pregnancy (Birch, 1989a).

BACKGROUND

Although some researchers see schoolgirl pregnancies purely in the consequential terms of poor health, poverty and low social status, it is important to state that 'the relationship between teenage mothers and disadvantage is complex as social, economic and environmental factors may often be a determinant rather than a consequence of adolescent motherhood (see Factsheet 5a, 1992). It is also these negative aspects which have at least as much, and in many cases more, adverse effects on a schoolgirl's ability to be a competent parent, than the effects of extreme youth and inexperience (Sharp, 1987).

Taking an overview of recent research (Miles *et al.*, 1979; Kiernan, 1980; Wilson, 1980; Russell, 1983; Coyne, 1986; Simms and Smith, 1986; Sharpe, 1987; Birch, 1991, Hudson and Ineichen, 1991; Factsheets 5a and 5b, 1992: Konje *et al.*, 1992), a 'typical' pregnant schoolgirl is considered to come from a large (average of five children), working class, single parent family where relationships are often unstable. Early parenthood is seen as the norm, where sisters and other close family and friends had also become parents at an early age. The girl's own mother was also likely to have been a young parent. Simms and Smith (1986) suggested that the girls were responding to the effects of a 'large family and early childbirth' sub-culture, even though their parents were not always pleased for their young daughters, rather than being a misfit creating a social problem. This young girl is also more likely to live in an area of high unemployment, where housing conditions are poor and overcrowded, and where there is a high level of poverty and social deprivation. The girl herself is seen as one who had gained little satisfaction at school, had under-achieved, was more likely to have been associated with crime and to have attended child guidance clinics. Although first pregnancies were unintentional, most expected to have more than one child. It was also noted that although most young girls did not intend to become pregnant, contraceptive uptake was poor (Miles *et al.*, 1979; Kiernan, 1980; Wilson, 1980; Russell, 1983; Coyne, 1986; Simms and Smith, 1986; Sharpe, 1987; Birch, 1991; Hudson and Ineichen, 1991; Konje *et al.*, 1992; Factsheet 5a, 1992). It must be clarified that this is a general conclusion and one which does not apply to every pregnant schoolgirl.

Early childbirth is seen as a response to a certain set of circumstances brought about by poverty and the resulting deprivation and reduced life chances. Having a baby is often seen as the only positive life experience that these young girls will achieve (Coyne, 1986; Birch, 1989a; Hudson and Ineichen, 1991). Having a baby at a young age was seen as being socially acceptable in Simms and Smith's study (1986) and was seen to afford these young mothers with greater status and satisfaction. Decisions are often made using limited judgement by the girls themselves who, by their very youth, will be making assessments on limited life experiences and from advice from family and friends with perhaps a similarly limited outlook (Hudson and Ineichen, 1991). In Simms and Smith's study (1986), they found that the schoolgirl's awareness of the social consequences of becoming a parent appeared to be 'non-existent'. Birch (1989a) considered that the absence of a father figure was a key factor in determining early parenthood, that in an effort to secure a paternal figure in her life the girl would perhaps move into sexual relationships.

In considering first sexual experiences, Christopher (1980) referred to two British studies (Schofield, 1965; Farrell, 1978). The information put together showed that, although more young people were admitting to sexual activity below the age of 19 years, the increase was still very small. In Schofield's study in 1965, it was found that 6% of boys and 2% of girls aged 15 years had experienced sexual intercourse whereas in Farrell's study in 1978, 26% of boys and 12% of girls had their first sexual experience before the age of 16 years (Miles *et al.*, 1979). More recent research indicates that this figure has risen as high as 41% (Factsheet 5a and 5b, 1992). Although this may be the case, it is still believed that young people are not generally 'promiscuous' (Hudson and Ineichen, 1991). The work of Sharpe (1978), Birch (1989a, 1991) and Dawson (1994) confirm this statement.

LONG-TERM EFFECTS OF DEPRIVATION

Birch saw schoolgirl pregnancy as part of a culture of poverty and deprivation. In considering the long-term effects, Birch referred to Kolvin's six indicators of deprivation, i.e. family disruption, parental illness, 'defective' care, social dependence, overcrowding, inadequate housing and poor parenting. When Birch applied these criteria to the girls in her study, she found that 82% of the girls and 96% of their babies were considered to be very deprived. Once locked into this cycle of deprivation, the effect is increased on the next generation. The downward spiral is brought about by a loss of education, followed by diminishing chances of finding employment and the inevitable life of poverty. This is compounded when, in an effort to acquire some financial stability, the young girl seeks a new partner, becomes pregnant again and steps further into financial problems (Birch, 1989b).

EFFECTS OF SOCIAL ISOLATION

Although most pregnant schoolgirls remain at home with a parent, they do suffer a measure of social isolation. Early parenthood inevitably leads to the young mother becoming isolated from her peer group and from the usual teenage activities and interests (Miles *et al.*, 1979). Those who tend to keep their babies are often young girls who find it difficult to maintain good, long-term relationships (Hudson and Ineichen, 1991). Girls who have strong supportive family networks are more likely to become successful mothers (McRobbie, 1989). This is borne out by our experiences at Arbour.

EFFECT OF THE MEDIA

There have been many social and economic changes in our society which have reduced the control and effects of the family, the church and the community. Ideals of personal fulfilment and identity have become more important. Sexual fulfilment is used by the media as one way to find satisfaction. Popular music, teenage magazines and advertising campaigns try to persuade us that teenage sexuality is acceptable. However, while young people are being encouraged to experiment with sexual activity at earlier ages, such behaviour is still seen as an adult activity (Miles *et al.*, 1979). The media portrays a romantic and exciting image of sexual experiences (Donovan, 1990). Young people absorb these images and endeavour to emulate them without fully appreciating the consequences. The reality is very different and these young girls find it hard to reconcile their life style with that portrayed in the media (Birch, 1989b).

SOCIETY'S RESPONSE TO THE SEXUAL ACTIVITY OF YOUNG TEENAGERS

Although, as Coyne (1989) points out, social taboos are not as strictly outlined as before and the age of sexual activity is falling, society's attitude towards teenage sexuality is still inconsistent. We give our young people conflicting messages as we ourselves have difficulty in coming to terms with the emerging sexuality of our 'children'. As Christopher (1980) points out, there is much discussion about the appropriate age of consent. Early sexual activity is present equally across all social and economic classes but the response to it differs between groups (Sharpe, 1987; Dawson, 1994). Working class girls are more likely to embark on a sexual relationship without seeking contraception first and are more likely to continue with a pregnancy (Russell, 1983; Sharpe, 1987; Dawson, 1994). Middle class girls are more likely to terminate pregnancies in favour of pursuing other long-term goals (Miles *et al.*, 1979). Farrell (1979) also found that those more likely to know about and use contraception were from the higher social groups. 53% of middle class girls were more likely to say they had used birth control compared with 32% of working class girls (Miles *et al.*, 1979). The response towards sexual activity is different between the working and middle classes. Middle class parents are more likely to talk to their children about sex and use medical terms, whereas working class parents find it difficult to discuss this with their children and often use slang words. Such words are considered to be offensive by our society (Christopher, 1980).

In a study carried out for the 'Alan Guttmacher Institute' on six comparable industrialised countries, it was found that, where there was a lack of 'openness' about sex, the teenage pregnancy rate was higher than in a country that was able to deal with such issues openly. Other factors present in countries with a low teenage pregnancy rate included easy access to contraceptive and abortion services, comprehensive sex education and liberal attitudes towards sex. This research refuted the claims that, where the above factors are present, sexual 'promiscuity' and an increased rate of teenage pregnancy is the result (Jones *et al.*, 1986; Factsheet 5a, 1992).

LEGAL STATUS

The legal position of a schoolgirl mother is very complex. As Hudson and Ineichen (1991) point out, being a mother and a schoolgirl are contradictory roles which must co-exist. Coyne (1986) suggests that it is this confusion which adversely affects their position within society. It is illegal for a boy of 14 years or older to have sexual intercourse with a girl who is under the age of 16 years but because the girl is considered to be unable to give consent, it is the boy who is seen as guilty of an offence. However, when that same young person becomes pregnant, she is considered able to decide the fate of the fetus. Schoolgirl pregnancy provides proof that an illegal act has taken place and as Phoenix (1991) points out, this highlights a number of moral issues which our society finds difficult to accomodate. The minimum legal age for consent to sexual intercourse is 16 years which is also the age at which marriage can legally take place (Wilson, 1980). This means that all children born to girls under the age of 16 are 'illegitimate' (Sharpe, 1987), although this status does not carry the stigma it once did.

With regard to contraception, there has been much controversy. The legal campaign and resulting protracted court room battles initiated by Mrs Victoria Gillick to make it illegal to advise or treat young people under 16 years without parental permission or knowledge, have not helped the situation. Consequently, the public and some professionals are not clear as to the legality of giving contraceptive advice and treatment. At present, such advice can be given, without parental involvement, at the discretion of the medical practitioner (see Factsheet 5e, 1992).

A schoolgirl's financial situation is also problematic. Legally, she is still classed as a child and therefore cannot claim income support in her own right for herself and her baby until she is 16 years of age. She can then apply for housing benefit, when it is appropriate. She is dependent on her parents claiming on her behalf if they, themselves, are already in receipt of this benefit. In her Camberwell study, Birch (1991) found that 57% of the girls' families were in receipt of welfare benefits. Such poverty is perpetuated because usually the only source of income for young mothers and pregnant 16 year olds is welfare benefit. In Clark's (1989) study, it was found that poverty was the greatest problem for the young mothers. She also found that guaranteed welfare benefit played no part in the decision whether or not to continue with the pregnancy.

Free milk tokens and a maternity grant are available to those in receipt of income support. This often means that, if the girl gives birth to her baby more than three months before her 16th birthday and her own parents are not in receipt of income support, she will not be able to claim the maternity grant. Although the state does not recognise officially that mothers under the age of 16 years exist, they provide the minimum of financial support for the babies. The young mothers are therefore entitled to claim child benefit and one parent benefit under the age of 16 years (Hudson and Ineichen, 1991). The irony here is that the costs and needs of parenthood remain the same whatever the age of the parent (Sharpe, 1987).

Housing and an inability to secure their own tenancy under the age of 16 years is also a problem and results in the young parent again having to rely on parental support to provide accommodation which is often of poor quality and already overcrowded.

These girls are also required to receive an education by law, but adequate provision is not always given and sufficient childcare is often not available to enable these young people to take up academic courses.

It is therefore highly probable that pregnant schoolgirls will move from parental dependency to state dependency and on to a life of severe financial hardship because when they need financial help most, they are denied such a resource. It has been argued that young mothers should be granted an unambiguous legal and social position within society and that greater financial and linked career opportunities should be provided.

EDUCATION

Research indicates that schoolgirls who become pregnant tend to have few academic aspirations and are more likely to be poor school attenders (Coyne, 1986; Simms and Smith, 1986; Birch, 1991). In Simms and Smith's study, it was found that 52% of pregnant teenagers had left school without any qualifications (see Simms ans Smith, 1986). This finding is also supported by the work of Kiernan (1980) who found that teenage mothers were more likely to show low academic abilities, lack ambition and tend to leave school at the minimum age. She also found that there was a lack of parental interest in their daughters' educational future. These parents were also less likely to have gained qualifications themselves while still at school (see Factsheet 5a, 1992).

De'Ath (1984) states that within individual schools a pregnant teenager is rare, which often makes it difficult for the school to meet that young girl's particular needs. Education authorities vary in their response. Some provide separate units, some offer home teaching, and others offer resources within an established mainstream school (Miles *et al.*, 1979; De'Ath, 1984; Simms and Smith, 1986). Dawson (1984) stressed the importance of equal opportunities being available for all pregnant schoolgirls within the education system. This means providing a number of options to suit individual needs and circumstances, with the appropriate co-ordinated back-up support services.

A schoolgirl's position is clearly defined in social and legal terms (Coyne, 1986). This causes problems, however, for pregnant schoolgirls, because in our societal framework a 'child' who becomes a 'mother' is a social and legal contradiction. In legal terms, a girl of school age must receive an education. She is not available to seek work and therefore is dependent on either her parents or the state.

Some argue that schoolgirl parenthood adversely affects academic performance and hence future employment (Miles *et al.*, 1979). Russell (1983) highlighted the 'lost educational opportunities' brought about by early pregnancy and the resulting withdrawal from school. In the survey carried out by Miles *et al.* (1979) it was found that 75% of pregnant girls had left school by the fifth month. Of these girls, 66% had received no education between leaving school and delivering the baby. 53% of those still under school age did not return to school after the birth. Only 25% of girls received home tuition during pregnancy.

Some of the research, however, seems to indicate that these young women have already voted with their feet and hence have already negatively affected their 'career prospects' (Birch, 1991; Hudson and Ineichen, 1991). In considering three studies carried out in Aberdeen, Wilson (1980) found that girls who became pregnant had already lost, or were losing, interest in their education by the age of eleven. Of those referred to the Arbour Project, most are already disaffected with their schooling and have usually been poor school attenders for some time before becoming pregnant. In either instance, it can be said that schoolgirl pregnancy can severely exacerbate an already undesirable situation. These girls often receive a poor education which usually leads to a reduced or non-existent future income, state dependency and subsequent existence at the poverty level for themselves and their baby (Coyne, 1986).

SEX EDUCATION

How much sex education a young girl receives at school depends very much on the attitudes and policies of the school's governing body. Although sex education is part of the national curriculum, how the subject is dealt with depends on their discretion. In 1988, government legislation deemed that parents should also be responsible for sex education (Phoenix, 1991). As far back as 1979, Miles *et al.* (1979) advocated that ideally, parents should be involved in the sex education of their children, whether it be at home or school. However, it must be remembered that working class parents particularly, have difficulty in discussing sexual matters with their children (Sharpe, 1987). In addition, what is offered at school is often inadequate both in terms of content and the time of 'delivery'. Most girls are already sexually active before this subject is discussed in the classroom (Birch 1989a; Miles, 1979). This situation is further exacerbated by a high level of non-school attendance by fifth year (Year Eleven) pupils in general, and pregnant schoolgirls in particular. In the Camberwell study, Birch (1989a) found that 64% of pregnant girls had received no sex education at all and that 62% were persistent truants. She found that 87% of these girls received no sex education at home. The experiences of the girls at Arbour confirm these findings.

Most 'knowledge' about sex is obtained from friends and is often inaccurate (Sharpe, 1987; Birch, 1989). In her research, Sharpe (1987) found that middle class girls were more likely to learn about sex and contraception from their parents, whereas working class girls found out about these subjects from their peer group. This lack of knowledge often results in young girls not being aware that they are pregnant. The consequences of this are late abortions or pregnancies (wanted and unwanted) going to term with little or no antenatal care.

The evidence available dispels the myth that sex education encourages sexual activity. Young people experiment through a lack of knowledge. Unplanned pregnancies are the result. It is generally agreed that pregnant schoolgirls are not 'promiscuous' and although nearly all pregnancies are unplanned, they develop from a reasonably 'long'-term relationship (Sharpe, 1987; Birch, 1989a; Hudson and Ineichen, 1991). Recent research concluded that more sex education is needed to help reduce the rate of teenage pregnancies and that it should be aimed at 12–13-year-olds with particular emphasis on those in social classes 4 and 5. The type of sex education and the kind of 'social' conditions in which it is taught is also crucial. If young people are able to discuss these issues in open environments, within the home and school, they are more likely to accept their emerging sexuality and feel able to take control of effective contraception from the start (Donovan, 1990).

CONTRACEPTION

There is widespread concern about the fact that most teenage pregnancy is unintentional. Despite some knowledge of what is available and where, and that it is free (and has been so since 1973) (Birch, 1991), young women under 16 seem unable or unwilling to use any form of contraception (Konje *et al.*, 1992). In Simms and Smith's study (1986), it was found that while one of ten schoolgirls intended to become pregnant, only two used any form of contraception. These two girls had received sex and birth control education at school. In a retrospective study of 1660 pregnancies of young women in Hull, Konje *et al.* (1992) found that 92% had never used any form of contraception. These findings were confirmed by Sharpe (1987).

One reason which may contribute to the lack of use of contraception is the very nature of sexual activity in adolescents which, as well as being unplanned, is also 'infrequent' and 'irregular' (Dawson, 1994). In the Camberwell study, Birch (1989a) found that despite having one unplanned pregnancy, one third of the girls continued not to use contraception, or to use it ineffectively. Subsequent pregnancies following soon after the first where also found by Coyne (1986). Conception is rarely a deliberate act but is not actively avoided. Simms and Smith (1986) referred to an air of 'fatalism' expressed by girls. This is not the case for those over 16 among whom there is still a relatively high incidence of unplanned pregnancy but less marked. Younger teenagers are less likely to take responsibility for contraception than older teenagers (Hudson and Ineichen, 1991).

The belief systems which surround the lack of contraceptive use and teenage sexuality are considered by Birch. There are contradictory messages coming from peer group, parental, religious and societal pressure where it is 'OK' to get 'carried away', that good girls don't need contraception, but a girl's 'worth' is measured in terms of her fertility (Birch, 1988). It is important that young people should be allowed to admit to their own sexuality. As long as they are conditioned to believe that sexual activity is wrong and that by seeking contraception they are admitting to an immoral and 'illegal' act, such young people will continue to rely on taking chances and not accepting responsibility. Refusing contraception, or dissuading young people from using it, will not stop schoolgirl pregnancy (Sharpe, 1987). Our society does not make it easy for young people to make use of contraception. As a result, we discourage those who have reached sufficient maturity to consider this issue by offering little encouragement and support for them to do so (Christopher, 1980).

The lack of control by the teenager is seen by Birch as a major factor explaining why they do not take up contraception. In her study, only 7% of pregnant London schoolgirls had used contraception. She points out that this lack of control extends to the whole of the girl's life. She is not accustomed to being able to make decisions for herself, for adults do not allow her to do so (Birch, 1988).

Wilson (1992) considered the issues surrounding the phenomenon that despite high availability of abortion services and family planning, the teenage birth rate had not gone down. He concluded that such factors as education, employment, cultural beliefs, family pressures, peer pressure and financial prospects were as important as the availability of adequate abortion and contraception facilities on the incidence of teenage pregnancy (Wilson *et al.*, 1992).

Society's double standards also perpetuate this model of 'it's OK to get carried away' because although it is acceptable for boys to be sexually active in our society, it is not so for girls. Girls are therefore reluctant to make responsible decisions on birth control (Coyne, 1986; Birch, 1988; Hudson and Ineichen, 1991). Planned sexual activity by young women is not socially acceptable.

UNEMPLOYMENT

Alternatives to teenage motherhood are considered to be a completed education followed by employment. The economic recession and the resulting shrinking labour market was considered by Coyne (1986) to play some part in school age mothers continuing to opt for parenthood. This is aggravated by the apparent inability of young women to fully appreciate the link between qualifications and career opportunities (Kiernan, 1980). McRobbie (1989) carried out a small study with 12 girls from the Birmingham area. She found that, similar to other studies, these young mothers were under-achievers at school, having opted out of education by their last year. Subsequently, when trying to enter a rapidly shrinking labour market, they found that there was a greater need to have gained some academic qualifications while at school. The result is that for those who do seek work, all that is available is poorly paid, repetitive, part-time or short-term work (Birch, 1989b). From a young woman's point of view, in a society where the chances of gaining a fulfilling career is small, early parenthood is at least no worse than the prospect of an adult life of unemployment and state dependency.

In Lambeth, Birch (1991) found that the areas with the highest rates of teenage pregnancy also had the highest levels of unemployment. The route of reaching adulthood through employment is now denied to a section of young women. Marriage was another path to adult status for young women but most young girls today do not view this as an option (Phoenix, 1991). There is less incentive to take preventative measures to stop pregnancy occurring. Without further appropriate vocational training and the provision of adequate and affordable childcare, becoming pregnant answers their immediate, short-term needs (Hudson and Ineichen, 1991). On a more positive note, research on 30 young mothers (aged 13–18 years) showed that having a baby did spur some on to succeed, whereas, without this incentive of providing for a baby, they may not have done so (Sharpe, 1987).

HOUSING

Birch (1991) found that 44% of the young women in her Camberwell study lived in unsatisfactory housing. Chronic overcrowding, where brothers and sisters often have to share bedrooms, was compounded by the arrival of a new baby. This is confirmed by the experience of the girls at Arbour, where in most cases the girls themselves are too young to apply for their own council or Housing Association tenancy and have to rely on parental support to provide them with accommodation. The only alternative, if family or friends are unable to help, is for the young girl to be placed in the care of the local authority. Suggestions that schoolgirls become pregnant in an effort to acquire housing is not substantiated by our experience at Arbour or by any recent research (Clarke, 1989). It needs to be restated that in legal terms these girls are too young to hold a tenancy in their own right and in Liverpool, where Arbour is based, it is very difficult for any young person under the age of 17 to secure a tenancy.

SUMMARY

Although our Western industrial society does not encourage schoolgirls to become pregnant, it does little to provide satisfactory reasons 'why not', or alternative life styles or opportunities. This, coupled with inadequate sex education and poor knowledge of contraception, exacerbates the situation. The age of a young pregnant teenager is not considered to be a problem in itself, but it does create difficulties within 'our' social, moral, economic and legal context. A pregnant schoolgirl becomes, at once, both a 'child' and an 'adult' and, in our society, we do not have a social or legal framework in conjunction with the necessary comprehensive support systems to cope with this phenomenon. As professionals, we have to be aware of the social context within which these young girls are situated and the circumstances to which they are reacting and be realistic as to the type of intervention and the subsequent outcome.

REFERENCES

Annual Report. *Brook Advisory Service* 1991/92.

Birch D, 1988: That old black magic? Belief systems in teenage pregnancy. *Journal of Adolescent Health and Welfare* 1(4), 45.

Birch D, 1989a: School pregnancy. In Studd J (ed.), *Progress in Obstetrics and Gynaecology,* January 7, 75–90.

Birch D, 1989b: Schoolgirl pregnancy – a culture of poverty. *Journal of Adolescent Health and Welfare* 2 (1), 13.

Birch D, 1991: *Are you my sister Mummy?* London: Youth Support.

Christopher E, 1980: *Sexuality and birth control in social and community work.* London: Temple Smith.

Clark E, 1989: Young single mothers today: a quantitative study of housing and support needs. *National Council for One Parent Families.*

Coyne AM, 1986: Schoolgirl mothers. *Health Education Council: Research Report* 2, 1–145.

Dawson N, 1989: Report on the 1987 survey of education provision for pregnant schoolgirls and schoolgirl mothers in the L.E.A.'s of England and Wales. *Journal of Adolescent Health and Welfare* 2(1), 1–5.

Dawson N, 1991: LMS – Lost maternal schooling? *Teenage Parenthood* 3, 1–3.

Dawson N, 1994: *The decision making process and personal constructs of pregnant schoolgirls and schoolgirl mothers.* Bristol: Unpubl. PhD thesis.

De'Ath E, 1984: Teenage parents: review of research. *National Children's Bureau February 1984*; Highlight No. 59.

Donovan C, 1990: Adolescent sexuality. *British Medical Journal* 300, 13.

Farrell C, 1979: In Miles M *et al.* (eds.), Pregnant at school – joint working party on pregnant schoolgirls and schoolgirl mothers. *National Council for One Parent Families.*

Hudson F, Ineichen B, 1991: *Taking it lying down.* Basingstoke: Macmillan.

Jones EF, *et al.,* 1986: *Teenage pregnancy in industrialised countries.* New Haven and London: Yale University Press, 233–236.

Kiernan K, 1980: Teenage motherhood – associated factors and consequences; the experience of a British cohort. *Journal of Biosocial Science* 12, 393–404.

Konje J, *et al.,* 1992: Early teenage pregancies in Hull. *British Journal of Obstetrics and Gynaecology* 99, 969–973.

McRobbie A, 1989: Motherhood, a teenage job. *The Guardian* 5 September.

Miles M, *et al.,* 1979: Pregnant at school – joint working party on pregnant schoolgirls and schoolgirl mothers. *National Council for One Parent Families*, 1–52.

Office of Population Census and Surveys. *Abortion Statistics 1983–92*; AB series Nos 10–18.

Office of Population Census and Surveys. *Birth Statistics 1983–92*; FM series Nos 10–20.
Phoenix A, 1991: *Young mothers?* Cambridge: Polity Press.
Russell KJ, 1983: Schoolgirl pregnancies – medical, social and educational considerations. *British Journal of Hospital Medicine* **29**, 159–166.
Schofield M, 1985: *The sexual behaviour of young people.* London: Longmans.
Sharpe S, 1987: *Falling for love.* London: Virago.
Simms M, Smith C, 1986: Teenage mothers and their partners – a survey in England and Wales. DHSS Report, **15**, London: HMSO, 112–119.
Teenage pregnancies, 1992: Family Planning Association, *Factsheet 5a.*
The legal position regarding contraceptive advice and provision to young people, 1992: Family Planning Association, *Factsheet 5e.*
Wilson F, 1980: Antecedents of adolescent pregnancy. *Journal of Biosocial Science* **12**, 141–152.
Wilson SH, *et al.*, 1992: Teenage conception and contraception in the English regions. *Journal of Public Health Medicine* **14**(1), 21–23.
Young people: sexual attitudes and behaviour, 1992: Family Planning Association, *Factsheet 5b.*

CHAPTER 23

Psychological aspects

MARION CHEESBROUGH ————————————————————

INTRODUCTION

Adolescence is a period of rapid physiological and psychological change, when, in Western societies at least, the adolescent renegotiates his or her role within the family, in school and work, and with peers and society in preparation for adult life. It is thus a time when different identities can be explored (Erikson, 1959). Moreover, the teenage years are crucial in terms of academic achievement and/or establishment in the workforce, which in turn promotes financial independence. Together these factors pave the way for adolescents to leave their family of origin, establish their own household, and enter into mature reciprocal relationships.

Becoming a parent similarly requires substantial adaptation and change, and can likewise be construed as a developmental crisis, not only for the individual but also for their partner and family of origin. However, when the developmental challenges of adolescence and parenthood occur simultaneously, they place demands on the individual that may be diametrically opposed (Sadler and Catrone, 1983). For example, the adolescent's attention is necessarily focused on the self as she explores and develops her adult identity, whereas the extreme dependency of the human neonate demands that the new parent's attention should be focused almost exclusively on the baby. Adolescence requires an avoidance of a premature role and identity assumption, parenthood requires from the mother the immediate assumption of a maternal role, and often precludes the continuation of other roles e.g. student or employee. Adolescence involves a move away from the family of origin whereas parenthood often requires the teenager to remain in her parents' home because of poverty and a need for social support and childcare assistance. This need to remain at home and care for her child often further restricts the adolescent's developmental opportunities by restricting peer contact. Finally, the adolescent who becomes pregnant is faced with the dual task of coming to terms with her emerging sexual identity, both physical and emotional, and the demands of bodily changes consequent upon being pregnant.

WHY DO TEENAGERS BECOME PREGNANT?

As with all other major life events, the significance of pregnancy and child-birth is culturally determined. Thus, being pregnant as a teenager has very different antecedents and implications in non-Western societies. This account concentrates on the experience in Europe and the United States. Even in Western societies there have been major changes. Whereas a generation ago unwed pregnancy was viewed as a relatively common part of a courtship sequence that almost invariably resulted in marriage, in the 1990s single motherhood is common in all age groups. Indeed, the social and political concern about teenage motherhood may have less to do with a perceived increase in its prevalence, which has not in fact occurred, and more to do with the demands that single motherhood places on society's resources (Furstenberg, 1991). There are likely to be many differences within and between countries, reflected in varying rates of adolescent pregnancy and childbearing. However, the dearth of non-American research makes these differences difficult to evaluate.

There is extensive evidence that despite widespread sexual activity among teenagers, pregnancy is not a random event, and social, educational and psychological factors are all implicated.

For some teenagers who become pregnant, there are interpersonal difficulties which originate in the early relationship between the teenager and her own mother. Becoming pregnant may be an attempt, albeit unconcious, to resolve these difficulties. Thus the teenager is hypothesised to have been an infant who received inadequate mothering, which resulted in her feeling that the mother could not be relied upon to satisfy her basic needs, whether they were for physical care or emotional support and intimacy. Infants have been observed to exhibit specific patterns of 'attachment' behaviour when in need of comfort and security (Ainsworth *et al.*, 1978). This behaviour is a reflection of the quality of caretaking and the mother–child relationship. It is not a characteristic of the child, although it is thought to become a 'prototype' for future relationships. The patterns of attachment that reflect feelings of insecurity in the infant constitute risk factors for future development, particularly in the sphere of interpersonal relationships. Pregnancy may (subconsciously) be seen as a way of reconstructing a more satisfying early mother–child relationship.

There is mounting evidence that would support this theory. Teenagers who become pregnant are more likely to have themselves been born to teenage mothers (Furstenberg *et al.*, 1987), and teenage mothers have been shown repeatedly to have difficulties parenting their children. These factors, which are known to adversely affect parenting, make the daughters of these mothers particularly at risk of later teenage pregnancy. Thus, the highest rate of adolescent pregnancy in the daughters of teenage mothers was found when the mothers reported lifelong depression and had moved out of their own mothers' homes before their child was 26 months old (Horawitz *et al.*, 1991), thus depriving the child of an alternative source of emotional support. Looking more specifically at attachment patterns confirms the prevalence of difficulties in the relationships between the teenage mother and her own mother, and this is likely to be replicated in her relationship with her baby (Lamb *et al.*, 1987; Levine *et al.*, 1991). This would all be consistent with the hypothesis of early emotional deprivation predisposing adolescents to seek emotional closeness through early sexual activity and parenthood, and suggests routes by which early childbearing may be transmitted from one generation to the next. Finally, a group of general practitioners in the south of England observed and evaluated 147 unselected consecutive patients presenting with 'unwanted' pregnancies, many, but not all of whom, were adolescent, and independently arrived at the same conclusion (Tunnadine and Green, 1978).

The idea of an apparently 'undesirable' behaviour or symptom representing a solution rather than a problem is particularly useful when thinking of entire family functioning. Thus the prime developmental task of adolescence is becoming independent, and pregnancy may, unconsciously, be used to achieve this end. The pregnancy can suceed in this by forcing the parents to recognise that the teenager has grown up, by forcing their hand in throwing the teenager out, or by providing an alternative child for the grandmother to care for, possibly preventing the grandparents from being left alone together to face an empty marriage. Paradoxically, teenage pregnancy can serve the opposite function, cementing families together and preventing real independence of the teenager, as a premature attempt to leave home via pregnancy with an unsuitable partner leads to a rapid dissolution of that relationship and return of the teenager and her baby to the family of origin.

A minority of girls who become pregnant have already been formally identified as having a psychiatric or psychological disorder, most commonly a conduct disorder, of which sexual acting out may be a symptom. Sexual activity in the context of alcohol and drug abuse can result in pregnancy, and very rarely a major psychiatric disorder, such as a manic episode in a girl with manic depressive psychosis, may result in impulsive sexual activity and pregnancy. Although rare, all of these will have major consequences for management.

In a minority of girls, pregnancy is a consequence of rape, whether this be by a stranger or a known adult, as in intrafamilial child sexual abuse (CSA). While the former may be instantly recognisable and accompanied with much overt distress in the victim and her family, the detection of the latter requires clinicians to be constantly alert to this possibility. It probably represents particularly severe and enduring abuse and carries particularly grave risks for the mother and child. A recent study showed pregnant teenagers to have exceptionally high rates of abuse. In the year preceding pregnancy, 33% had been physically or sexually abused, and in 22% it continued during pregnancy (Parker, 1993). This was very rarely disclosed to medical staff.

PSYCHOLOGICAL CONSIDERATIONS IN THE MANAGEMENT OF THE PREGNANT TEENAGER

General Considerations

In general, older pregnant adolescent girls differ little in the kinds of problems they encounter from those encountered by pregnant adult women, once the problems associated with socioeconomic factors have been accounted for (Wolkind and Krug, 1985). However much of the discussion below will still be relevant to them, as all these women and their children remain vulnerable, although it is by virtue of social deprivation rather than by young motherhood.

Children under 16 who become pregnant, however, are in a different category. Pre-existing disadvantage, both socioeconomic and familial, is more severe and antecedent, and consequent psychological disorder is more common. What's more, there are legal and childcare considerations. It is likely that both the teenager and, if she continues with the pregnancy, her baby will be substantially disadvantaged.

Teenagers typically present late for antenatal care, yet are more in need of care and monitoring than mature women who are less at risk. They are likely to be confused and frightened by what is happening and may be truly ignorant about basic reproductive facts. Denial, in the sense of an unconscious refusal to accept a difficult reality, is commonly seen in an initial reluctance to recognise and accept the fact of being pregnant at all, 'I hoped it would go away if I didn't mention it'. Sometimes, especially in very young girls, denial is extreme and even at delivery the girl appears to be unaware that she has been pregnant. Other girls may consciously conceal their pregnancy for fear of the consequences (Hudson and Ineichen, 1991). Many have had previous adverse encounters with authority figures, for example at school, and expect criticism or punishment. Anxiety impairs their ability to recall explanations and instructions, which has clear implications for satisfaction and compliance with advice or treatment.

The characteristics of the service may be critical in determining their utilisation by teenagers and a separate clinic geared to teenagers and conducted after school hours may promote better compliance (Lena *et al.*, 1993). Good communication between all involved is essential. The teenager has the same rights to confidentiality as any other patient, and respecting this will help to gain her confidence. Regular contact with the same sympathetic professional will help her to feel more accepted and understood and, therefore, more able to take in and comply with advice. Work with adolescents requires tolerance, patience and time and staff members may not be equally suited to it. For some girls, the gender of the member of staff will be important and, especially where abuse is an issue, a chaperone may be reassuring for the girl and essential for the member of staff to protect themselves from possible misunderstanding about appropriate and inappropriate contact in different settings.

It is important to keep in mind both the individual patient and others who influence her, particularly her family and other professionals. The family of the pregnant girl is crucial in a variety of ways. First, an understanding of the family dynamics may well be a prerequisite to understanding how the girl has arrived in this predicament and will guide staff involved in helping the girl make necessary decisions. Second, facilitating the family's support of the girl is likely to be a cost effective strategy, as understanding and help from a family member, often the mother, will help the girl negotiate the pregnancy and, if she continues with it, the delivery (Lena *et al.*, 1993). Thereafter, studies have shown grandmothers to be one of the main sources of support (Wolkind and Krug, 1985; Furstenberg *et al.*, 1987), and a critical determinant of outcome for the baby (Cooley and Unger, 1991). Finally, if pregnancy is the outcome of abuse or gross parental neglect, a duty rests with all professionals involved to share their concerns with the appropriate authorities. In the United Kingdom this would be the Local Authority Social Services Department.

While the family is often a source support for the pregnant girl, it can simultaneously be a source of stress to her, even in the absence of gross dysfunction. Other members of the family, particularly the girl's mother, have been shown to suffer considerable stress themselves. Most families will benefit from contact with a social worker, but obstetric staff also need to be prepared to see parents, to discuss the girl's care and to enlist their help.

Some teenagers in difficulty amass a large network of other professionals, who may not always work together in a co-ordinated way. Others receive very little support at all. The younger adolescent should be allocated a social worker who can also act as the girl's advocate, offer practical and emotional support and liaise with and co-ordinate the activities of others who might help the girl. This may be by arranging 'network' meetings where professionals get together to plan the care of the teenager and, if she continues with the pregnancy, to ensure that the girl's plans for the future of the baby are appropriate. Professionals can thus support each other in providing care, for example, by ensuring clinic attendance. The role of each professional involved should be clearly communicated to the girl and her family. If the girl is under 16, there is a requirement in Great Britain that her educational needs should continue to be met. To this end, an educational psychologist may be involved and, in some areas, special educational resources have been made available. Continuation of education is a predictor of favourable outcome for mother and child but can act as a barrier to antenatal care. Establishing links with school-based medical services may be a solution (Cartwright *et al.*, 1993).

In dealing with teenagers, there is a constant balance to be kept between recognising their immaturity and their adolescent developmental needs, and addressing that more adult part of them that they will need to call forth to meet the challenge of premature parenthood.

Pregnancy Resolution

As soon as pregnancy is confirmed the teenager must be told in as sympathetic and unhurried manner as possible, allowing time for discussion. It is probably better if, initially at least, the teenager is alone, although she may choose, and should be permitted, to be accompanied at antenatal appointments and particularly, during delivery by someone she finds supportive. She will need help in deciding what to do about the pregnancy. When counselling her, professionals should bear in mind pre-existing social and psychological factors, as well as the possible consequences of her decisions.

Psychological aspects of termination of pregnancy

The decision of whether or not to seek a termination of pregnancy is probably the first to be made, and of all pregnancies in teenagers in England and Wales, more than half end by therapeutic abortion. Ideally, the decision should be that of the teenager herself, supported by her parents, staff and possibly her partner. When the girl is under 16 and there are disagreements about what should be done, or when the child is not able to understand the nature and consequences of the procedure, colleagues should be consulted and legal advice sought, as the legal position regarding the age at which a minor is able to give or withhold consent to medical treatment remains unclear (Sheild and Baum, 1994).

For some girls, the decision is straightforward. Termination of the pregnancy may be impossible either because of its advanced stage or because of overriding personal or religious prohibitions. For others, it will be the only conceivable course of action. The latter view is more likely to be taken by those doing better at school, who are from more affluent backgrounds, and whose mothers are either unaware of the pregnancy or, along with the partner, support of the decision to terminate. They are more likely to be very young, 14 or under, or over 18 (Jorgensen, 1993).

Other teenagers find this a difficult decision to make, and need time to think through the consequences of both alternatives with the relevant information available, e.g. state financial benefits or mother and baby homes. Specific enquiries should be made about fears, as many girls fear that they may be permanently damaged by an abortion, or that future pregnancies will be harmed.

If the decision to have an abortion is made, what are the likely psychological consequences for the adolescent? As with older women, transient, but at times marked, feelings of guilt can occur and it has been reported that guilt and depression may occasionally be reawakened with a subsequent pregnancy. However, more usually, there is an rapid improvement in mental state as feelings of misery, helplessness and desperation are resolved. In the long term, teenagers who have had abortions have no excess in psychiatric morbidity compared to those who had never been pregnant, and, in comparison to those who continued with the pregnancy, functioning is enhanced in both educational and interpersonal spheres (Jorgensen, 1993).

Psychological aspects of adoption

For girls who continue with the pregnancy, the question of adoption may arise, although, in the end, only about 5% relinquish their babies. The characteristics of these adolescent mothers conform to those who opt for abortion rather than those who keep their babies, and the rate of infant adoption has fallen since abortion was legalised. These girls are more often from higher socioeconomic groups with higher educational aspirations; have more often had, or know of others who have had, a good experience of adoption; are more influenced by parents than partner; and have a realistic view of the future that does not glamorise parenthood.

As with girls who opt for a termination of pregnancy, those who opt for adoption fare better than their child-rearing peers in terms of educational, social, financial and employment prospects. Both groups report being satisfied with their decision, although the adoption group are slightly less so. It is certainly true that while there is no evidence that teenagers who give up their babies have a higher rate of mental disorder than either childbearers or peers who have never been pregnant, some persist in feeling distressed and at times preoccupied with thoughts of the child they have given up.

Partners of teenage mothers

For some pregnant teenagers, the decision to continue with a pregnancy is made in the expectation of marriage to the father, either during pregnancy if the girl is legally old enough, or later. The fathers are often two to three years older and thus not teenagers themselves, but in other ways they resemble the teenage mothers in socio-demographic variables, ignorance about pregnancy and contraception, lack of preparedness for parenthood and lack of parenting skills. They also report high levels of stress and depression (Robinson, 1988). Less than half of the white teenage mothers marry, and even fewer black teenagers do so. The chance of the marriage being satisfactory, or even surviving, is low. However if it does, it offers the teenage mother by far the best chance of a satisfactory outcome (Furstenberg *et al.*, 1987), although of course this may well be related to better prior functioning.

Regardless of marital state, the involvement of the partner has been shown to have beneficial effects on the self-esteem and general satisfaction of the girl, and later, on the development of the child (Cooley and Unger, 1991). Thus, when the young couple remain together, fathers should be encouraged to support their girlfriends practically and emotionally. They are more often than not living near the poverty line themselves and do not provide financial maintenance.

Society has been more critical of teenage fathers than teenage mothers and young men who have got their girlfriends 'into trouble' expect this attitude from medical staff, so may have to be specifically invited to participate in supporting their partner and child.

Becoming a single parent

The final, and by far the most common, option for the teenager who continues with a pregnancy is to become a single parent, often with varying degrees of support, including co-parenting, from her family of origin. The implications of this decision, often made by default, will be considered below in the context of the determinants of outcome of teenage motherhood. The comments made above, about the need to involve and work with the family are particularly relevant when the grandparents are to provide a home for the teenage mother and her baby after the birth.

Psychiatric and Psychological Problems in Pregnancy

There is widespread evidence that throughout pregnancy and the puerperium, teenagers are especially susceptible to stress and feelings of helplessness, with low self-esteem, a sense of personal failure, despair and depression being common symptoms (Russell, 1982). While this is, in part, attributable to the girl's pre-existing psychological state, it is exacerbated by her current predicament and a general enquiry should be made at each visit.

These feelings can, and usually do, occur in the absence of formal psychiatric illness but they nevertheless need attention. Not only is the distress genuine and often ameliorated by discussion and practical support, but also there is an increased risk of deliberate self-harm in pregnant teenagers, both attempted and completed suicide (Appleby, 1991). Furthermore, the identification of personal adjustment difficulties in pregnant adolescents may also identify a group at especially high risk of later parenting problems (Passino *et al.*, 1993).

Whenever symptoms are reported, a fuller assessment is needed. This is time consuming, particularly as other members of the family may need to be seen and may well necessitate a separate appointment. The girl should be gently encouraged to discuss her problems. Iinitially, at least, it may be helpful to ask 'open' questions (for example, 'how have things been recently?') and to avoid too many direct questions. Suicidal feelings should be explicitly enquired about. Social, family and partner problems are likely to be prominent, but the clinician needs to be alert to symptoms of co-existing depressive illness, as pregnancy has been shown to be an important risk factor for major depressive illness in adolescence (Reinherz *et al.*, 1993). Symptoms have to be considered in context, but include pervasive misery and an inability to find enjoyment in anything; appetite or sleep disturbance; loss of energy, motor agitation or retardation; loss of interest; impaired ability to concentrate or feelings of self-reproach.

When there is concern about a pregnant teenager, a prompt referral to the adolescent mental health services should be made. Child and adolescent psychiatrists are medically trained as well as having expertise in the assessment and management of psychological and psychiatric disorders and can therefore weigh up the risks and benefits of treatment in pregnancy. In most circumstances, psychotropic medication is not indicated even when there is depressive symptomatology because some of these drugs, if taken in overdose, have significant risks for mother and fetus. However, for the few who have clear depressive illness they can be very useful when used alongside psychotherapeutic interventions. For most, the appropriate intervention will be social work involvement and psychotherapy, either for the individual or with the family.

As well as problems arising during pregnancy, a pre-existing disorder may require psychiatric involvement, as may problems arising after delivery. There is no overall reported excess of puerperal psychiatric illness in adolescents, and immediate management is the same as that given to older women. However, the occurrence of even mild dysphoria is likely to threaten the already precarious coping and early parenting of teenage mothers. Occasionally, an adolescent can be so overwhelmed by events that she decompensates and behaves in a bizarre manner that is difficult to distinguish from psychosis. Again specialist involvement is essential.

Whenever there is significant postpartum dysfunction, whether psychiatric or otherwise, an assessment of the parenting ability of the girl and of the supports available to her must be made in order to ensure the safety and welfare of the child. In the United Kingdom, this usually involves a multidisciplinary case conference convened by the local social services department.

THE OUTCOME OF ADOLESCENT MOTHERHOOD

The Outcome for the Adolescent Mother

The developmental outcome for mothers is variable and influenced by multiple interrelated factors. The pre-existing disadvantage of teenagers who become pregnant is typically accentuated by parenthood. These girls are much less likely to complete their education than those who delay childbearing, and those who dropped out of school while pregnant are unlikely to return to any form of training or education in the next 5 years. They are less likely to be employed, and if they are working, are unlikely to remain in one job for longer than a year. They are more likely to be living in poverty and on state benefits than their non-childbearing sisters (Furstenberg *et al.*, 1987; Phoenix, 1989).

Teenagers who become parents are likely to do so without the support of the baby's father (Hudson and Ineichen, 1991), indeed they are less likely to ever be married than those who delay childbearing. If they do marry, the relationship is unlikely to endure. Furstenberg *et al.* (1987) found that by the time the mothers were in their early thirties only 16% were married to the father of their first baby. However, many women had had further children, often while still teenagers. At 5-year follow up, only one in five were reliable contraceptive users. Indeed Furstenberg *et al.* (1987) found that the lives of teenagers who became pregnant were pervasively characterised by disruption and disorganisation in almost all spheres, not only in the period soon after the birth of their first child, but at 5-year follow up.

It is perhaps not surprising that girls who become pregnant as teenagers find it difficult to manage their child's and their own lives. Pre-existing factors such as socioeconomic disadvantage and difficulties in managing interpersonal relationships persist, and the additional stresses of bringing up a young child, or often children, without the support of a partner are superimposed. Brown and Harris

(1978) have shown these to be potent risk factors for depressive illness in a community sample of mothers (of any age), and it is not surprising that teenagers have elevated levels of misery, unhappiness and depression. Maternal unhappiness or mental disorder interacts with excessive numbers of life events, such as breakdown of relationships, frequent house moves, childcare and employment crises and poverty. While these events are clearly not independent they act, together with resultant emotional and behavioural problems in the children, as a vicious spiral from which it is difficult for the teenager to extricate herself and her family.

The work by Furstenberg *et al.* (1987) is significant because nearly 75% of the original sample of 404 childbearing teenagers was followed up 17 years after the original study, when most of the women were in their 30s. It provides evidence of not only the vulnerability of this group but also its resilience. While educationally these women were not able to equal their counterparts who had delayed motherhood, more than half did return to school or training, often when their youngest child went to school. Longer term follow up also revealed a steady improvement in their functioning, in relation to independent living, independence from state financial support and in holding down a job. It must be noted though that in none of these areas were the study women able to match controls. By the time they were in their 30s, almost all the women had learnt to control their own fertility, particularly by abortion and sterilisation, and only 13% had been pregnant in the preceding 5 years. Their difficulties with interpersonal relationships endured however. More than 20% had never married, and only 26% were in a first marriage. Thus, although the prospects for the teenage mother who elects to keep her child may not be quite as bleak as previously envisaged, and a substantial part of the disadvantage, particularly in older adolescents, is related to factors other than early childbearing, these girls face a difficult and uncertain future. Most teenage mothers feel they have been disadvantaged by their early parenthood and wished that they had delayed childbearing (Phoenix, 1989; Furstenberg, 1991; Hudson and Ineichen, 1991).

The Outcome for the Child

This account focuses on the determinants of psychological outcome following teenage pregnancy itself. The children of very young mothers (under 16s) are more likely to suffer obstetric adversity, such as prematurity (see p. 383) with or without enduring handicap, and this has implications for psychological outcome for the child and his/her family, as is the case when the mother is older. This risk may well act synergistically with those of young motherhood itself.

Just as the backgrounds of many adolescent mothers renders them at risk even before they became pregnant, so is some of their children's increased risk by virtue of the same socioeconomic factors. Studies have shown that children of adolescents have poorer developmental outcomes than children of older mothers, in terms of lower IQ, lower educational attainment, and lower overall lifetime income. The older a teenager is when she becomes a mother, the better the prospects are for both her and her child. For the over 16s, controlling for socio-economic factors removes much of the difference, although there is a some residual effect, for example, in verbal ability and prevalence of conduct disorder. The under 16 group fare worse in all areas. There may be several mechanisms whereby premature parenthood itself increases risk.

One important strand of influence is the teenager's feelings about being pregnant (as indicated by having considered abortion, delay in seeking antenatal care, etc) and depression. This is related to her attitudes to the child and her ideas about parenting (Haskett *et al.*, 1994), and to the sensitivity of her handling and quality of interaction with the child. This is reflected in the attachment behaviour of the child to the mother and is associated with the level of co-operation of the child and developmental progress (Melhuish, 1989).

Numerous studies have shown that teenagers have more difficulties in these areas than older mothers. Teenagers in general, and under 16-year-olds in particular, are more generally unhappy, hold less positive and accepting views of pregnancy, and have unrealistic expectations of their child's abilities (Haskett *et al.*, 1994). They also exhibit less sensitive handling behaviour, less involvement and verbal interaction, less variation in daily routines and more rigidity, more restriction and more punishment (Garcia Coll *et al.*, 1987). Teenage mothers are commonly physically intrusive, for example by pinching and poking their babies (Lamb *et al.*, 1987). Their children are at increased risk of child abuse, although it should be noted that most teenage mothers do not physically abuse their children (Haskett *et al.*, 1994).

While the children of adolescents are at increased risk of emotional and behavioural problems and educational difficulties (Furstenberg *et al.*, 1987; East and Felice, 1990), the heterogeneity of outcome should be stressed. Furthermore, in any individual case the contribution of the baby cannot be ignored. There is extensive evidence that some babies, by virtue of their temperamental characteristics or other individual factors, are more difficult to rear, and while this situation may be manageable for well-supported mature parents, for adolescents, it may develop into a downward spiral of increasing dissatisfaction with the maternal role, depression and parenting difficulties.

The degree and type of support a teenage mother receives may be critical in determining whether the increased risk to her child's development is expressed (Wolkind and Krug, 1985). Research shows support to be related to socioeconomic and cultural factors. For example, low income African–American families tend to have no male partners and grandmothers are prominent, although this pattern is, not surprisingly, also found with younger teenage mothers. For both older and younger teenagers, residence with the grandmother is often an economic necessity. Where the grandmother undertakes childcare, she contributes to the overall cognitive stimulation of the home, enabling the older adolescent to complete her education, to be more responsive to her child and for both mother and baby to have a better developmental outcome. The developmental outcome is negatively affected by the grandmother's presence when she does not provide childcare and when younger adolescents remain at home for a long time, although possibly this is because these teenagers have a greater degree of pre-existing disturbance which precludes independent living. Child development is promoted by grandmother childcare rather than mere presence, and although initially advantageous this has costs, both in terms of fatigue and depression in the grandmother, and later on in terms of family functioning (Cooley and Unger, 1991). Thus, there may be confusion about lines of authority and responsibility which leads to lack of consistency and confusion for the child. Caretaking by the grandmother may facilitate a lack of involvement between the teenager and her child and may cause problems when either the adolescent mother or her mother wishes to renegotiate the situation later on.

Support from a partner, not necessarily the father of the baby, during pregnancy and soon after delivery has a somewhat different effect (Unger and Wandersman, 1988). It seems to contribute little materially, but to be associated with overall life satisfaction in the mother thereby promoting her childcaring abilities. Continued presence of the father is rare even for older adolescents, but when contact is maintained, the father's play with the child promotes social and cognitive development and family stability may be enhanced (Cooley and Unger, 1991). Again it is the quality of the father's involvement and not merely his presence that is critical, as high rates of marital discord and breakdown have been documented, and parental conflict is known to have a deleterious effect on child development.

Most of the studies on the children of teenagers concentrate on infancy and early childhood, and little work has been done to determine whether early difficulties persist. Furstenberg's follow up of children of teenage mothers when they were between 15 and 17 showed them to have suffered more frequent separations from their mothers, inconsistency in primary caregiver, absence of father figures and difficulties in terms of academic achievement. There is an excess of emotional and behavioural problems, including juvenile delinquency for boys in particular. Perhaps the most striking finding, however, is the contrast between the efforts made by the once teenage mothers to steer their children away from premature parenthood and the striking excess of early sexuality and pregnancy in their children. In America, 15% of children of teenager mothers repeat the pattern (Jorgensen, 1993), and in Furstenberg's study the figure was as high as 26% for girls. These childbearing children of former adolescent mothers have bleaker educational and financial prospects than their mothers did (Furstenberg *et al.*, 1987), and their adverse life events, such as reception into care, suggest their children will be more disadvantaged (Wolkind and Krug, 1985).

PREVENTION OF TEENAGE PARENTHOOD

While many authors recently have argued that, for older adolescents particularly many of the adverse outcomes of motherhood are not directly attributable to the age that childbearing occurred (Phoenix, 1989), few would contend that teenage motherhood is not a difficult and arduous path to take and would not be better delayed.

Primary prevention has focused on health education, giving sexual and contraceptive information, dealing with interpersonal relationships and fostering realistic perceptions of parenthood. Contraceptive services need to be readily available and accessible, as do services for teenagers who become pregnant.

Specific programmes have also been developed, some targeted at populations that are at particular risk of becoming pregnant, such as sisters of adolescent mothers (East and Felice, 1992), while others are aimed at preventing repeat pregnancies in particularly vulnerable groups such as the very young or mentally retarded (Levy *et al.*, 1992). Some aim to improve the parenting of adolescent mothers (Causby *et al.*, 1991). These are generally school-based educational programmes. Participants of these programmes are more able to cope in such areas as childcare, infant health, continuation of maternal education and prevention of repeat pregnancy when compared with controls who receive no intervention. As they are school-based, they may, however, not be addressing the most vulnerable groups who drop out of school altogether.

Premature pregnancy and parenthood results from, and contributes to, social and emotional disadvantage and deprivation, and is thus perpetuated from one generation to the next. While specific projects have an important role to play, if we are really going to tackle the problem of teenage motherhood, we will have to address these wider issues.

REFERENCES

Ainsworth MDS, Blehar MC, Waters E, Wall S, 1978: *Patterns of attachment. A psychological study of the strange situation.* Hillsdale NJ, Lawrence Erlbaum Associates.

Appleby L, 1991: Suicide during pregnancy and in the first postnatal year. *British Medical Journal* **302**, 137–140.

Brown G, Harris T, 1978: *The social origins of depression. A study of psychiatric disorder in women.* Chapter 16: A model of depression. London: Tavistock, 264–270.

Cartwright PS, McLaughlin FJ, Martinez AM, *et al.* 1993: Teenagers' perceptions of barriers to prenatal care. *Southern Medical Journal* **7**, 737–741.

Causby V, Nixon C, Bright JM, 1991: Influences on adolescent mother–infant interactions. *Adolescence* **26**(103), 293–304.

Cooley ML, Unger DG, 1991: The role of family support in determining developmental outcomes in children of teen mothers. *Child Psychiatry and Human Development*, **21**(3), 217–234.

East PL, Felice ME, 1990: Outcomes and parent–child relationships of former adolescent mothers and their 12-year-old children. *Journal of Developmental and Behavioral Pediatrics* **11**(4), 175–183.

East PL, Felice ME, 1992: Pregnancy risk amongst the younger sisters of pregnant and childbearing adolescents. *Journal of Developmental and Behavioral Paediatrics* **13**(2), 128–136.

Erikson EH, 1959: Identity and the life cycle. Monograph. *Psychological Issues*, **1**(No 1). New York: International Universities Press.

Furstenberg FF, 1991: As the pendulum swings: teenage childbearing and social concerns. *Family Relations*, **40**, 127–138.

Furstenberg FF, Brooks-Gunn J, Morgan SP, 1987: *Adolescent mothers in later life.* Cambridge: Cambridge University Press.

Garcia Coll CT, Hoffman J, Oh W, 1987: The social ecology of early parenting in caucasian adolescent mothers. *Child Development* **58**, 955–963.

Haskett ME, Johnson CA, Miller JW, 1994: Individual differences in risk of child abuse by adolescent mothers: assessment in the perinatal period. *Journal of Child Psychology and Psychiatry* **35**(3), 461–476.

Horowitz SM, Klerman LV, Kuo HS, Jekel JF, 1991: Intergenerational transmission of school-age parenthood. *Paediatrics* **87**(6), 862–868.

Hudson F, Ineichen B, 1991: *Taking it lying down. Sexuality and teenage motherhood* Section 1: What teenagers do. Basingstoke: Macmillan Education Ltd, 5–125.

Jorgensen S, 1993: Adolescent pregnancy and parenting In Gullotta T, Adams G, Montemayor R, (eds), *Adolescent sexuality.* Sage Publications, Inc., 103–141.

Lamb ME, Hopps K, Elster AB, 1987: Strange situation behaviour of infants with adolescent mothers. *Infant Behaviour and Development* **10**, 39–48.

Lena SM, Marko E, Nimrod C, Merritt L, Poirier G, Shein E, 1993: Birthing experience of adolescents at the Ottawa General Hospital Perinatal Centre. *Canadian Medical Association Journal* **148**(12), 2149–2154.

Levine LV, Tuber SB, Slade A, Ward MJ, 1991: Mothers' mental representations and their relationship to mother–infant attachment. *Bulletin of the Menninger Clinic* **55**(4), 454–469.

Levy SR, Perhats C, Nash-Johnson M, Welter JF, 1992: Reducing the risks in pregnant teens who are very young and those with mild mental retardation. *Mental Retardation* **30**(4), 195–203.

Melhuish EC, 1989: Maternal psychological state and infant development with mothers under twenty: a research note. *Journal of Child Psychology and Psychiatry* **30**(6), 925–930.

Parker B, 1993: Abuse of adolescents: what can we learn from pregnant teenagers? AWHONNS *Clinical Issues in Perinatal Womens Health Nursing* **4**(3), 363–370.

Passino AW, Whitman TL, Borkowski JG, *et al.* 1993: Personal adjustment during pregnancy and adolescent parenting. *Adolescence* **28**, 97–122.

Phoenix A, 1989: *Young mothers.* Cambridge: Polity Press, 145–176, 217–247.

Reinherz HZ, Giaconia RM, Bilge P, *et al.*, 1993: Psychosocial risks for major depression in late adolescence: a longitudinal community study. *Journal of the American Academy of Child and Adolescent Psychiatry* **32**(6), 1155–1163.

Robinson B, 1988: *Teenage fathers.* Lexington Books, 8–12.

Russell J, 1982: *Early teenage pregnancy* Edinburgh: Churchill Livingstone.

Sadler LS, Catrone C, 1983: The adolescent parent: a dual developmental crisis. *Journal of Adolescent Health Care* **4**, 100–104.

Sheild JPS, Baum JD, 1994: Children's consent to treatment. *British Medical Journal* **308**, 1182–1183.

Tunnadine D, Green R, 1978: *Unwanted pregnancy – accident or illness?* Oxford: Oxford University Press, 102–103, 181–183.

Unger DG, Wandersman LP, 1988: The relation of family support to the adjustment of adolescent mothers. *Child Development* **59**(4), 1056–1060.

Wolkind S, Krug S, 1985: Teenage pregnancy and motherhood. *Journal of the Royal Society of Medicine* **78**, 112–116.

Index

Note: page numbers in *italics* refer to tables. Page numbers in **bold** refer to figures.